The
FORMATION
of
NERVE CONNECTIONS

The

FORMATION

of

NERVE CONNECTIONS

a consideration of neural specificity
modulation and comparable phenomena

R. M. GAZE

*Division of Developmental Biology, National Institute for Medical
Research, Mill Hill, London, England*

1970

Academic Press · London · New York

ACADEMIC PRESS INC. (LONDON) LTD
Berkeley Square House
Berkeley Square,
London, W1x 6BA

U.S. Edition published by
ACADEMIC PRESS INC.
111 Fifth Avenue,
New York, New York 10003

Library of Congress Catalog Card Number: 72-129786
International Standard Book Number: 0-12-278550-9

PRINTED IN GREAT BRITAIN AT
THE UNIVERSITY PRESS
ABERDEEN

PREFACE

This book was written in the second half of 1969, while I was on academic leave from the University of Edinburgh. When I started to write I thought that the task was fairly straightforward. I now realize that it was not. During the period of writing, and associated with the attacks of thought that the writing brought on, my views on the mechanisms involved in the formation of nerve connections underwent a form of metamorphosis. However the post-metamorphic views are themselves subject to rapid change and development and the end of all this, of course, is not in sight.

One reason for certain difficulties that I have had in writing this book is that much of the work discussed is still being done. This is particularly noticeable in Chapter 4, where I deal with retinotectal connections. Indeed, the farcical situation arose where early drafts of this chapter had to be withdrawn because they became out of date—were overtaken by events—before my friends had a chance to read them.

I should like to thank all those who have helped me to prepare this book. In particular, the members of the Neurobiology Research Unit in the Physiology Department at Edinburgh University, all of whom have assisted me (and the experimental work) in most immediate fashion. It is, perhaps, somewhat invidious to particularize; but I would like to offer my special thanks to Dr. M. J. Keating, who, wittingly, caused me to rewrite whole sections of the script, and to Dr. Joan Feldman. Others who have given me the benefit of their critical advice have been Dr. M. C. Prestige, Dr. K. Straznicky and Dr. Lorne Mendell. Finally, I should like to thank Professor P. D. Wall for his comments on Chapter 3, and Professor Lewis Wolpert for a critical reading of Chapter 4. In all cases, needless to say, I am solely responsible for the final result.

MAY 1970   R. M. GAZE

v

CONTENTS

1. INTRODUCTION

The fact that it is possible to write a useful textbook of anatomy indicates that there are extensive similarities between animals of like kind. These similarities are obvious when we deal with the gross structure of the body and their existence points to control mechanisms which must guide the development of form in each individual. No two animals are identical in structure but if they are of the same species the similarities greatly outweigh the differences. The same phenomenon of similarity between animals of the same kind exists in regard to the nervous system. It is possible here again to make an anatomical chart which has general validity from one animal to another. Obviously the degree of resolution offered by such an anatomical chart must be limited; at the level of fine detail we may expect to find differences between individuals. But in general it is true that certain parts of the brain are known to be interconnected and certain nerve pathways always run from here to there.

The existence of similarities in neural structure between animals of a similar kind (and also, to a lesser extent, between animals of dissimilar kinds) indicates that the inter-neuronal relationships formed during development are not random; they are patterned. And this in turn leads us to seek the factors, which must be presumed to exist, leading to the development of these neuronal patterns. We are interested, in other words, in pattern formation in morphogenesis, and specifically in neurogenesis.

The existence of a species-specific anatomy is thus the problem facing us; and we may now ask how relevant is the available anatomical evidence, since the answer to this question may indicate the degree of resolution that will be required of any mechanisms we may propose. It will become obvious through the discussions later in this book that much of the anatomical information on nerve connections has been obtained by inference from the study of function; and one of my purposes will be to indicate how unreliable such inference may be. Thus I will have two main reasons for questioning the structural information that is presently held to be correct: the first is to attempt to find out whether the connections that supposedly exist have relevance for neural function and if so, what this relevance is; the second is to investigate, in those few cases that I am able

1*

to consider, what connections actually exist and how they developed.

An example from the field of functional anatomy may help to demonstrate the nature and extent of this double problem. In frogs, the retina always connects with (among other regions) the contralateral optic tectum; and furthermore the ganglion cells in the nasal half of the retina appear always to connect with the caudal part of the tectum. We do not know, however, the degree of resolution of the retinal map on the tectum. It would be reasonable to ask whether a ganglion cell in one particular retinal position always connects with one particular tectal cell. In general we can ask, with respect to any neural connections, with what precision they are formed; whether this represents an area-to-area localization, a cell-to-cell connection, or even a selectivity at the level of axon terminal-to-dendritic spine. In most cases the answers to even these general questions are not known; and the evidence, as we shall see later, may be conflicting. Since our present area of interest is the formation of nerve connections it is relevant to ask what precisely *are* the connections that are formed. Throughout this book we will have to return repeatedly to this question since unless we find answers to it, the further question of the control of the formation of these connections becomes meaningless.

I shall discuss the factors controlling the formation of nerve connections in two main situations, embryogenesis and adult nerve regeneration. These two situations are very different; during embryogenesis nerve cells are developing as well as growing processes; the target tissue (nervous or nonnervous) towards which a developing axon grows, is itself developing and in many cases the further development of the target is partly dependent upon the proper ingrowth of the connecting axons. There are also various inductive interactions to be considered between the elements of the neurogenetic system. In adult neural regeneration, on the other hand, we are dealing (in most cases) with a reconnection of two already differentiated tissues; inductive interactions may be expected to be minimal, if they exist at all; and the fibres will in most cases be growing along pathways that are partly preformed by the original fibres. Despite these major differences between neurogenesis and adult fibre regeneration we may hopefully look for similar mechanisms controlling the selective formation of nerve connections in the two situations. It is quite possible, of course, that the controlling factors are very different in the two cases; but as a working hypothesis, and to prevent the multiplication of entities, we assume initially that what directs fibres during embryogenesis may also direct them in later life.

In classical experimental embryology the main operative tools that have been used are selective ablation and the recombination experiment. In the former case the experimenter removes a certain part of an embryo, or organ, and later observes the effect on further development. With luck the effect may be both startling and illuminating, as when a piece of the prechordal plate is removed in the embryo and this leads to a failure of separation of the two eyes (Mangold, 1931) or absence of a chiasma (Silver, 1961). In the recombination experiment the experimenter transplants pieces of embryo from one site to another or from one embryo to another, to observe the effect on development. Possibly the best known example of this sort of approach is the induction of the nervous system by the roof of the archenteron.

Recombination of embryonic tissues, used in this way, has revealed the wide field of inductive interactions and thus accentuates the interdependence of various parts of the organism during development. Recombination has also been extensively used, however, in the study of neurogenesis; and here the use is rather different. There are two ways of looking at such a recombination experiment on the nervous system. One involves studying in the usual fashion the inductive interactions that may occur. The other involves analysis of the "wiring diagram" of the parts concerned. In this case we treat the nervous system as a piece of electronic machinery; it has processing elements (cells, synapses) and wires (processes). If an enthusiastic but ignorant amateur wanted to investigate the functioning of an electronic black box, and his only tool was a soldering iron, he could alter the wiring somewhat and hope to be able to deduce from the result certain information. He could switch round inputs A and B, for example, and find out if the device still worked properly. Or he could mix up inputs and outputs. And if the thing *still* worked properly he would at least know it was more complex internally than he had previously assumed. Or if the result of a systematic alteration in the wiring was a systematic alteration in the function, then he could start making educated guesses as to *how* the one led to the other.

Let us consider, as a most trivial example, the following situation: there is a large, rambling old house with a bell-push in each room. The bells ring in the servants' quarters and each bell indicates which room has been "excited". The experimenter wants to find out how this system may work; so he carefully removes the bell-push from room A, takes it right to the other end of the house and wires it up in place of the bell-push in room X. He then pushes the button that he has just grafted into a new situation and sits back and waits for action. Five types of result may occur, perhaps more: (1) Nothing—he has made a mistake in the way he wired it up, or the graft did not take; (2) Everything—frantic activity on the part of the servants, who are confused as to the origin of the message; (3) The servants go at once, and consistently, to a particular room, other than A or X; (4) The servants go straight to room X where the button (from room A) was pushed. This behaviour would perhaps suggest that the nature of the bell-push was not very significant but that the wire to which it was connected was; (5) The servants go straight to room A (from which the bell-push had been taken). This last pattern of behaviour, or that of No. 3, would really make the experimenter sit and think. Each of these situations has its parallel in the neural recombination experiments and it may thus be seen that the possibilities for entertaining speculation are manifold.

Although this volume is concerned with the mode of formation of nerve connections, for obvious reasons it will not be possible in any finite work to consider *all* nerve connections even in a fairly small nervous system. The numbers are too great. I therefore intend to take the only path open to me and deal exclusively with certain classes of connectivity. Hopefully, certain generalizations will emerge that have a more general validity then the necessarily restricted survey from which they were drawn. The areas of neural connection that will concern me are those dealing with what I will call the *primary sensory inputs* to the nervous system and the *primary motor outputs*, as well as some types of intracentral connections. By primary sensory input I intend the main sensory projections from receptor to centre; for instance the retina-brain path; the auditory and olfactory paths, and the cutaneous sensory input. By primary motor paths I intend the Sherringtonian "final common pathway" or motor neurone. Lastly I will discuss evidence on the formation of connections drawn from a more central part of the nervous system and will contrast the findings from the intercentral pathways with those from the primary inputs and outputs. It will at once be apparent that I intend to be very restrictive in the scope of my survey. This is necessary. Whole areas of the nervous system will be completely ignored. Partly this is because I can only discuss topics I know something about; and partly because most of the work on the formation of connections has been done on the systems that I include.

More markedly than with the other bodily systems, our ideas on how the nervous system functions have changed in the past thirty years and are changing now. And since our understanding of the detailed structure of the nervous system is still so rudimentary, the currently-held views on nervous function at any time considerably influence our ideas on how the system is connected. Ideally we might hope to analyse the neural structure and then deduce from this how it works; this approach has had very considerable success with what could be called the "plumbing" of the body. Such an approach is unlikely to be completely successful in the case of the nervous system for several reasons: in the first place it is too complex—there is too much of it and we cannot, as yet, deal with the numbers involved; in the second place we have only a rather hazy idea of what the nervous system is *for*. Obviously we know quite a lot about certain of the functions of the nervous system; but on the other hand we have difficulty in even defining some of its activities. Consideration of the phenomena of language, and the difficulties attendant upon any attempt to define "intelligence", is sufficient to indicate that the functioning of the brain as an information-handling device is of an altogether different order of complexity to anything we have so far studied. In this situation I find that the chronological approach to the investigation of neural connectivity is the least confusing and this is how I shall consider most of the experimental evidence.

The evidence to be presented suggests, at least to me, that the control mechanisms directing the formation of nerve connections may be rather different according to whether we are dealing with the primary inputs and outputs or with intracentral connections. In the former case it seems that connections are laid down according to a genetically determined plan and, once the appropriate development stage of "determination" has been passed, these connections are fixed, immutable. The system is prewired and quite independent of function. The situation may be very different when we consider intercentral connections; there is now good evidence that the formation and maintenance of some of these is dependent on neural function.

We may consider the nervous system to consist of three phases or components: the input, the centre and the output. Electronic, or rather computing, analogies readily spring to mind. Indeed, in many cases the analogies are rather close. In a modern small laboratory computing system we have the central "works" consisting of the computing machinery itself, and we also have separate peripheral units for input (e.g. a tape reader) and for output (a printer). In some systems it is possible to plug in separate and distinct types of input or output, so long as they are compatible with the arrangements in the central console. In a nervous system also we have a central computing mechanism which is connected to inputs and outputs. And in the nervous system we can also plug in various types of input or output: we can alter the arrangements existing.

We may consider what might happen if we had a computer, the central facility of which was very large and fast, but with a small, slow and generally inadequate input system. We present it with a problem and the problem is slowly ground through the single-channel input into the machine, which eventually comes up with the answer. If now we throw away the inadequate input stage and plug in one comparable in ability to the machine itself, we might expect to be able to obtain the answer to our problem much faster—and perhaps even a better answer. Similarly with a nervous system; we have an animal with rather inadequate visual input; so we remove the original eye and replace it with a larger (?faster) eye from a different species. The system works (Stone, 1963), the animal sees, and there is some evidence (though not more than a passing suggestion) that the quality of the eye may be reflected in the quality of the visual performance.

However, one major difference between the nervous system and the computer in this situation is that, when a large eye is grafted in place of a small one, it gives rise to marked changes (increase in tectal size and cell number) in the centre. Again, it must be remembered that the eye-graft usually has to be done during embryonic or larval life, while both eye and centre are susceptible to change. A nearer analogy for the computer might be to graft a different input mechanism during the construction of the machine. But before we could take this analogy further we would have to be dealing with a self-organizing computer system.

Again, we may give a computer two modes of output; one a typewriter, the other an artificial voice, each powered by appropriately patterned electrical impulses. If now we switch connections and feed the "voice" output onto the typewriter we may blow it up, or get no result; or we may get a most nonsensical output. And similarly, the typewriter output, if fed into the voice loudspeaker, would give an uninterpretable series of noises. In a comparable situation a nervous system does rather better. We may switch "arm" output for "leg" output and we still obtain a meaningful result; but now the "arm" appears to move as a "leg" or vice-versa (Székely, 1963).

One of my main themes in this book is that, before we can usefully investigate *how* nerve connections form, we should know a little about *what* connections are formed. And the importance of this latter knowledge, to me, stems from my belief that structure and function are intimately related in the nervous system; and that any deep comprehension of neural function will require accurate knowledge of neural connectivity. This is a most exciting time in the study of the brain and its functions because there is considerable and increasing interaction between neurophysiologists, psychologists and those concerned with modelling various of the functions of the brain. The study of the nervous control of movement is complex but poses few problems at the conceptual level; this is not the case with the study of sensory mechanisms or intellectual processes. In these fields part of the difficulty lies in being sufficiently precise in our definitions of what we are investigating. And one of the main advantages of the cybernetic approach is that it requires precision of statement to permit an "effective procedure" in model building.

Recombination experiments performed over the last few years force us to question the "conventional wisdom" of neurophysiology. Biological science, more markedly perhaps than religion, suffers from dogmatic assertion. It suffices for a biological assertion to be eye-catching for it to pass into the realm of biological dogma; a good example of this is the so-called "convexity detector" in the frog retina (Lettvin *et al.*, 1959) which detects a stimulus of small size but not necessarily convex (Gaze and Jacobson, 1963b). As Galbraith has it (1958), although truth may rarely overtake falsehood, it has winged feet compared with a qualification in pursuit of a bold proposition.

In the study of the formation of nerve connections observation has to precede analysis. And here lies one of our main difficulties; the nervous system is an information processing system and as such eminently suitable to having logical statements made about its functioning. Ever since the first reports of "homologous response" in transplanted amphibian limbs (Weiss, 1922), we have had a continuing stream of assertions as to the logical requirements for the proper functioning of the observed systems. But the trouble with logical statements about the nervous system is that, for them to have biological as well as logical validity, the premises must be correct. And from 1922 up to the present time experimenters have been busily occupied in revising the premises. This process is a continuing one of course, and recognition of the temporary nature of so many biological "facts" suggests the advisability of a certain amount of caution in the construction of intricate logical edifices on the basis of the "known structure" of the nervous system. To paraphrase Galbraith (1958), the shortcomings of science are not original error but uncorrected obsolescence. Much of the rest of this book will thus be devoted to what may perhaps be called "logical archaeology", or the excavation of ever deeper layers of neurological dogma in the hope that eventually we will reach biological reality.

2. NEUROMUSCULAR CONNECTIONS

Vertebrate skeletal muscle contracts only when it receives an adequate excitation from its motor nerves. In lower vertebrates (amphibians, fishes, birds) there are different varieties of skeletal muscle, with different speeds of contraction. The fast fibres are "twitch" fibres—they give a twitch contraction in response to a single impulse arriving by the appropriate nerve; the slow fibres are mostly non-twitch fibres and require repetitive stimulation from the appropriate motor nerve to initiate a contraction. The mode of innervation of these separate types of muscle is quite distinctive when investigated histologically (Gray, 1957; Bone, 1964), histochemically (Hess, 1960; Dubowitz, 1967) or electrophysiologically (Kuffler and Vaughan Williams, 1953a,b; Hunt and Kuffler, 1954; Takeuchi, 1959; Hnik *et al.*, 1967). Even so, it is a valid generalization to say that a skeletal muscle contracts only on receipt of an adequate motor excitation via its motor nerves.

The observations to be discussed in this chapter relate to the mode of control and mode of innervation of vertebrate skeletal muscles by the spinal cord. But before we can usefully investigate these relationships it will be as well to enquire somewhat into the nature and meaning of motor coordination.

In a normal animal motor activity, whether reflex or "voluntary", is coordinated. By this we imply that there is a proper functional balance between the various muscles involved; they are brought into action with a timing and intensity of contraction that is commensurate with the movement being performed. Not only is the activity coordinated in this sense, it is also appropriate to the stimulus situation. When we itch, we scratch; when confronted by a lion, we either faint or run. We do not run or faint when we itch, nor do we scratch when we see the lion. In each case the action is appropriate to the situation. Again, when we itch on the belly we scratch the belly and when we itch on the flank we scratch the flank. In most cases it would be pointless to scratch the belly if the site of irritation was the flank and vice-versa. This matching of the motor response to the stimulus situation raises several problems of which the two most obvious are how does the motor apparatus know where the stimulus is? (this will be discussed in some detail in a later chapter); and how does the motor apparatus accurately apportion excitation to the great variety of muscles necessarily involved in such a complex action as scratching? To scratch, after all, does not merely involve waggling the nails or claws backwards and forwards in a certain position; it involves also all the preparatory movements required to bring the scratching instrument to the site affected, and these ancillary movements, in a cat, involve virtually the entire body musculature.

As has been pointed out by Weiss (1941) there is a striking disproportion between our knowledge of the physiological properties of the nervous elements involved and our understanding of the operation of the nervous system as the coordinator of these elements in the motor activity of the animal.

"A few explanations suggest themselves quite readily. The most obvious one is the infinitely greater difficulty and complexity of the task facing the student of the nervous system. This may be a challenge to inquisitive minds, but it certainly does not predispose the subject for mass attack by routine methods. So long as one clings to the study of elements, one is dealing with well-circumscribed units, a well-defined subject, presenting clear-cut problems, and one can call on familiar and approved methods of analysis. As soon as one raises the eye from the unit to the whole system, the subject becomes fuzzy, the problems ill-descript, and the prospect of fruitful attack discouraging in its indefiniteness. This may explain why a considerable number of able experimental workers prefer to circle around the focal problems at a respectful distance rather than heading straight at them. It also explains why discussions of central nervous function operate so much more liberally with words than with facts; for it is remarkable how general the tendency is in this field to cover up factual ignorance by verbalisms. The average attitude is somewhat like this: the 'whole' gets a large share of one's thought and talk, but the elements get all the benefit of one's actual work; here the problems seem to be so infinitely more tangible." (Weiss, 1941).

If we are correct in assuming that a skeletal muscle only contracts on adequate excitation via its motor nerve fibres, then the occurrence of a phase of contraction in one particular muscle indicates that some or all of the motoneurones supplying that muscle have discharged impulses. The motoneurones sending fibres to a particular muscle may be termed the motoneurone pool of that muscle; in some cases (e.g. cat) these moto-neurones comprise discrete groups within the spinal cord; in other cases (urodeles) the neurones supplying any one muscle are spread out widely through the spinal cord (Székely and Czéh, 1967). In either case activation of the muscle implies activation of the corresponding neurones.

In a movement-sequence such as walking, an animal employs its limb in a certain, highly reproducible, fashion. A newt walks with a gait that involves flexion, extension, abduction, adduction of the various limb joints in predictable order. Thus according to our previous proposition, this movement-sequence indicates a corresponding discharge-sequence in the appropriate motoneurones. The movements of a newt's limbs while walking can be illustrated by using cinephotography and preparing diagrams from the film; a complete cycle of the walking sequence can then be shown as in Fig. 2.1. This illustration, taken from the work of Weiss (1941), shows the method devised by this author for indicating sequences of muscular activity and thus of the corresponding central nervous discharges.

Such a diagram is called a "myochronogram" by Weiss and is obtained by analysis of slow-motion pictures. Weiss assumes that, for instance, when the forearm is bent against the upper arm, this indicates that the central nervous system has activated chiefly those neurones innervating the biceps muscle, and this is shown on the myochronogram as contraction of this muscle. For the sake of ease of interpretation, Fig. 2.1 shows only the movements of six major muscles acting on the shoulder and elbow joints.

Thus if the myochronogram be accepted as a valid method of indicating the "time-score" of muscular contractions during walking, such a record as that of Fig. 2.1 shows that the various major muscle groups are activated in an orderly sequence in one cycle of the movement; and this in turn indicates a corresponding orderly sequence in the discharge pattern of the spinal motoneurones. We will return later to this question of the adequacy of cinephotography for the determination of the timing of motoneurones.

If muscle contraction is brought about by ordered sequences of moto-neurone discharges from the spinal centres, with each motoneurone pool coming into action at an appropriate part of the movement cycle, what will be the result of surgical alteration of the innervation pattern of the muscles concerned? Experiments aimed at testing this situation have been per-formed by Weiss over a period of many years and more recently by several others. The pioneering experiments of Weiss have been reviewed by that author in a most comprehensive and detailed fashion in two papers (Weiss, 1936; 1941).

Weiss (1941) considers that theories of coordination can be divided into three classes: *preformistic, heuristic* and *systemic*. The preformistic (or *preformistic-structural*) concept refers to stereotyped, preformed anatomical connections between neurones in the centres, and between these neurones and the peripheral muscular effectors. This concept of coordination is based on observations of reflex activity and suggests that the adequacy of a response is a result of the correct anatomical construction of the neuro-muscular apparatus. That is, the body has its coordination built-in. While there is no doubt that such built-in coordination mechanisms do exist in animals, the question is, as Weiss (1941) points out, whether or not these preformed mechanisms can be generalized to account for *all* coordination. Built-in coordination is very appropriate for simple movement systems

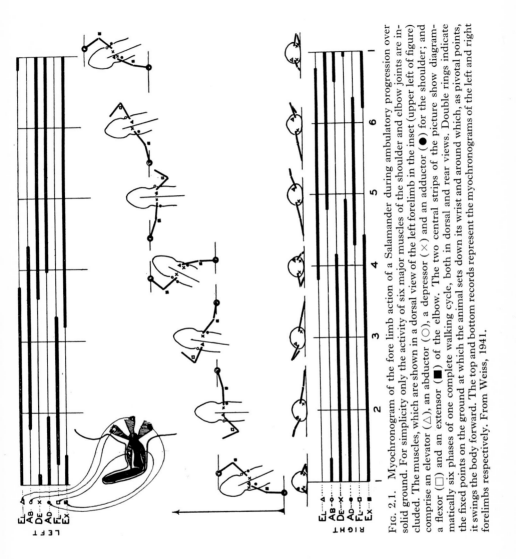

FIG. 2.1. Myochronogram of the fore limb action of a Salamander during ambulatory progression over solid ground. For simplicity only the activity of six major muscles of the shoulder and elbow joints are included. The muscles, which are shown in a dorsal view of the left forelimb in the inset (upper left of figure) comprise an elevator (△), an abductor (○), a depressor (×) and an adductor (●) for the shoulder; and a flexor (□) and an extensor (■) of the elbow. The two central strips of the picture show diagrammatically six phases of one complete walking cycle, both in dorsal and rear views. Double rings indicate the fixed points on the ground at which the animal sets down its wrist and around which, as pivotal points, it swings the body forward. The top and bottom records represent the myochronograms of the left and right forelimbs respectively. From Weiss, 1941.

involving a strictly limited number of degrees of freedom of motion; however in many cases we are trying to account for coordinated activity in more complicated motor situations, as with a ball-and-socket joint, where more than one degree of freedom of movement is possible. In such a situation the functional groupings of muscles about a single joint will change with the movement being effected; no longer is there a simple dichotomy between flexors and extensors, agonist and antagonist. With a ball joint any two muscles may operate facultatively as agonists or antagonists and the controlling centres are presented with a problem of multiple choice involving the selection of a definite combination of muscles out of a large number of possible combinations. As Weiss (1941) states:

> "... it will be well to keep in mind what Herrick, that most judicious student of the anatomy of the central nervous system, had to say in this connection (1930, p. 645*): 'No complication of separate and insulated reflex arcs, each of which is conceived as giving a one-to-one relation between stimulus and response, and no interconnection of such arcs by elaborate switchboard devices can conceivably yield the type of behaviour which we actually find in higher vertebrates. . . . These facts are regarded as incompatible with the traditional dogmas of reflex physiology, with its precisely localized and well-insulated reflex arcs and centers of reflex adjustment. . . . The mechanisms of traditional reflexology seem hopelessly inadequate.'"

In this passage Weiss is quoting Herrick in 1941. Such a statement could hardly be justified now, in the post-Ashby, intelligent machine era. Numerous groups of people are busy at this time designing automata to do just what Weiss and Herrick were dismissing as unlikely, if not impossible. Even now, however, we have to admit that the problem of multiple-choice offered to the centres by complex joints and multiples of these do pose major problems for the student of coordination. ⟨Only nowadays the question we have to ask is not whether such activity is *possible* on a preformist-structural basis, but whether this is how the system actually works.⟩

Weiss' second class of theory dealing with coordination is the *heuristic*. By this term he means any theory which submits that the common appropriateness for the body of motor effects has been developed ontogenetically under the moulding action of practice and experience. The essential point of the heuristic concept is that the *effectiveness* of a response confers selective value, and hence stability, on the originally tentative grouping of the muscles through which it is brought about. As with the preformistic-structural concept, we will have cause to return to this idea later when discussing alternative explanations for the experimental findings to be described.

Weiss' third and final class of theory concerning coordination is what he calls "*systemic*". Under this concept its proponents would concede to the

---

* *Proc. natn. Acad. Sci. USA,* **16**, 643–650.

nervous system a certain primordial dynamic ability to respond to any change in the stimulus situation by a total response of maximum adequacy for the organism as a whole. This concept, so vague as to be almost meaningless, owes more to teleology than to observation and I do not propose to consider it further.

We are then left with the other two major groups of hypotheses, preformistic-structural and heuristic, to account for the existence of coordinated activity in motor systems. And to differentiate between these should be quite possible on an experimental basis. Indeed, this is what all the fuss has been about over the past 45 years. Much experimentation, some of it highly ingenious, has been done (most of it by Weiss) and still the arguments continue as to mechanisms.

Weiss (1941) stated, rather plaintively, that one might have expected the issue to have long been settled one way or the other. And now, 28 years later, the whole problem is back in our hands for reconsideration. Weiss thought, of course, that he had himself settled the question of the origin of neuromuscular coordination in the lower vertebrates by the various experiments we are about to discuss. Yet once again it has turned out that this was an over-confident assessment of the situation; the logic was in most cases impeccable; only some of the premises were wrong.

The appropriate mode of experimental approach to the problem of differentiating between preformistic and heuristic mechanisms of the development of coordination was outlined by Weiss in 1941:

"If coordination is preformed in self-differentiated central impulse patterns, which yield adequate peripheral effects only by virtue of what may be called evolutionary precedent and in the individual case amounts to predesign, they should prove stable and conservative even if experimentally prevented from producing appropriate functional effects. If, on the other hand, functional effectiveness is all that counts in shaping the patterns of coordination, one should expect any experimental reduction of that effectiveness to be followed by corrective modifications of the impulse patterns—[evidence of plasticity and of lack of intrinsic organisation.]. . . A crucial experiment, therefore, must aim at disrupting the monotony of central-peripheral correspondence. It must upset either the discharge pattern of the centres or the play of muscles or the distribution of nerve connections in such a manner as to make the established central impulse patterns yield incongrous effects for the body. If, thereafter, the body recovers more efficient use of the affected part— either instantaneously by systemic reaction, or gradually by heuristic procedure—the systemic or heuristic theories would score. If, on the other hand, corrective changes fail to occur and the nervous system continues to operate the part according to the old standard scheme of innervation now rendered inadequate, this would be incontestable proof of the *preformation* of coordination in form of definite central impulse patterns which do not produce appropriate effects, depending on whether the effector system for whose operation they are predesigned is intact or disarranged".

OBSERVATIONS ON "HOMOLOGOUS" OR
"MYOTYPIC" RESPONSE

The suggested mode of approach here is thus a variety of the recombination experiment and the observations began with some work of Weiss (1922) on the motor function of supernumary transplanted limbs in amphibia. In these experiments Weiss transplanted limbs in larvae of Salamandra maculosa after limb innervation had occurred and limb function had started. It was found that the transplanted limbs, provided that they were placed within the general region of the limb-segments of the spinal cord, would become innervated and show coordinated motor function. In each case the transplanted limb was found to show "homologous response" with the normal limb; that is, when the normal limb flexed, so did the transplant; when the normal limb extended, so did the transplant, and so forth and so on, for all observed movements. These experiments were repeated and extended by Weiss over the next few years and the results were published, in English, in a series of papers from 1926 to 1937 (Weiss, 1926; 1937a; 1937b; 1937c; 1937d.) In particular, the phenomenon of homologous response, and the whole question of the origin of coordination, has been reviewed by Weiss in a most stimulating and lucid fashion in two papers which have rightly become classics in this field (Weiss, 1936; 1941). Homologous response has also been shown to occur in urodele limbs that had been transplanted as buds in the embryo (Detwiler, 1925); in anuran limbs transplanted in embryo (Hughes, 1964); in birds where the limb anlage was transplanted in embryo (Székely and Szentágothai, 1962); and possibly in the human as a result of intrauterine maldevelopment (Weiss, 1935).

Weiss' original experiments on homologous response were performed on small animals (larvae of Salamandra maculosa) and only responses of the limb as a whole could be well seen. In his later work this author used large axolotls and newly metamorphosed toads and was thus able to extend his observations to the level of individual muscles. The results of this work can be summarized as follows: if a limb is transplanted into the vicinity of another limb and thus receives its new innervation from the appropriate limb-level of the spinal cord, each muscle in the transplanted limb will, when actively moving, function simultaneously with the homologous muscle in the adjacent normal limb and with the same degree of intensity (syndynamic response). This phenomenon has been called "homologous" or "myotypic" response in the transplant (Weiss, 1926).

Myotypic or homologous response in the muscles of a transplanted limb may be seen with great regularity in urodele limbs transplanted under these conditions and the homologous function occurs in all cases, no matter what the topographic relationship of the transplanted limb to the body and to the normal limb may be (Weiss, 1926). Thus if the transplant comes from the opposite side of the body and is placed near the normal limb in dorso-dorsal orientation, the result is a mirror-image arrangement as shown in Fig. 2.2. Homologous response in such a case indicates simultaneous activity in like muscles of the two limbs and, due to the symmetrical disposition of the normal and the transplanted limbs, their locomotor effects cancel each other (Fig. 2.3). This type of behaviour appears to rule out any adaptive or "learning" mechanism causal in the development of the homologous response.

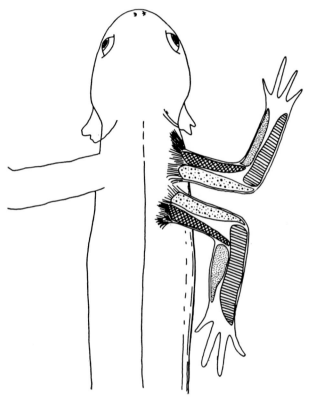

FIG. 2.2.   Diagram to show the mirror-image arrangement of muscles in a normal right limb and a supernumary left limb transplanted near by with reversed rostrocaudal orientation. Muscles of identical names are indicated by identical shading. From Weiss, 1950.

In spite of the functionally maladaptive nature of this sort of symmetrical "scissors" movement, no changes were observed with time that could suggest any modification of the movements as a result of experience (Weiss, 1937d). The uselessness, or even the positively disadvantageous nature of some such limb transplants is well illustrated in some further variations on this theme by Weiss. If, instead of grafting a left limb beside a normal right limb, the two limbs are cross-transplanted (Fig. 2.4) the resulting

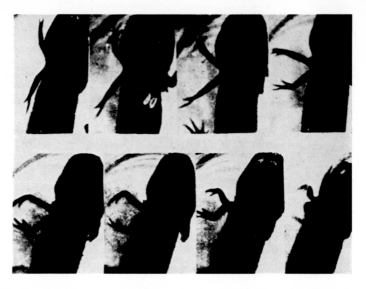

FIG. 2.3. Sequence from a motion picture of a salamander with a pair of limbs of opposite polarity at the left shoulder, performing exact mirror-image movements. From Weiss, 1950.

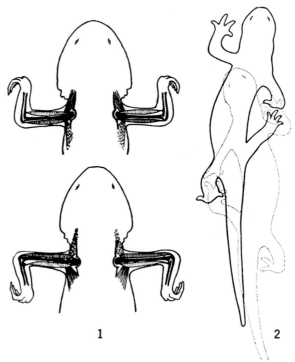

1   2

FIG. 2.4. (1) Diagram showing the anatomy and muscular arrangements in the forelimbs of (top) a normal animal; (bottom) an animal with exchanged forelimbs. ┊ ┊ ┊ adductor muscle (m. pectoralis); ≡ abductor muscle (m. deltoideus). ||||||| extensor of the elbow (m. anconeus); :::::: flexor of the elbow (m. humero-antibrachialis): (2) Diagram showing the method of progression of the salamander (after Braus). The dotted contour indicates the initial phase, the full contour the end phase of one step during which the left foot and the right hand have retained their places on the ground. From Fig. 1, Weiss, 1937, *J. comp. Neurol.* **67**, 272.

anatomy of the forelimbs is the reverse of normal in the rostrocaudal direction. In this situation the muscles of the transposed (reversed) limbs, while going through precisely the same cycle of activity which their synonymous muscles would go through in the normal limbs, move the body backwards instead of forwards (Fig. 2.5). Actual regression only occurs if other means of progression, such as the tail and hindlimbs, have been removed or paralysed. If the hindlimbs are present however, the effect is one of constant struggle between hind and forelimbs with the net result that the animal swings back and forth without moving from the spot. Some such animals were kept for more than a year without showing any sign of altering this maladaptive behaviour (Weiss, 1941).

In certain cases, when partial ankylosis has rendered part of the transplanted limb immobile, homologous response may be seen in the remaining mobile portion; or, when some of the limb muscles are missing, as when defective regeneration has resulted in the elbow of the transplant inserting directly in the host's body wall, the mobile transplanted forelimb remains inactive during contraction of the normal upper arm muscles but shows homologous response when the forearm muscles of the normal limb contract (Weiss, 1937a). In these cases homologous response is manifested in fragments of transplanted limbs; the reverse situation may also occur when multiple limbs are implanted within a small area (Weiss, 1937a). When this is done, the movements of the multiple transplants, inasmuch as they move at all, show myotypic response. However it appears that there is an upper limit to the number of limbs at one site that can be effectively and completely innervated by the host; when four limbs were present at one site, in no case was the function of all four complete (Weiss, 1937a) and a partial reason for this failure is probably the mechanical and traumatic upset at the site of implantation, resulting from having such a grove of limbs sprouting from one shoulder. It seems generally to be impossible to secure adequate nerve supply for more than two transplants in addition to the normal limb (Weiss, 1936).

Myotypic response in transplanted limbs may also occur when the donor and the host are of different species. Limbs taken from *Amblystoma punctatum* and grafted onto the much larger *A. mexicanum* (Weiss, 1937a) showed homologous response with the host limb. Heteroplastic transplantations of comparable sort have also been reported by Hertwig (1926, see Weiss, 1937a) and they show that homologous muscles of different species are more closely related in the one respect which determines their response to the central nervous system than are any two non-homologous muscles, even of the same individual. In some such heteroplastic transplantations there is a considerable size-discrepancy between the transplant and the host limb. There may be up to 1:10 ratio of body volume (Weiss, 1937a) and despite this inequality, which must be partly reflected in the muscle masses involved in the contractions, the movements of the transplant and

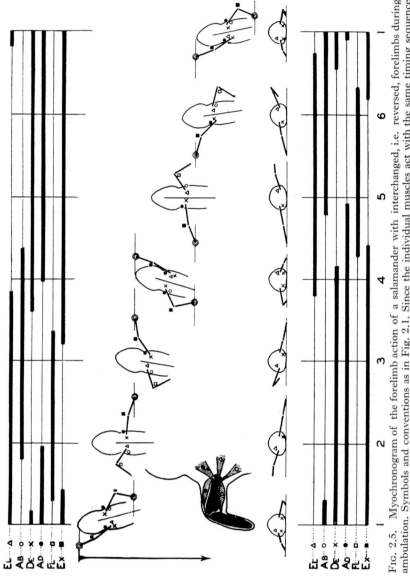

FIG. 2.5. Myochronogram of the forelimb action of a salamander with interchanged, i.e. reversed, forelimbs during ambulation. Symbols and conventions as in Fig. 2.1. Since the individual muscles act with the same timing sequence as they had done when they were still operating normal legs with unreversed musculature, instead of progression the result is regression. From Weiss, 1941.

the normal limb are homologous. Since in any movement of a joint several muscles are involved, it appears that corresponding movements, or eventual angular positions of the limb, in the normal and in the transplant, can only be achieved if the ratio of intensities of contraction of the muscles engaged in the movement is similar in the normal limb and in the transplant. Yet the absolute tensions developed by the small muscles of the transplant will presumably be much smaller than those developed in the normal limb. In an autoplastic transplant, where the limb is approximately the same size as the normal limb, homologous response is "syndynamic"; that is, each muscle in the transplant contracts not only simultaneously with the corresponding muscle [in the normal limb] but also to the same extent. This cannot be so where limbs of considerably different size are concerned, and the way in which the "syndynamic" nature of homologous response is scaled-down in small limbs would be worth investigating.

When the muscles in a transplanted limb show homologous response it appears that the central nervous system is calling them into action by name, so to speak. When the biceps in the normal limb contracts, so does the biceps in the transplant; when the triceps in the normal limb contracts, so does the triceps in the transplant. And so on, for all the individual muscles examined. This is evidence that the central nervous system "knows" which muscle is which in the transplanted limb. But there is another way in which muscles can be excited, apart from by descending impulses from the spinal cord. This is by means of the myotatic or stretch reflex, which may be very strictly localized to the muscle excited. Stretch reflexes involve, in mammals, a two-neurone arc, where impulses coming up from stretch receptors in a particular muscle are fed as a monosynaptic excitatory input to the motoneurones supplying the same muscle— the tightest form of neuronal coupling possible. The organization of reflex excitation of the limb musculature appears to be quite different in the frog, where afferents from the muscles themselves are incapable of giving rise to motoneurone firing and thus muscular contraction (Simpson, 1969). Monosynaptic EPSPs are recordable from frog motoneurones but they do not, by themselves, lead to discharge of the cell; reflex firing of frog moto- neurones is, on the other hand, readily brought about by "natural" stimulation of localized regions of skin (Simpson, 1969). When the level of excitatory input to the motoneurone is high enough (in *Xenopus*), as for instance it may be with subliminal cutaneous input, then it is possible that a muscle stretch reflex may occur (Holemans *et al.*, 1966; Meij *et al.*, 1966; discussed by Simpson, 1969). Thus it seems that what occurs in anurans is monosynaptic facilitation of the motoneurone rather than monosynaptic excitation as in the cat. The status of the stretch reflex in urodeles has not been investigated; yet localized responses to muscle stretch may be seen in muscles of transplanted limbs; and in this case reflex excitation of one particular muscle in the transplant is accompanied by similar activation of the corresponding muscle in the normal limb (Verzar and Weiss, 1929; Weiss, 1937a). Weiss noted that such reflexes are only seen in the presence of adequate tonic excitation as a background, so the situation in urodeles may be comparable to that in the anurans. This suggests that in a transplant showing homologous response, not only does the centre correctly identify the muscle in the motor connections formed but the muscle is also correctly identified by the sensory fibres as well. Since Simpson (1969) has shown, however, that the motoneurone EPSPs evoked in frogs by cutaneous stimulation are characteristic for the skin region stimulated, it is possible that the "joint-specific" reflexes obtained by Weiss (Verzar and Weiss, 1929; Weiss, 1937a) were at least partly specific for inputs other than the muscle afferents. That limb sensory innervation, however, is not *necessary* for the appearance of homologous response was shown by experiments involving the deafferentation of the forelimb region before transplantation of a limb into the district (Weiss, 1937c).

There are two further experimental modifications that require comment at this time. The observations mentioned so far have involved transplantation of limbs and in such cases it is possible only in the most general way to determine the innervation of the transplant. To make the analysis of function in reinnervated limbs more penetrating it would be necessary to know with precision the origin of the nerve supply. This has been done in some experiments where the transplanted limbs were innervated solely by a branch of the inferior brachial nerve, cut at elbow level. In this situation the transplant was innervated wholly by a lower-arm nerve containing, presumably, exclusively fibres for wrist and finger muscles. Transplants supplied in this fashion showed homologous response in *all* muscles, including those of the shoulder and upper arm (Weiss, 1936).

The second experimental modification is a variant on that just described. Weiss (1930a,b; 1931) achieved a method for the transplantation of individual muscles in young adult anurans whereby the muscles could remain alive and functional and could be innervated by a preselected and precisely determined nerve supply. In such cases many of the transplanted and foreign-innervated muscles showed homologous response with the normal muscle of the same name. We will consider these results in more detail later when we discuss possible mechanisms for the phenomenon of homologous response.

OBSERVATIONS ON THE MECHANISM OF THE HOMOLOGOUS RESPONSE

Before we discuss the possible mechanisms which may underlie the homologous response of transplanted limbs and muscles it will be as well to ask first whether there exists in fact anything requiring explanation. The observations on myotypic or homologous response have been available for over 40 years and yet they have made very little impact on the world of neurophysiology. This comparative lack of interest taken in these findings by neurophysiologists is surprising. Perhaps it is partly to be explained, as Weiss (1941) suggests, by the well-known preoccupation of physiologists with the constituent elements rather than with the system as a whole. An alternative explanation could be that the observations are misleading, the phenomenon of homologous response does not actually exist, and all right-thinking neurophysiologists realize this.

Unfortunately the factual basis for the reports of myotypic response has been inadequately revealed by most of the experimentation on the subject. Much the greater part of the evidence has come (and continues to come) from visual or photographic observation of the contracting muscles. It was by this means that Weiss constructed his myochronograms. And in all such cases the precision of the observations has been less than is required to provide an adequate framework for the complex logical edifice that has been constructed to account for the supposed findings.

The precise timing (and, to some extent, the intensity) of contraction of a muscle *can* be estimated by cinephotography; but only if the muscle is observed in an adequately isolated condition. As soon as the muscle is observed in its natural surroundings, playing its part along with several other muscles in ordering the movement of one or more joints, photography becomes at best an inadequate method for determining the phasing of activity. Weiss (1931) has attempted to get round this difficulty by recording the mechanical activity of individual transplanted muscles in newly-metamorphosed anurans. And while mechanical recording is here preferable to photography, the techniques then available (thread, levers, smoked drums) were too crude to permit adequately precise determination of phase and strength of contraction.

Most of the discussion about homologous response has centred on the timing of the contractions in the transplant and the relationship of this timing to activity in the normal limb. In this situation the tacit assumption is made that the muscular contraction is brought about by nerve impulses. If this is so then the ideal method for comparing the timing of neuronal discharges would be to record directly the compound action potentials from the appropriate motor nerves in the normal limb and in the transplant. This has not so far been attempted, as far as I know, largely because of the very considerable technical difficulties involved. Firstly there is the dauntingly small size of the muscles concerned and thus of their nerves; then there is the difficulty that always attends multiple recordings, where problems increase exponentially with the number of recording channels being used; and finally there is the difficulty associated with movement of the animal, although it is possible that this could be obviated by neuro-muscular blocking agents.

A more direct, and therefore more satisfactory, method of timing the activity in the various muscles concerned is to use electromyography. Here we are still confronted with difficulties of muscle size and we also have the problem of movement artifact, which can make interpretation of the records difficult. However by use of fine (50μ diameter) insulated wires, twisted together in pairs, with several pairs threaded through a tubular silk suture to keep them together, it has proved possible to record from up to eight muscles simultaneously in a urodele limb (Székely, 1968) with the type of result shown in Fig. 2.6 and there seems to be no reason why this method should not be extended to take in even more muscles simultaneously. Preliminary results obtained by the use of this method (Székely, 1968) have raised some doubts about the validity of the previous observations on homologous response. Electromyographic recordings made in freely moving animals showed that, while some of the homologous limb muscles (e.g. extensor ulnae) were active simultaneously in both normal limb and transplant, other homologous muscles (e.g. brachialis, extensor digitorum communis) contracted with a considerable phase-shift relative to each other. Since the phase-shift was of the order of 100–300 msec, it was too small to be detected by watching the animal, and the movements of the normal and grafted limb appeared to be synchronized (Székely, 1968). Obviously, further investigation is needed, using electromyographic recording, before we can say to what extent, with what precision, homologous response obtains in transplanted limbs. Yet even at the present time we are able to say, since the available photographic evidence is adequate for this purpose, that there does exist a problem. The homologous response that may be seen after limb transplantation is sufficiently remarkable for us to ask how the nervous system does it.

THE INNERVATION OF THE TRANSPLANTED LIMB

The simplest way to account for coordinated function, or myotypic response, in a transplanted limb would be (a) in the case of a replacement graft, for each nerve fibre in the host limb nerve supply to find its way to the appropriate muscle; or (b) in the case of a supernumary graft, for each of the host limb nerve fibres to branch and for the branches to find their way to the appropriate muscle in the transplant. Under these circumstances properly coordinated function in a replacement graft and myotypic response in a supernumary graft would automatically follow from the anatomical distribution of the nerve fibres.

Normally the urodele forelimb is supplied by the 3rd, 4th and 5th spinal roots. In the case of a replacement graft, the entire forelimb nerve supply of the host is available to innervate the transplant. But when the graft is supernumary, limb innervation occurs from those fibres in the vicinity of the implant which have been cut, by accident or by design, at the time of operation. In a series of experiments involving replacement

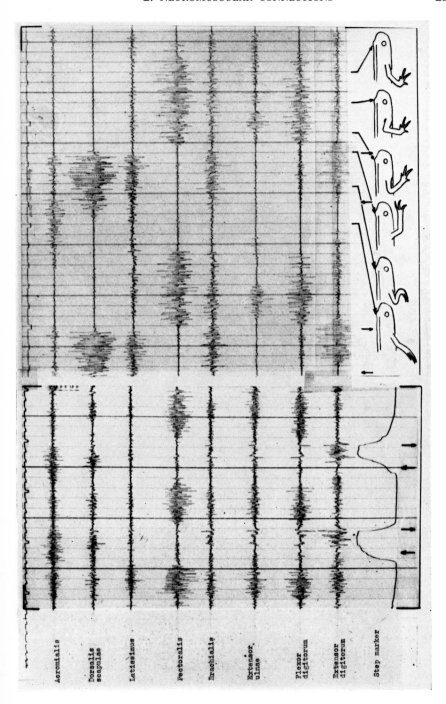

FIG. 2.6. Simultaneous electromyographic recordings from various forelimb muscles in a newt. Record supplied through the courtesy of Dr. G. Székely. From Székely, Czéh and Vörös, 1969.

autografts in *Amblystoma*, Detwiler (1920) excised a forelimb bud and reimplanted it from one to seven segments caudal to its proper position. He noted that with a caudal shift of one or two segments, the limb still became innervated by the normal 3rd, 4th and 5th brachial segments of the cord. Removal of the limb bud further caudally resulted in innervation by more caudal segments, but coordinated limb function was still seen in some of the limbs, so long as they received innervation from at least one of the three brachial nerves. When the limb was innervated exclusively by non-brachial nerves, it no longer showed coordinated function. These experiments suggest, what has since been confirmed by the active group of Hungarian embryologists whose work will be mentioned later, that the limb-segments of the cord require to be connected with the limb for the latter to function properly. This conclusion was pointed nicely by later experiments by Detwiler and Carpenter (1929) in which limbs were so placed as to be innervated by the 5th, 6th and 7th spinal nerves. Such grafts generally show coordinated movements (Detwiler, 1936) and severing the 6th or 7th nerves, the 5th remaining intact, had no effect on limb function; whereas severance of the 5th nerve terminated coordinated movement in the limb. It thus seems likely that in these cases the whole functional innervation of the limb was dependent on fibres from the 5th nerve, one of the normal limb supply. Weiss also reports cases where he innervated a graft, this time a supernumary limb, from the 5th nerve only; and this spinal nerve made functional connections with all the limb muscles present (Weiss, 1937b). Interestingly, the 5th nerve has been described as the "weakest" of the three (Weiss, 1936) in that its transaction in an otherwise normal animal causes no appreciable functional defect in the limb.

Since the normal innervation of the forelimb is by 3, 4 and 5, it seems odd that an apparently normal functional innervation can be achieved by 5 alone. One feels like asking what the other two are for. But here we have to consider the nature of spinal nerves and segmental arrangements in the urodeles, which is very different from that in mammals. Székely and Czéh (1967) have shown, by observation of muscle contractions following localized electrical stimulation within the cord, that in axolotls most limb muscles are represented in each of the three brachial segments (Fig. 2.7). A similar conclusion may be reached from the earlier work of Nicholas and Barron (1935) who found that electrical stimulation of any one of the three plexus nerves gave contractions in muscles over the whole length of the arm; and from the experiments of Thompson (1936), who found degenerating fibres present in all muscles examined after sectioning any one of the three limb nerves. On this evidence we must say that each of the three segmental nerves, that normally together supply the limb, contains a skeleton supply of fibres adequate in kind for all the muscles of the limb. Thus it is not so surprising that a limb can be adequately innervated by

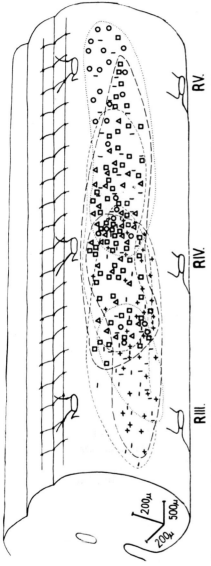

FIG. 2.7. Distribution of limb motoneurones in the spinal cord of the axolotl. A grid of 100 $\mu \times 500\ \mu$ squares on the surface of the spinal cord indicates the sites of stimulation. The electrode was inserted at the intersection points of the grid, and advanced in 20 μ steps. The symbols represent the places of lowest threshold in evoking muscle contractions, as projected to the lateral surface of the cord. Note the distortion of the micron scale.

— — — shoulder $\left\{\begin{array}{l} + \text{ Protractors and Elevators} \\ \square \text{ Retractors and Depressors} \end{array}\right.$

– – – – arm $\left\{\begin{array}{l} — \text{ Flexors} \\ \triangle \text{ Extensors} \end{array}\right.$

· · · · · · forearm $\left\{\begin{array}{l} | \text{ Flexors} \\ \bigcirc \text{ Extensors} \end{array}\right.$

After the work of Székely and Czéh (1967); from Székely, 1968.

only one of the segmental nerves but the mechanism whereby this takes place has still to be elucidated.

The number of fibres in each of the three brachial nerves was counted by Weiss (1937b) on the normal side and on the side carrying one or more transplants. Although there was considerable fluctuation between counts in different roots on the normal and the operated side, the extremes of difference between the total numbers of left and right limb fibres ranged only from $+30\%$ to -9.8%, a variation that would also be found in normal animals. That is, the total numbers of motor fibres produced within the spinal cord on the two sides was comparable. Direct counts of the numbers of spinal cord cells on the two sides have confirmed that in these animals the addition of an extra limb does not lead to increase in cell numbers on the affected side (Detwiler, 1936).

Thus the addition of one or more extra limbs to the periphery causes no appreciable increase in the total number of limb fibres proximal to the plexus (Weiss, 1936). Yet the final number of fibres present in each limb is strikingly close to normal (Weiss, 1937b) and this increase in the number of fibres occurs solely by branching of the existing fibres during their regeneration. The tendency of transplanted limbs to become filled with nerve fibres up to their normal capacity is very intriguing and suggests the existence of some form of control by the periphery of the number of regenerating fibres admitted (Weiss, 1937b). It is worth noting here that, while the cord cell counts are probably reliable, this does not necessarily apply to the fibre counts. These latter were performed by light microscopy, using myelin staining (Weiss, 1937b). Weiss estimated that the total number of fibres, including unmyelinated fibres, would be greater by less than 25%. While this could be so, it requires checking with the electron microscope, in view of the fact that light-microscopic estimates of the number of unmyelinated fibres may be wrong by more than a factor of ten (compare the results of Bruesch and Arey, 1942, who used light microscopy on frog optic nerve fibres, with those of Maturana, 1959, who used the electron microscope). In this context it would also be useful to know whether, although the numbers of root fibres are comparable to normal, these fibres are the same ones as were originally present. It may be that, following inadequate peripheral connection, certain fibres regress and are replaced by new outgrowth. If we are seriously to consider preferential reinnervation of muscles by their appropriate nerve fibres, then it becomes most relevant that we should know the *extent* of branching at or near the nerve lesion, since the number of ingrowing branches should be sufficient to allow considerable numbers of fibres to fail to find their right muscles.

Weiss (1937b) based his estimates of the number of fibres present in the transplant on counts performed on myelin-stained sections. These counts showed that, for instance, in a transplant innervated by the 5th nerve, in order to account for the normal number of fibres in the grafted limb, each fibre entering the limb would have to branch approximately six times as extensively as it would do under normal conditions. However, these estimates seem to have been made on fairly long-term, functioning grafts; in other words, when the reinnervation has already reached a fairly stable state. But the initial regeneration of these fibres will be, in all probability, unmyelinated. We have therefore *no* indication of the initial extent of branching during the ingrowth of the regenerating fibres and it would be most worthwhile to examine this electron microscopically. Collateral nerve sprouting, which is highly relevant to any mechanism of reinnervation in transplanted limbs, has been extensively reviewed by Edds (1953); and Shawe (1955) has shown that, in the rabbit, extensive sprouting occurs around the level of the nerve lesion, with the numbers of fibres present below the nerve crush reaching a maximum at 50 days; many of these branches had disappeared by 100 days. Myelination was seen to proceed from about 10 days onwards and about half the early axons failed to myelinate and disappeared. In an electron microscopic study of axon sprouting in partially deneurotized nerves in the rat, Causey and Hoffman (1955) found that the normal tibial nerve in this animal contains very few unmyelinated fibres but that as early as 24 hours after resection of L5, groups of small (0·1 micron) fibres are to be seen in the nerve. With increasing time after operation greater numbers of such bundles of unmyelinated fibres could be seen and in some fields the collaterals outnumbered the surviving myelinated fibres by 7:1.

Weiss (1937b) argues strongly against [selective reinnervation] as the explanation of homologous response in transplanted limbs and muscles. One of the bases of his argument is that there are about 40 muscles in the urodele forelimb and that, according to observations on the phenomenon of homologous response, each of these can be independently activated by the spinal cord. On the basis of selective reinnervation we would therefore have to postulate 40 different types of motor nerve fibres, one for each muscle (but see comments at the end of the chapter), and each type would have to be capable of reaching and connecting exclusively with its appropriate muscle type (Weiss, 1937b). As we will see later, exclusivity of the sort envisaged is not an initial requirement for selective reinnervation. If we leave this point aside for the present and continue to the next part of Weiss' argument, we find that he is prepared to concede as possible the existence of so many different specificities among the nerve fibres, but rejects the idea of specific ingrowth. The choice made by the ingrowing nerve fibres would have to be made (Weiss, 1937b) at the point where the nerve fibres enter the limb, indicating that the regenerating fibres were able to identify and follow their proper paths from this point. At the site of nerve entry there is frequently to be found a meshwork of nerve fibres which could perhaps be interpreted as an attempt of the growing fibres to find their appropriate pathways. This interpretation is refuted by the observation that the neuroma frequently disentangles itself into a series of parallel bundles at a level far proximal to the most proximal end of the degenerated peripheral fibres. Thus the ingrowing fibres would be grouped long before reaching the level at which selection was supposed to occur.

In a further argument, Weiss (1937b) takes up the numbers of fibres involved. In one animal showing the homologous response in a transplant innervated by the 5th nerve, some 900 fibres were found to innervate the graft. Assuming that 60% of these are sensory we are left with 360 motor fibres of which some 120 go to the trunk muscles, leaving 240 for the limb itself. With 40 different muscles, and allowing for some branching, we would get a figure of approximately 15 fibres per muscle. Weiss thinks that the numbers are so small that they leave little margin for error on the part of the fibres and that the massive overproduction of branches that would presumably be necessary to allow successful reinnervation of this sort to occur has never been seen. It is relevant to mention, however, that one would not perhaps *expect* to see such massive branching when it occurred, using the myelin-staining methods of Weiss. All such branches will be unmyelinated at first and it is very likely, in view of the work of Shawe (1955) and Causey and Hoffman (1955) referred to previously, that those fibres which fail to connect adequately may regress, leaving only those that have effected satisfactory connections. If thus one had extensive initial branching, such that members of each "class" of neurones found their way into each of the regenerating fascicles, the eventual picture could be somewhat similar to that described.

There is some evidence against the idea of specific initial reinnervation, however, that is rather better than that already mentioned. The work I refer to involves the innervation of transplants by distal limb nerves (Weiss, 1937b) and the innervation of individual transplanted muscles by preselected foreign nerves.

The transplants discussed so far were mainly innervated by fibres coming from the region of the limb plexus supplying the adjacent normal limb. In such cases it is not possible in any one instance to specify the original destination of the fibres which eventually innervate the transplant. And if the innervation is directly from one of the three limb segment nerves, the evidence of Nicholas and Barron (1935) and of Thompson (1936) indicates that a complete set of limb nerve fibres would be present in any case. If, however, the innervation of the transplant is taken from one of the distal nerves in the normal limb, then we may be reasonably sure that the fibres contained therein are properly destined for distal limb muscles and *not* for muscles of the upper arm. This was done in several animals by Weiss (1937b). The nerve selected was the inferior brachial (normally supplying the flexor muscles of the forearm at this level) or one of its branches. The nerve was cut at the level of the elbow and looped back to innervate the transplant. The graft then gave homologous response and electrical stimulation of the supply nerve as it entered the transplant resulted in contraction of the entire musculature of the limb, including the muscles of the upper arm and the extensors of the forearm. Histological examination confirmed the restricted source of the innervation. In this situation therefore, we have nerve fibres, or, to be more precise, a nerve, which originally innervated a restricted region of the forelimb and which eventually successfully innervated an entire limb graft. This observation would seem to preclude initial selective reinnervation since the adequate fibres would not be present in the chosen nerve supply. However, in view of the importance that attaches to this experiment, from the point of view of the modulation hypothesis (see p. 33), we would be justified in requiring more convincing proof that *only* the designated nerve had reinnervated the limb.

The second experimental situation where the innervation of a transplant can be accurately known involves the transplantation of individual muscles to a foreign site and their selective innervation by a preselected, foreign nerve (Weiss, 1930a,b; 1931). These observations were made on small (3–5 cm) toads, *Bufo viridis*, and Weiss devised a method for the successful autotransplantation of selected muscles from the hindlimb to a site on the lower back of the animal. The isolated muscle would then be supplied with a nerve chosen by the experimenter, in particular a nerve containing no fibres for the muscle in question. For instance, for transplanted upper thigh muscles nerves were brought from the lower thigh; and for lower thigh muscles the nerve from the antagonist was chosen. In some cases one of the spinal nerves supplying the hindlimb (8th, 9th and 10th roots) was used to innervate the transplanted muscle. Muscle activity in response to various forms of "natural" stimulation was recorded mechanically, using levers and a writing drum.

The results of these experiments are extremely interesting: they are fully described in a paper in Pflügers' Archiv (Weiss, 1931). There were two major classes of result: Group A (13 animals) showed specific myotypic response in the transplant (Fig. 2.8) and no response synchronous with the simultaneously recorded control muscle; group B (13 animals) showed predominantly the phenomenon of myotypic response in that these contractions were most marked, but this group of animals also showed non-specific contraction in that the transplant would, in addition to the major contraction of a myotypic nature, contract along with all the other muscles to some degree (Fig. 2.9). There was also some small amount of evidence suggesting that the number of non-specifically reacting muscles declined with increasing time after the operation: of 10 animals recorded between 50 and 100 days after operation, 3 were in group A and 7 in group B; whereas of 14 animals recorded between 100 and 150 days after operation, 10 were in group A and only 4 in group B. As Weiss (1930b) remarks, the numbers of animals are too small to be conclusive; they may, however, show a trend for increasing homology of response with increasing time.

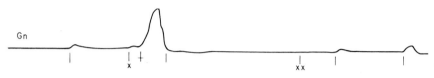

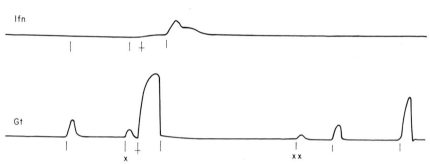

Fig. 2.8. Function of transplanted gastrocnemius, innervated by the n. peroneus. Upper curve, normal gastrocnemius; middle curve, normal iliofibularis; lower curve, transplanted gastrocnemius. Response to multiple stimulations of the ipsilateral forelimb. In this case, one of Weiss' Group A (see text), the transplanted muscle acts homologously with the control gastrocnemius. From Weiss, 1931.

In further experiments Weiss (1936) denervated one limb of a young toad and then supplied it with innervation from one of the nerves of the other limb. Initial reinnervation of the limb muscles was associated with a well-marked stage of unspecific contraction, when any activity in the limb was associated with a general contraction of all the reinnervated muscles. Eventually some homologous response appeared in these animals, many weeks later. In the absence of more detailed reports of the experiments it is perhaps reasonable to postulate that the initial mass response was due to innervation of the musculature by branches of the (unmodulated) deviated nerve; whereas the later partial appearance of homologous response could have been due to reinnervation by the appropriate fibres.

In an attempt to trace individual nerves to their precise terminations, Weiss (1937b) employed electrical stimulation in cases of limb transplantation. If nerve-branching from the nerves supplying the normal limb plays a part in the innervation of the transplant, and if both branches, that in the normal limb and that in the transplant, make functional connection, one would expect electrical stimulation of one of the branches to result in

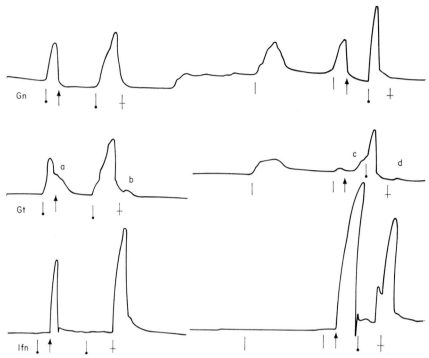

Fig. 2.9. Function of transplanted gastrocnemius, innervated by n. peroneus. Upper curve, normal gastrocnemius; middle curve, transplanted gastrocnemius; lower curve, normal iliofibularis. Stimulation applied to ipsilateral forelimb. In this case, one of Weiss' Group B (see text), the homologous response of the transplanted muscle is interrupted by unspecific contractions, simultaneous with those of the iliofibularis, at a, b, c, d. From Weiss, 1931.

contractions in both limbs, brought about by a form of axon reflex. In two experiments, responses attributed to axon reflexes were in fact seen; these were only obtained in the one direction of conduction and not the other, and the response in each limb was from different muscles. Weiss took these findings to mean that some bifurcated fibres ended on different muscles in each limb. Unfortunately the interpretation of these electrical stimulation experiments is not so obvious as one would like, for at least two reasons: firstly, the area being stimulated was very small and it would be extremely difficult to rule out stimulus escape to nearby structures; this did in fact happen, since muscles adjacent to the point of stimulus were in some cases directly excited. Secondly, even if stimulus escape did not occur, the experimental findings do not necessarily indicate branched fibres connecting each with more than one type of muscle. As may be seen from Fig. 2.10 if we consider some of the branches to be abortive, a different interpretation of the results is possible.

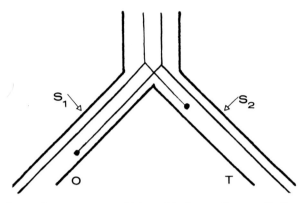

F IG. 2.10. A neural arrangement which could give an "axon reflex" as observed by Weiss (see text), but with a different explanation. The branched nerve trunk contains two axons as shown, which themselves branch; but one branch of each ends blindly. In this situation, stimulation at point S_1 (original limb) would give rise to an "axon reflex" in the transplant (T)—but contractions in the two limbs will be in different muscles and mediated by different nerve fibres; stimulation at S_2 (transplant) would give no "axon reflex" in the reverse direction.

Axon reflexes have been demonstrated in human motoneurones, following peripheral nerve lesions (Fullerton and Gilliat, 1965). These authors stimulated the median or ulnar nerve at the wrist and recorded the electromyogram from the appropriate small hand muscles. Normal subjects show a direct, or M wave followed by a much smaller (5% of M) F wave; the M-wave latency represents the conduction-time from wrist to muscle (2–4 msec), whereas the F wave is partly due to antidromic excitation of motoneurones, being linearly related to the length of the arm, and having a latency of 24–32 msec. Patients with high peripheral nerve lesions often show intermediate muscle responses and these appear to be due to axon reflexes, since (1) the latency is decreased by stimulating more proximally; (2) the latency is usually too short to permit conduction up to the cord and back again; (3) increasing the stimulus strength alters the timing—it shortens the latency markedly—presumably due to direct stimulation of both branches, thus giving now a direct M wave for each; (4) this interpretation seems to be confirmed by the result of stimulation at two positions, when proximal stimulation gave decreased latency for the weak stimulus (afferent arc only stimulated), but increased latency for the strong shock (efferents stimulated direct). These axon reflexes were only seen in patients with peripheral nerve lesions and they would indicate branching at or near the site of injury. No comparable evidence has yet been produced for the amphibian experiments described here.

INTERPRETATIONS OF THE HOMOLOGOUS RESPONSE

From the results of his early experiments Weiss (1926) was led to conclude:

(1) Homologous response occurs in transplanted limbs and muscles.

(2) The homologous or myotypic response occurs in all circumstances and no matter what the topographical relationship of the transplant may be to the body and to the normal limb, i.e. it may occur even though the functional result is grossly maladaptive.

(3) The innervation of the transplant is from multiple branching of fibres occurring near the site of implantation.

(4) The ingrowth of fibres that occurs is non-selective, it being a matter of chance on what muscles the particular branches of the nerve fibres eventually form their end-organs.

(5) Each motor ganglion cell in the implantation region is connected with a number of different muscles of different kinds. This, Weiss thought, had to follow from (a) the lack of hyperplasia in the motor centres after transplantation, (b) the great amount of branching at the site of implantation, and (c) the observation that a distal limb nerve, of limited fibre composition, could effectively innervate a whole limb.

(6) Although connected with the same ganglion cell and receiving their excitation from the same ganglion cell, each of the muscles concerned is capable of contraction without the others, as shown by the homologous response.

From these various points Weiss reached the conclusion that the muscle *does not respond to every excitation conveyed to it from the ganglion cell*. This consideration led him to propose his well-known *Resonance Principle* to account for neuromuscular coordination and its development. Each muscle was considered to have its own specific form of irritability and could be excited only by the appropriate impulse pattern. Central coordination consisted in the combining of excitations for the various muscles that were to function at a given moment. All the component excitations (impulses, patterns of impulses) were conveyed through *each* of the fibres of the motor root, to the periphery, where the particular muscles responded to their specific excitation components. Thus the muscles were held each to play the part of a selective filter which would respond, or "resonate", only to the appropriate pattern of excitation coming, along with that for all the other muscles, down the motor nerve fibre.

The key point in this resonance hypothesis was that the muscle itself did the selecting from the grand total of excitations heading similarly down each and every motor nerve fibre. This would imply that, whenever a particular muscle is activated in a reflex contraction, the same patterns of impulses are also going to other muscles in the same group which do not contract. This point was investigated by Wiersma (1931) who recorded, in

2*

frogs, either the electrical activity in the sartorius nerve and simultaneously the mechanical activity of the triceps femoris and the ileofibularis, or the electrical activity in the nerve to the cruralis and simultaneously the mechanical contractions in triceps femoris and sartorius (Fig. 2.11). The

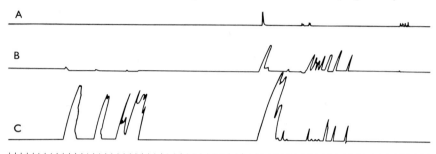

Fig. 2.11. Experiment demonstrating the incorrectness of the original neuromuscular resonance hypothesis. Mechanical recordings made from the triceps femoris (B) and sartorius (C) indicate the reflex activity of these muscles in response to adequate cutaneous stimulation. Despite the presence of activity in these two muscles there are no action potentials recordable from a nerve branch going to a muscle that is not involved in the reflex responses (A: electrical recording from nerve to cruralis). Initially, the sartorius contracts in response to a mild stimulation, but no electrical activity is seen in the n. cruralis; then both sartorius and triceps contract simultaneously and electrical activity is recorded in the crural nerve; next contractions of both sartorius and triceps occur, but in the absence of activity in the crural nerve; and finally, in response to contralateral cutaneous stimulation, the crural nerve gives a discharge but no response occurs in either of the two muscles recorded. The experiments were done on spinal frogs. From Wiersma, 1931.

results were not in agreement with Weiss' resonance theory: when the sartorius contracts to mild reflex stimulation, no impulses are seen in the nerve to the cruralis; when triceps contracts, there need be no impulses in nerve to cruralis; and when impulses occur in nerve to cruralis, there need be no contraction in either muscle recorded.

These observations disposed of the original resonance theory and Wiersma proposed that, instead of the muscles, the motor neurones themselves did the selecting. There remains, however, the problem of accounting for the homologous response in transplanted limbs. If the spinal centre has already selected the appropriate impulses and distributed them to certain motor neurones, then those motoneurones must connect with the proper muscles in order to give a coordinated homologous response. Weiss therefore altered his argument somewhat and postulated that each muscle had its own specificity, an intrinsic property of the muscle itself, and this specific character "modulated" the nerve fibre which connected with the muscle. The process of modulation was thought of as a centripetally-travelling specification of the nerve fibre by the muscle and was now taken to embrace the whole motor unit, including the motor neurone in the cord (Weiss, 1936). The nature of the modulation effect was (and is) quite unknown but was presumably some biochemical change induced in the nerve fibre by effective contact with the muscle in question. Thus a fibre ending on a gastrocnemius muscle would become modulated as a gastrocnemius-specific fibre; this modulation would extend right up to the motor neurone itself. In 1936 (Weiss) the concept was that a gastrocnemius-specific motoneurone in the cord would admit only gastrocnemius-specific impulses. With some modification, notably a slight shift of emphasis from "specific impulses" to specific intracentral connections (Sperry, 1941), this remains the view of most authors up till the present era. Figure 2.12 illustrates a recent synthesis of Weiss' ideas on the subject of modulation. The specific character of supernumary muscle B modulates the (randomly ingrowing) neurones that innervate it and the modulation

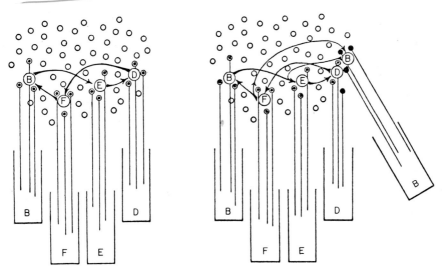

FIG. 2.12. Diagram showing the functional relationship between a supernumary muscle B and the coordination pattern FBED. A supernumary muscle B is grafted in the vicinity of muscle D and the graft eventually becomes innervated. The normal order of contraction of the original muscles B, F, E, D is FBED, as indicated by the arrows between the motoneurone pools. Supernumary muscle B is found to contract synchronously with normal muscle B; and since the muscle contraction merely serves as an indicator of the activity in its motoneurones, it appears that the motoneurones newly connected with the graft B have become functionally linked with those innervating the regular muscle B, as shown in the right half of the figure. From Weiss, 1950.

process, working up at the motoneurone level, induces the formation of new functional connections with the neurones supplying the original muscle B. Thus myotypic response can occur.

The discussion of neuromuscular coordination in this chapter so far may well give the impression that there is really only one writer in the field. The emphasis on the experiments and interpretations of Weiss is however not excessive in view of the fact that he started the observations on homologous response and has been the most prolific and ingenious investigator involved in the further analysis of such behaviour. There have been others working along similar lines however, notably R. W. Sperry and his collaborators and these workers have been responsible for the most recent *volte-face* in the somewhat confused study of myotypic response. In 1947 Sperry investigated the motor effects of section and regeneration of the oculomotor nerve in frog tadpoles and salamander larvae, both in mid- or late-larval stages. Section of the main oculomotor trunk was followed by motor recovery but not by recovery of coordination. The eye movements after regeneration of the nerve were abnormal and suggestive of a mass contraction of the eye musculature. There was little improvement in this abnormality with the passage of time and thus these experiments suggested that the misregenerated fibres had, mainly, retained their original central reflex timing without adjustment to their new motor terminations. There was, however, some evidence of partial restoration of coordination in that eye movements in the vertical plane appeared to be in the right direction and phase after regeneration. The overall failure to recover coordinated activity was not due merely to the effect of nerve section as such, since when the nerve branches supplying the individual muscles were cut and allowed to regenerate, functional recovery was excellent.

Quite different results were obtained when the operations were done in much younger frog tadpoles (18 mm length). Animals of this developmental stage already have compensatory eye movements, and in this case functional recovery after operation was eventually complete in all cases. The early stages of recovery, during the first $2\frac{1}{2}$ weeks after operation, were similar to those in the older animals: abnormal eye movements were seen. These younger tadpoles however showed continued improvement in coordination over about 7 weeks until the re-establishment of properly coordinated eye movements in all three planes was complete. In his interpretation of these results, Sperry was unable to decide whether selective muscle reinnervation or myotypic respecification of the regenerating nerves was responsible for the good recovery in early tadpoles; but he did note that regeneration here would be combined with the initial outgrowth of new motor axons and that this could play a part in the recovery process.

In further experiments, this time on the recovery of coordinated behaviour in fin muscles of the fish *Sphaeroides spengleri* after section of their nerve (Sperry, 1950), good recovery of muscular coordination was found after nerve regeneration. In this case Sperry discounted the possibility that selective reinnervation might have occurred and favoured instead myotypic respecification of the regenerating nerve fibres followed by synaptic reorganization in the spinal centres on a chemoaffinity basis. Thus up to this time (1950) there appeared to be very little reason to question the now-classical doctrine of "specific muscle energies" or myotypic respecification of nerves by their muscles. The first suggestion that another, quite different, mechanism might be involved in the restoration of co-ordinated motor function, came in a paper by Sperry and Deupree (1956). These authors studied return of motor function in fishes after a variety of nerve lesions. Simple section of the nerves supplying the pectoral fin in *Sphaeroides testudineus* was followed after a few weeks by gradual recovery of fin movements, which from the beginning seemed to be properly timed. Eventually the restored function appeared to be normal. When this experiment was repeated on *Histrio histrio*, a species with a very specialized pectoral fin, the morphology and movement patterns of which are ana-logous to, and almost as complex as, those of the tetrapod limb, good but not perfect motor coordination was eventually restored. In other experiments, good functional recovery occurred in *H. histrio* after reinnervation of the pectoral fin by a considerably reduced nerve supply. Reinnervation of the pectoral fin by pelvic fin nerves in *H. histrio* resulted in initially abnormal movements which showed the beginning of more normal coordination over a period of three weeks or so. In adult *S. testudineus* section of the oculomotor nerve was followed, within 28 days, by only weak twitches of the reinnervated muscles, the excursions of which were so small that it was not possible to determine the direction and timing of the contractions.

In their discussion of these results, Sperry and Deupree suggested that the failure of the pelvic-to-pectoral nerve crosses to give good functional recovery could be due to (*a*) failure of the regenerating fibres to form adequate connections with the foreign muscles, (*b*) incapacity of the pelvic fibres to undergo the respecification required to suit the pectoral muscles, (*c*) lack of adequate synaptic readjustment in the spinal centres. Some, at least, of the pelvic fibres were able to establish functional connections with the pectoral musculature, since the pectoral fin showed some reflex movements. But the recovered pectoral movements remained weak and the muscles showed some atrophy, which suggested that the pelvic fibres did not form connections as readily with pectoral as with pelvic musculature. In the case of the oculomotor regenerations, the results approached the functional picture that would be expected if only those axons that happened to connect with their original muscles were able to form functional con-nections. Sperry and Deupree saw in these results a degree of functional incompatibility between motor fibres and strange muscles to which they do not normally connect.

These results raise again, in a rather inverted fashion, the whole question of selectivity of ingrowth as a possible factor in the myotypic response. Functional incompatibility between nerves and foreign muscles suggests functional compatibility between nerves and their proper muscles. The question of selective reinnervation in these cases was taken up again and answered definitively, in two of the most important papers to appear in this field for many years, by Mark (1965) on the cichlid pectoral fin and by Sperry and Arora (1965) on the cichlid oculomotor system. These papers both show essentially the same result in two different situations: (1) section of the main nerve trunk may be followed by regeneration and the full recovery of motor coordination. Since re-educative adjustments could be excluded (Sperry, 1958; Mark, 1965), the recovery of motor coordination could be accounted for either by selective restoration of the original pattern of innervation or by non-selective reinnervation accompanied by myotypic respecification. To distinguish between these alternatives it sufficed to ensure misregeneration of the nerve. (2) After deliberate misdirection of the nerve subdivisions into the wrong muscles, with stringent precautions to prevent the fibres getting back to their proper destinations, abnormal and non-coordinated function was found in all cases. The nerve-crosses in these oculomotor experiments are shown in Fig. 2.13.

Sperry and Arora (1965) noted in their report of the experiments on the oculomotor nerve that the weak and abnormal responses obtained after misregeneration contrasted markedly with the excellent strong recoveries obtained after section of the main nerve trunk or following section of a nerve subdivision and reimplantation into its own muscle.

These results, and the comparable results of Mark (1965) on the pectoral fin musculature, indicate clearly that in these experimental situations the coordinated function that is restored following section of the main nerve trunk is a result of selective reinnervation of the denervated muscles. Myotypic respecification of the neurones, with alteration of their discharge-timing to suit randomly-formed foreign neuromuscular connections clearly does not occur. For when the fibres are forcibly made to innervate the wrong muscles, the motor phasing is abnormal. The results lead us to assume that, following section of the main trunk, the fibres regenerate beyond the scar and either find their original paths distal to the site of section or else they employ a shotgun approach and all fibres innervate all possible muscles, with the final selection being done at muscle level. The observation (Sperry and Arora, 1965) that there was no detectable abnormality of timing in the early stages of recovery suggests that the fibres had already sorted out on a pathway basis before reaching the muscles. And the ability of the muscle to select appropriate fibres from a mixture of appropriate and inappropriate ones was shown by experiments in which simultaneous implantation into a muscle of a foreign nerve along with the proper nerve was performed (Sperry and Arora, 1965). In this case when function was tested 12 days after operation the restored function of the appropriate nerve was strongly dominant in all cases. In another series of fish the same procedure was adopted except that regrowth of the original nerve was delayed by repeatedly crushing it far proximally near the junction with the main trunk. When functional testing indicated that reinnervation by the foreign nerve had occurred, the original nerve was

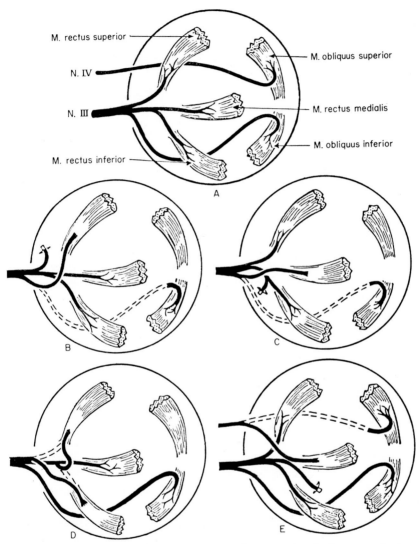

FIG. 2.13.   Surgical interchange among motor ocular connections in *Astronotus*. Designation of muscles with normal innervation is shown in A. The abducens nerve and muscle,
not involved in the transplantation, are omitted. B, inferior oblique nerve crossed into
superior rectus muscle; nerve of superior rectus deflected into orbital septum. C, inferior
oblique nerve crossed into medial rectus muscle; nerve of medial rectus deflected to
septum. D, nerve of superior and inferior rectus muscles interchanged. E, superior
oblique nerve cut and crossed into medial rectus muscle, nerve of medial rectus deflected
into septum. For results, see text. From Sperry and Arora, 1965.

allowed to regenerate into the muscle. Under these conditions the original nerve again gradually acquired dominant control of the muscle and contractions mediated by the foreign nerve could no longer be demonstrated after 2 weeks. Thus inappropriate motor neurones can and do innervate the muscle but are functionally displaced when appropriate neurones are allowed to grow in. *does innervation by inappropriate neurons ever result in co-ordinated movements.*

Obviously, in the light of these results it becomes necessary to re-examine the whole question of homologous responses and myotypic respecification of neurones by the muscles they innervate. But first a word of caution: the restoration of pectoral muscle function after nerve regeneration was initially taken to be an example of myotypic respecification (Sperry, 1950); further study showed it to result from selective reinnervation of the muscles, since when this was prevented by controlled deflection of the nerve fibres, abnormal function resulted. But in the previous descriptions of myotypic response, by Weiss, controlled innervation of a muscle by a foreign nerve still resulted in homologous response (Weiss, 1931; 1936). And furthermore, earlier work by Arora and Sperry (1957) on neuromuscular coordination in the fish *Astronotus* had led them to conclude that, in the innervation of the jaw muscles, selective reinnervation did not occur, while modulation did. The experiments involved section and controlled cross-union of the nerves to the elevators and depressors of the jaw, and properly coordinated function was seen even when the cross-union appeared to be adequately controlled. After regeneration of the nerves, the coordinated function of the muscles was investigated by separating right and left halves of the mandible and observing their separate movements. After nerve cross-union the movements of the affected half-mandible were in most cases properly timed.

One type of observation (Arora and Sperry, 1957) would, however, throw some doubt on the existence of modulation in these experiments: two animals showed impaired movement of the affected half-mandible, and when the nerve on the normal side was cut, the other half-mandible (that is, on the previously operated side) remained locked in a closed position. Examination revealed that in these animals the elevator nerve had grown back into its own stump, along with the crossed depressor. If modulation had occurred in this situation, then *both* innervating nerves should have taken on the timing of the normal jaw elevator muscle; and the jaw should have been able to fall open during the periods when normally the depressors should have been working. The fact that in these animals the jaw stayed locked shut would suggest that the elevator muscles were receiving excitation in *both* phases of the normally reciprocal cycle, and thus that modulation had not occurred. It is perhaps surprising that the work and conclusions of Arora and Sperry (1957) hardly received mention in the later paper by the same authors (Sperry and Arora, 1965).

There is here therefore (Arora and Sperry, 1957; Sperry and Arora,

1965) a conflict of observations: either we are dealing with two separate situations, with different explanations, or else one of the observations is wrong. And in this context it is worth noting that Mark (1965) initially attempted to do his nerve deflection experiments on salamanders but was forced to abandon these animals in favour of fish because his anatomical checks showed that nerve fibre sprouting was so profuse that he could not exclude the possibility that a significant number of fibres had, by devious routes, regained connection with their original muscles. Indeed, Sperry and Arora (1965) also remark that in fishes, the original nerve showed a marked tendency to grow back into its own muscle in their cross-transplantation experiments.

Mark (1965) has suggested a working hypothesis to account for the restoration of coordinated motor function in amphibians and fishes and the failure of such restoration to occur in mammals. He points out that in these lower vertebrates multiterminal, polyneuronal innervation of striated muscle fibres is of common occurrence (Bone, 1964; Takeuchi, 1959). Specific selective reinnervation of muscle may then occur in cases where each muscle cell is normally innervated by several nerve endings. The selection by the muscle of the appropriate nerve contacts would take place by some form of competition between sprouts of different central origins, as shown by the experiments of Sperry and Arora (1965). In those cases where a muscle fibre is normally innervated by only one nerve fibre, as is the rule in mammals, contact of one fibre with a muscle cell appears to preclude the formation of further functional contacts by other fibres. The first nerve sprout to arrive at a denervated muscle fibre, irrespective of its central origin, would thus form an end plate and take command of the whole muscle cell. With multiterminal polyneuronal innervation of muscle fibres, however, the development of one ending on a muscle fibre during reinnervation would presumably not prejudice the chances of other endings developing subsequently on the same cell; thus there would be scope for competitive interaction between different nerve fibres and the muscle fibres which would lead eventually to selection of a majority of correct nerve fibres innervating each muscle.

VARIETIES OF NEUROMUSCULAR CONNECTION AND THE EFFECTS IN DIFFERENT ANIMALS OF REGENERATING NERVE FIBRES INTO MUSCLE

Following the observations of Mark (1965) and Sperry and Arora (1965) on the selective reinnervation that may occur during regeneration of muscle nerves, it is worth our while to look into the question of selective reinnervation in various neuromuscular situations.

(a) In fishes, the innervation of swim-muscles has been extensively reviewed by Bone (1964). The situation is somewhat confused in that widely differing neuromuscular relationships are to be found in different types of fish; but two kinds (at least) of muscle fibre have been described, those in some cases being described as red and white or slow and fast fibres. The former terms refer simply to the colour of many of the fibres and the latter terms to the speed of *contraction* of the fibres. The existence of polyneuronal multiterminal innervation has been described and the terminations on slow muscle fibres are of the "en grappe" type. Neuro-muscular transmission has been investigated electrophysiologically in fishes by Takeuchi (1959); he recorded intracellularly from fast (white) and slow (red) muscle fibres in pectoral fin muscles of the snake fish, *Ophiucephalus argus*. Junctional potentials could be recorded from any point on the surface of *both* types of fibre, indicating (since junctional potentials are not propagated) that each type has multiterminal innervation. Furthermore, the amplitudes of junctional potentials were graded with stimulus strength, showing (since any one junctional potential following a nerve impulse in a single fibre is all-or-none) that both types of muscle fibre have polyneuronal innervation. Conducted spike action potentials were set up in white muscle fibres following junctional activation but this was not so in the red muscle fibres. Lastly, as mentioned previously, Mark (1965) and Sperry and Arora (1965) have shown selective reinnervation to occur in the fish neuromuscular system.

(b) In amphibians there exist slow and fast skeletal muscle fibres and their physiological properties have been investigated, in the frog, by Kuffler and Vaughan Williams (1953b). The fast muscle fibres are "twitch" fibres and show conducted action potentials while the slow muscle fibres are "non-twitch" or "graded-contraction" fibres which show non-propagated muscle potentials (Kuffler and Vaughan Williams, 1953a).

The innervation of these different types of frog muscle fibre is likewise quite distinct. The slow, graded muscle fibres are innervated by small-diameter motor nerve fibres and the fast, twitch muscle fibres by large-diameter nerve fibres (Kuffler and Vaughan Williams, 1953a; Gray, 1957; Hess, 1960). The mode of innervation of the two types of muscle fibre is again quite distinct (Fig. 2.14); the twitch fibres are innervated by "en plaque" endings while the slow muscle fibres receive "en grappe" connections.

Since in frogs some muscles are composed of purely fast twitch fibres (e.g. sartorius) while others contain mixtures of fast and slow muscle fibres (e.g. posterior semitendinosus), it is possible to examine the effects of altering the innervation of one type of muscle fibre by nerve cross-union experiments. Close and Hoh (1968) did this in the toad *Bufo marinus*. They found that fast twitch muscle fibres could become reinnervated by the small motor nerve fibres and slow graded muscle fibres could become innervated by the large motor nerve fibres. They found no evidence that such cross-innervation caused any alteration in the characteristics of the

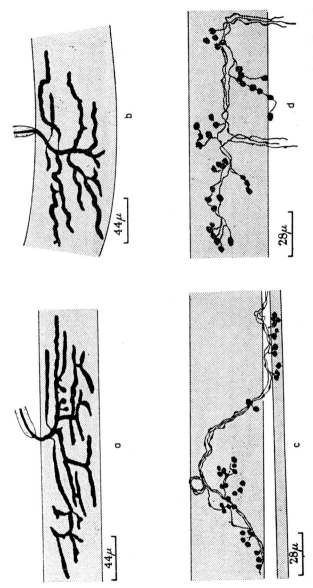

FIG. 2.14. Extrafusal end-plates of frog skeletal muscle. a and b, "twitch" end-plates characteristic of the "large" axon system. c and d, "grape" end-plates supplying "tonic" fibres, characteristic of the "small" axon system. Camera lucida (methylene blue and osmic acid). From Gray, 1957.

muscle fibres concerned. These authors also observed that there was a difference in the facility with which nerve fibres from one muscle appeared to innervate the other muscle; posterior semitendinosus nerves only partially innervated the sartorius muscle whereas sartorius nerves completely innervated the posterior semitendinosus muscle. There thus appeared to be some kind of incompatibility between the posterior semitendinosus nerve and the sartorius muscle; and the latter showed a remarkable preference for its own nerve.

The failure of Close and Hoh (1968) to find evidence of transformation of muscle fibre characteristics after cross-innervation contrasts with the findings of Miledi and Orkand (1966), who crossed the sartorius nerve to the iliofibularis muscle in the frog. The sartorius, a fast twitch muscle, normally gives only a transient twitch contraction on prolonged depolarization with acetylcholine; the iliofibularis, which contains slow as well as twitch fibres, normally gives a prolonged contraction on treatment with acetylcholine and this lengthy contraction is a function of the slow muscle fibres. The cross-innervated iliofibularis, supplied with a sartorius nerve, gave only a brief contraction when depolarized by the action of acetylcholine, suggesting that in this characteristic at least, the cross-innervation had affected the response of the muscle fibres.

There is thus some evidence, from the work of Close and Hoh (1968) of selective reinnervation in the frog. And Miledi (1960) has shown that, in this animal, regenerating motor axons tend to form end-plates at the correct positions in the muscle. There are as yet, unfortunately, no adequate studies on the intimate mechanism of reinnervation in the urodeles.

(c) In birds there exist slow and fast muscle fibres. The muscles that have received most attention recently have been the chick anterior latissimus dorsi (ALD), which is a slow muscle with multiple end-plates of the "en grappe" type, and the posterior latissimus dorsi (PLD), which is mainly a fast muscle with single "en plaque" end-plates (Zelena et al., 1967; Hnik et al., 1967). These two muscles differ also in their electrical characteristics: in the fast PLD, single shocks to the nerve produce synchronous propagated muscle action potentials whereas in the slow ALD, single shocks to the nerve result in only local, non-propagated potentials in the muscle.

Selective reinnervation of chick slow or fast muscle by its original motor supply during regeneration was shown by experiments of Feng et al. (1965). These authors used the ALD and PLD muscles, the nerves of which run in a common trunk but can be partially separated into a pure ALD branch and a mixed PLD one containing a small ALD component. This arrangement made it possible to provide conditions for random regeneration after section of the main trunk; and also allowed separate stimulation of the original nerve branches in the central segment after regeneration. In one group of experiments the central stump of the common trunk was joined to the peripheral stump of the PLD branch only; and in a second group the central and peripheral stumps of the sectioned nerve trunk were joined together. In normal chicks stimulation of the separated ALD branch gives contraction in ALD only while stimulation of the impure PLD branch gives a small contraction in ALD as well as causing PLD to contract. After regeneration, if reinnervation were non-selective, in animals after the first type of operation, stimulation of either the ALD or the PLD branch should have equal effect in making PLD contract; while in animals after the second type of operation, stimulation of the pure ALD branch should make both ALD and PLD contract to approximately the same extent, and stimulation of the PLD branch should do likewise. In fact the results were very different from expectation. Four of six animals with the first type of operation gave no response in PLD when the ALD nerve branch was stimulated; and in the other two animals stimulation was only minimally effective. Of 13 animals with the second type of operation there were eight in which reinnervation was entirely selective and five in which there was only a very feeble cross-innervation of PLD by ALD nerve (Fig. 2.15).

In other cross-union experiments (Zelena et al., 1967; Hnik et al., 1967), the "slow" nerve to ALD was joined to PLD, the "mixed" nerve to PLD was joined to ALD, and a "pure twitch" nerve, from anconeus scapularis, was implanted into the denervated ALD. The transfer of a slow ALD nerve to the fast PLD muscle resulted in changes in the electromyogram and end-plate configuration. Some 4–6 months after operation only end-plate potentials could be recorded from the (normally) fast PLD muscle in response to single shocks to the nerve. In agreement with this change, the end-plates in PLD after cross-union were of the "en grappe" type. Cross-union of the PLD nerve to the slow ALD muscle gave no marked changes from its previous characteristics. Since the PLD muscle is to some extent a mixed one, with both slow and fast components, its nerve will carry fibres appropriate for each type of muscle tissue. Despite this the target ALD muscle remained mainly innervated by "en grappe" endings (Hnik et al., 1967). When the slow ALD was reinnervated by fibres from the nerve to anconeus scapularis, a pure twitch muscle, both the endings close to the site of implantation of the nerve, and the electrical characteristics of the fibres so innervated, became transformed into the fast variety.

(d) In mammals there are slow and fast muscle fibres. In contrast to the situation in amphibians and fishes, however, in mammals both fast and slow extrafusal muscle fibres appear to be "twitch" fibres and are innervated by the large-diameter motor axons. The mammalian small-nerve motor system supplies intrafusal muscle fibres.

All mammalian limb muscles seem to be of the slow variety at birth

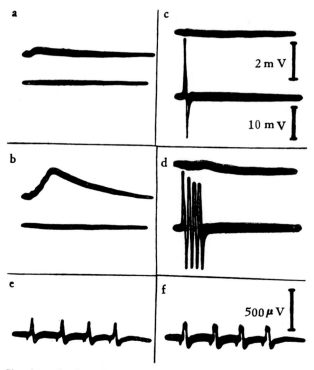

FIG. 2.15.   Showing selective reinnervation of ALD and PLD each by its own nerve branch during regeneration of the mixed nerve; observations made 118 days after operation. The records on the left (a, b, e) and on the right (c, d, f) were obtained on stimulation of the pure ALD and the impure PLD nerve branch respectively. a, b, c, d: pairs of simultaneous records from ALD (upper) and PLD (lower). Note the different amplifier sensitivity for ALD and PLD. In a and c, single shock; in b and d, 4 shocks at 214/sec. Note that stimulation of the pure ALD nerve branch elicits response in ALD only, while stimulation of the PLD nerve branch calls forth response chiefly in PLD. e, f: action potentials from the regenerated PLD nerve set up by separate stimulation (4 shocks at 214/sec) of the ALD(e) and PLD(f) nerve branches in the central stump. From Feng *et al.*, 1965.

and differentiation of the adult type fast and slow characteristics takes place within the first few weeks of independent life and is dependent upon effective contact with the appropriate part of the nervous system (Buller *et al.*, 1960a). Cross-union of a fast-muscle nerve into a slow muscle results in alteration of the contraction-characteristics of the target muscle in the direction of the muscle donating the nerve; and similarly when the cross-union is performed in the reverse direction (Buller *et al.*, 1960b (cat); Close, 1965 (rat)). These transformations of muscle type may occur following operation in infancy or even in adult life.

Thus the characteristics of the innervating nerve fibres control the muscle contraction time; some influence is passed from nerve to muscle and it is of considerable interest to find out whether any comparable

influence is exerted the other way round, from muscle to nerve, since this
is the direction of action of the postulated myotypic respecifying factors.
Motoneurones innervating slow muscles normally have a much longer
after-hyperpolarization following the discharge of an impulse than do the
motoneurones supplying fast muscles (Eccles *et al.*, 1958). Yet the after-
hyperpolarizations recorded from soleus (slow) motoneurones after they
had innervated flexor digitorum longus (fast) for over 20 weeks, showed no
signs of complementary quickening although the target flexor digitorum
longus muscle had slowed its contraction time considerably as a result of ✓
the nerve transfer. Nor was there any appreciable change in the conduction
velocity of the cross-united nerve fibres (Buller *et al.*, 1960b). These
negative findings do not imply, of course, that no modulation of the nerve
fibres has occurred. In regard to the time characteristics of the innervating
motor neurones, however, no modulating influence by the muscle could
be detected. The change in the contraction time of the cross-innervated
muscle is associated with a corresponding change in the myoglobin content
(the colour changes—Eccles, 1963) and in the histochemical pattern of
enzyme distribution in the muscles concerned (Dubowitz, 1967).

⟨Attempts to demonstrate selective reinnervation of mammalian muscles
by their appropriate motoneurones have been unsuccessful.⟩ Weiss and
Hoag (1946) endeavoured to give the original and the foreign nerve fibres
an equal chance to reinnervate a rat muscle by placing them in the two
limbs of a forked artery and allowing them to regenerate towards the distal
stump of the nerve in the parent stem of the Y-shaped artery. They found
that under these conditions the two nerves appeared to innervate the
muscle at random, the original nerve having no systematic advantage over
the foreign one. This question was again tackled, with variations (and
improvements) in technique, by Bernstein and Guth (1961). They concluded, following a variety of experimental approaches, that there was no
evidence of selectivity in the regeneration of the plantaris and soleus nerve
fibre constituents of the sciatic or tibial nerves in rats. In addition to these
experiments there is of course the large amount of clinical evidence on
regenerating neuromuscular connections. The earlier work on connection-
specificity has been admirably reviewed by Sperry (1945a).

INVESTIGATIONS INVOLVING SPINAL CORD
TRANSPLANTATIONS

The experiments considered so far have approached the problem of
neuromuscular connection specificity by means of various ingenious
alterations to the peripheral connection pattern; the spinal cord was not
deliberately altered but the connections of the spinal motoneurones with
the muscles were disrupted and allowed to reform either in a randomized
fashion, as when limbs are transplanted, or in a carefully controlled way,
as when certain muscles were given innervation by preselected nerves.

It is, however, possible to approach the question of neuromuscular specificity from the other end of the "final common pathway"—by operation
on the spinal cord itself. What would happen if a group of motoneurones
supplying a certain muscle were to be transplanted to a different part of
the spinal cord? Would they still be able to achieve innervation of the proper
muscle? or would they then innervate a different muscle, and if so, would
the discharge-timing of the motoneurones remain appropriate to the
original muscle or would it change to suit the new target organ? It is not,
of course, feasible to do such an experiment for a whole variety of reasons,
most of which will be obvious. But a somewhat similar approach has been
used, with great success, by members of the very active Hungarian school
of neuroembryologists. These experiments have involved the transplantation of limbs to abnormal sites and in some cases transplantation of multi-
segmental pieces of the spinal cord *anlage* as well.

It has been well established that limbs innervated by spinal cord
segments that normally do not supply limbs, do not show coordinated
movements (Detwiler, 1920; 1936 (urodeles); Miner, 1956 (anura);
Székely and Szentágothai, 1962; Straznicky, 1963 (chicks)). This fact, taken
along with the results of his investigations on spinal cord transplantation,
has led Székely to propose (1963) that there exists a specific limb-moving
apparatus in those regions of the cord that normally innervate limbs, the
brachial and lumbosacral segments. Limbs transplanted to the thoracic
region become innervated by thoracic segments of the spinal cord; sensory
innervation of such transplanted limbs may be demonstrated in frogs
(Miner, 1956) and in chicks (Székely and Szentágothai, 1962), but motor
innervation by the thoracic segments is abortive. Székely and Szentágothai
(1962) noted that the supernumary limbs (chick) remained motionless and
contained no muscle at all; degeneration of muscles, however well innervated, began on the 10th day of incubation and by the 13th day
practically all muscle tissue was degenerating. Since maturation of the
neuromuscular end-plates is not completed until about the 12th day or later
(Drachman, 1968) it seems that neuromuscular innervation of these
thoracically-innervated limbs never achieved completion before muscular
degeneration set in. The muscular atrophy following thoracic innervation
in these transplanted limbs was not simply a consequence of the abnormal
siting of the limb, since Straznicky (1963) has shown that comparable
atrophy occurs in a normal chick forelimb when the brachial segments of
cord had previously been removed and replaced by thoracic segments.
Control innervation of a normal forelimb by transplanted brachial segments
from a donor in place of the brachial segments of the host resulted in
normal neuromuscular activity. Somewhat similar lack of movement, with
muscular atrophy and joint ankylosis has been reported for urodeles
(Székely, 1963).

Thoracic segments, therefore, cannot successfully innervate limb musculature. Brachial and lumbosacral segments, however, can do so; and most interesting results have been obtained when leg-moving segments ✓ were transplanted in place of arm-moving segments, or when brachial or lumbosacral segments were transplanted to the thoracic region and there given an extra limb to innervate. In urodeles (*Pleurodeles* and *Triturus*) Székely (1963) grafted brachial segments into the thoracic region, between stages 24–35 of embryonic life, and also transplanted nearby a pair of forelimbs or a pair of hindlimbs. Despite the fact that such transplanted limbs, when innervated by thoracic segments, remain non-functional, atrophic and ankylosed, when innervated by transplanted brachial segments the limbs performed coordinated walking movements in good synchronization

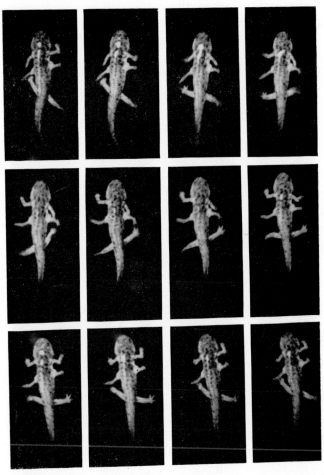

Fig. 2.16. Moving picture series illustrating the locomotion of an animal (*Pleurodeles waltlii*) in which the 8th, 9th and 10th spinal cord segments have been replaced by the 3rd, 4th and 5th (brachial) segments. The supernumary limbs (middle pair) are moving synchronously with the normal forelimbs on the same side. From Székely, 1963.

with the normal forelimbs (Fig. 2.16). Similarly when the extra limbs were hindlimbs, they showed good movements which were synchronized also with the normal forelimbs. When the host's lumbosacral segments had been replaced by brachial segments, limb transplantation was not necessary since the host's own hindlimbs were able to indicate the functional effect of the transplanted cord segments. In this case there was a tendency for the hindlimb to move in parallel with the forelimb on the same side, i.e. the hindlimb tended to show a forelimb rhythm. The parallel coordination between normal forelimb and brachially-innervated hindlimb was not so obvious in these experiments as in the previous group of experiments and cinephotography revealed a considerable delay in the rhythm of the hindlimbs (Fig. 2.17). Despite this lag, which increased with each cycle

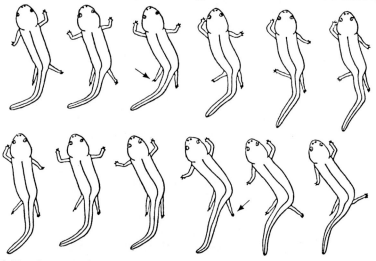

FIG. 2.17.   One complete locomotor cycle redrawn after a cinematographic film demonstrating the time delay and rhythm-shift of the hindlimbs innervated by grafted brachial cord segments. The movement of the left hindlimb starts in the third phase (arrow), lagging two phases behind the forelimb movement and reaches its maximum in the fifth phase. The right forelimb starts moving in the seventh phase and is accompanied three phases later (arrow) by the hindlimb which reaches the maximum in the last phase. In the following cycle these delays become even greater and parallel coordination gradually shifts into diagonal coordination. The animal was moving in shallow water. *Pleurodeles waltlii*. From Székely, 1963.

until the hindlimbs came into phase with the rhythm that would have been seen in normally-innervated hindlimbs, the parallel coordination usually resumed suddenly and the two limbs on the same side would again move in parallel, camel-gait fashion, until the increasing lag of the hindlimbs again threw the fore- and hindlimbs out of phase. Székely commented that observation of several such cases led him to conclude that there was a tendency for the transplanted brachial cord segments to maintain a forelimb rhythm in the hindlimbs.

The converse of these two groups of experiments was also performed. That is, thoracically-placed supernumary limbs were innervated by transplanted lumbosacral segments; and in other animals the host's own brachial segments were replaced by transplanted lumbosacral segments. When supernumary limbs were innervated by transplanted lumbosacral segments two types of result were obtained. In three animals out of 21 the supernumary limbs gave movements synchronized with the corresponding hindlimb (Fig. 2.18). In the remaining 18 animals the transplanted limbs

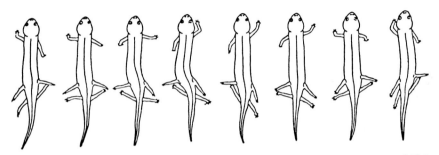

FIG. 2.18.   Ambulation of a *Triturus vulgaris* over solid ground. The 11th, 12th and 13th segments have been replaced by heterotopic lumbosacral segments in the 38th (Glücksohn, 1932) embryonic stage. The supernumary hindlimbs are moving synchronously with the normal hindlimbs on the same side. Redrawn from a cine film. From Székely, 1963.

showed more or less delay relative to the normal hindlimbs. In cases where the host's brachial segments were replaced by grafted lumbosacral segments good parallel coordination developed between the forelimb and the hindlimb of the same side (Fig. 2.19). Székely also noted that, apart from minor discrepancies, the character of the movement depends largely on the nature of the segmental apparatus and not so much on the limb itself. This control of the nature and extent of a limb's movements is naturally limited by the anatomical structure of the limb itself, but within these limitations the motility of, e.g. a forelimb with lumbosacral innervation is similar to that of a hindlimb. The nature and extent of the various time-lags observed are also of great interest and deserve to be more fully studied with electromyographical methods. Preliminary attempts in this direction were reported by Székely (1968) when he found electromyographic evidence for phase shifts of the order of 100–300 msec between the timing of certain muscles in transplant and normal limb.

Straznicky (1963) has shown that, in the chick, the exchange of brachial cord segments between embryos on the third day of incubation (stages 15 and 16 of Hamburger and Hamilton) permits normal wing function, whereas replacement of brachial segments by thoracic segments results in immobile, atrophic, ankylosed wings. In these birds also, the replacement of the brachial cord segments by lumbosacral segments led to peculiar

coordinated movements of the wing occurring in parallel with the movements of the leg on the same side. This parallel movement was confined
to the shoulder joint, the other joints remaining immobile although they
were not ankylosed and the musculature was apparently well innervated.
Those wings which showed parallel movements with the legs showed no
sign of the normal wing reflexes after stimuli that elicit these in normal
animals.

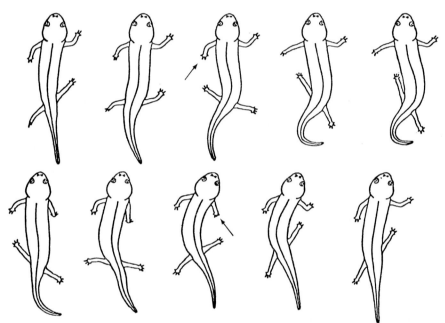

FIG. 2.19.   Characteristic "camel-gait" walking cycle of a *Pleurodeles waltlii* in which the
brachial segments have been replaced by lumbosacral segments. The movements in the
elbows are restricted and the left forelimb is somewhat rotated, so that its lower surface is
directed mediocaudally. There is a delay of two phases in the motion of the forelimbs
(arrows), they reach, however, the maximum of protraction simultaneously with the
hindlimbs on the same side. Such pattern of coordination could be seen in several con-
secutive cycles. Movements performed in shallow water. Redrawn from a film. From
Székely, 1963.

Taken together, these ingenious experiments of Székely and Straznicky
certainly indicate that there is some special organization in the limb-
moving segments which enables them, and only them, to innervate a limb
effectively. Limbs innervated by non-limb segments undergo profound
atrophy which may be prevented by innervating the limb by a limb-
segment. This statement applies even if (Straznicky, 1963) the segments
used are appropriate for the wrong limb. This sustaining effect of limb-
segments thus shows no specificity in terms of arm or leg; on the other
hand, the nature of the movement generated depends on which segments
are used and not on the nature of the limb innervated.

The various parts of the spinal cord differ from one another in that only the limb segments are able (1) to evoke coordinated movement and (2) to sustain the limb musculature. We may ask at what stage during development does this difference arise. This question has been answered, for newts, by experiments performed by Straznicky and Székely (1967). These authors found, in their transplantation experiments, that the brachial segments were functionally determined by stage 20, at the time of closure of the medullary tube. If brachial and thoracic segments were exchanged earlier, during the medullary plate stage, the limb and trunk segments could replace each other in all functional respects. This means that at the medullary plate stage the thoracic segments are still not irrevocably determined as non-limb-moving segments. This had earlier been shown by Detwiler (1923). If the transplantation is done sufficiently early, the new brachial position of the thoracic segments leads to the development within these segments of the functional (and morphological) characteristics of brachial segments. This is an example of embryonic induction, where the development of the transplanted tissue is altered in direction by some influence exerted by the immediate environment, Straznicky and Székely (1967) performed medullary tube transplantations in *Pleurodeles* of stages 20–27, from the closure of the medullary tube to late tail bud stage. In their first group of experiments the three brachial segments were replaced by thoracic segments taken from other embryos of the same age. After having their limb movements analysed the animals were killed before metamorphosis and the limb innervation investigated histologically. The results of these experiments showed that limb movements failed in proximo-distal sequence as the medullary tube transplantations were performed at increasingly older embryonic stages (Fig. 2.20). When the operation had been done at or before stage 23 almost complete limb activity was obtained. Defective shoulder movement occurred in 7 out of 16 animals operated at stage 24. With operation at stage 25 movement was normal at the wrist only, in 7 out of 10 cases. The shoulder remained motionless when the operation was done at stage 26 whereas movements of the hands were less affected. Operation at stage 27 resulted in motionless limbs except for one animal (out of 9) in which slight wrist movement occurred. These results show that the fibres in the latter cases had grown down through the musculature of the upper arm to reach their destinations and this argues strongly against any form of modulation as the mechanism involved in establishing appropriate neuromuscular connections during development.

The capacity of thoracic segments to adapt to their new brachial environment, to be induced to form a limb-moving system, gradually diminishes with increasing age at operation and this failure manifests itself in proximo-distal sequence in the limb. The failure could be due to decreasing inductive influence of the brachial environment or to decreasing competence in

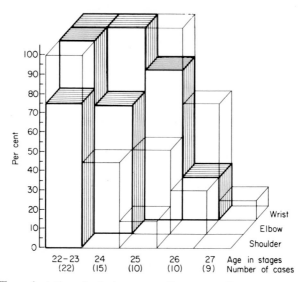

FIG. 2.20. Transplantation of spinal segments. Stereogram illustrating the motility of the different joints in animals operated in increasingly older stages. Columns drawn with heavy and thin lines represent complete and defective movements, respectively. The vertical axis indicates the percentage of cases in which the represented movements occurred. On the first horizontal axis the ages of operations and (in parentheses) the number of observed cases are given. The second horizontal axis refers to the three joints of the forelimb. From Straznicky and Székely, 1967.

the graft or to both these factors. However in further experiments the authors transplanted thoracic segments from donors of stage 22 into hosts of stage 28 and only one out of 18 animals gave normal limb movements. This would suggest that the environmental inductive influence is becoming inadequate at stage 28. Further, when thoracic segments were taken from embryos of stage 24 and grafted into hosts of stage 22, three out of six cases had normal limb movements. This is a better result than that obtained when stage 24 segments were grafted into hosts of the same age and it indicates that the grafts of stage 24 embryos are still highly competent for "brachial" transformation.

The proximo-distal failure of movement in these experiments was accompanied by decreased numbers of ventral root fibres as the operations were performed on older embryos (Table I). Not only were the total numbers of root fibres diminished following the later operations, but also fibre counts at various levels of the limb nerves showed that the muscles of the upper arm and shoulder received fewer of the remaining fibres than did the muscles of the forearm and hand. The authors interpret this finding as indicating a form of preferential pathway selection by the remaining fibres. Table I shows that the fibre counts for brachial roots 3 and 4 (root 5, which also contributes to limb innervation, has been ignored in the Table

Table I

The number of fibres in the brachial ventral roots after transplantation of thoracic segments in the place of brachial segments at various developmental stages. From Straznicky and Székely, 1967

Stage at at operation	Animal no.	Fibre counts in ventral root		Average fibre counts for groups[a]		Motility		
		root 3	root 4	root 3	root 4	shoulder	elbow	wrist
Normal	1	415	470	436	431	+	+	+
	2	468	496			+	+	+
	3	471	351	*866*		+	+	+
	4	385	406			+	+	+
	1	354	281	408	387	±	+	+
	2	539	503			±	+	+
	3	419	405	*795*		−	+	+
23	4	320	358			−	+	+
	1	433	329	343	343	±	+	+
	2	292	318	*686*		−	±	+
24	3	304	382			−	−	+
	1	257	202	221	171	−	−	+
	2	231	168			−	−	+
25	3	240	157	*397*		−	±	+
	4	274	164			−	−	+
	5	129	162			−	−	±
	1	119	115	105	77	−	−	±
	2	69	81			−	−	−
26	3	124	—[b]	*128*		−	−	+
	4	123	188			−	±	+
	5	92	—[b]			−	−	±

The first row contains the data obtained from four normal animals. In the following rows the data of animals operated in successively older stages are shown.

[a] The figures printed in italics indicate the average fibre counts for roots 3+4.
[b] Only root 3 was present.

because in most cases it was very small and could not be found) decrease evenly over the grafted segments as the operations were performed at increasingly late stages. There was no evidence of a decreased fibre count in the craniocaudal direction with later operation, as might have been expected from the known craniocaudal distribution of motoneurones for the various limb muscles in mammalian and anuran spinal cords. The even decrease in each of the graft roots concerned suggests an even distribution of motoneurones, for any one muscle, over several segments of spinal cord, and this was in fact found by Székely and Czéh (1967) using microelectrodes to stimulate individual motoneurones (Fig. 2.7).

ELECTROPHYSIOLOGICAL INVESTIGATIONS OF MODULATION

As I have mentioned previously, there has been a remarkable dearth of investigations on myotypic respecification using up-to-date electrophysiological techniques. If modulation of a neurone by its target muscle occurs, and if this process involves alteration in the synaptic input to the motoneurone, then the ideal way to investigate this phenomenon is by means of intracellular recording from the motoneurone with observation of the monosynaptic EPSP activity of the cell. This experimental approach has been used by Eccles and his collaborators with interesting but inconclusive results.

Eccles *et al.* (1960) contrasted the existence of what may be called "plastic" changes (i.e. the effects described under the heading of modulation) in amphibians and fishes with the absence of such changes in mammals. These authors pointed out that the monosynaptic pathways from primary afferent fibres to motoneurones are particularly well suited to quantitative evaluation and can be used to assess the extent of any modulation changes that may follow nerve cross-union. The size of the excitatory post-synaptic potentials (EPSPs) recorded from a motoneurone give a good measure of the monosynaptic activation of that motoneurone. With few exceptions it turns out that the monosynaptic excitation from the afferent (Group 1a) fibres of a muscle is restricted to the motoneurones of that muscle and its immediate synergists. Thus to map the origin of the EPSPs in a motoneurone gives a direct test for any changes in central pathways that might result from a reversal of motoneurone function following cross-union. Eccles *et al.* (1960) cross-united the nerve to the peroneal muscles to the nerve of the medial gastrocnemius and, in other experiments, the peroneal and lateral gastrocnemius nerves. After cross-union of peroneal to medial gastrocnemius, 40% (41/102) of the peroneus motoneurones were monosynaptically activated from their acquired synergist, lateral gastrocnemius, whereas normally this aberrant connection was rare (6%; 3/52). There was also a large increase in monosynaptic activation from other post-tibial extensors. There occurred no similar change in the monosynaptic excitatory action on the medial gastrocnemius motoneurones innervating the peroneus muscles.

Eccles *et al.* (1960) also noted that in the cross-union of peroneal with medial gastrocnemius, both the medial gastrocnemius and peroneal nerves had diminished actions on the peroneal motoneurones (and on other motoneurones); they interpreted this finding as being due to the chromatolytic degeneration of a considerable proportion (about 2/3) of the Group 1 afferent fibres of peroneal and medial gastrocnemius nerves. The authors therefore suggested that the degenerating central terminals of these afferent fibres could have stimulated non-specific collateral sprouting of adjacent normal fibres which would then establish some of the aberrant synaptic connections observed. Eccles *et al.*, thought that any postulated non-specific sprouting of this nature was unlikely to account for more than a small proportion of the observed aberrancy of connections. However a further series of experiments was undertaken to evaluate the extent of collateral sprouting under comparable conditions. Eccles *et al.* (1962) induced degeneration of primary afferent fibres in the spinal cord by severing dorsal roots central to the ganglion or by severing muscle nerves in kittens. The central stump of each severed muscle nerve was reunited to its own peripheral stump so as to eliminate any central effects due to modulation. After extensive partial section of dorsal roots there occurred a substantial diminution of monosynaptic activation of all species of motoneurones in the vicinity. From this result the authors concluded that there was no evidence for any appreciable growth of new monosynaptic connections when about 2/3 of the primary afferent fibres had degenerated; or if there were any such sprouting, the sprouts were either abortive or connected to motoneurones of the same or synergic species. Essentially similar results were obtained following section and self-union of medial gastrocnemius and deep peroneal nerves: there was a large diminution in the effectiveness of volleys in the sectioned nerves and it was concluded that, again, the degeneration of a considerable proportion of the primary afferent fibres did not evoke from the residual intact fibres any appreciable development of collateral sprouts that made new monosynaptic connections to motoneurones.

In view of the findings of Eccles *et al.* (1962), that random collateral sprouting occurs to a very limited extent if at all under these conditions, the previous result of Eccles *et al.* (1960) gained added interest. These authors had observed that, after one type of nerve cross-union in the kitten (peroneal with medial gastrocnemius) there were marked changes in the pattern of monosynaptic innervation of the motoneurones, and these changes were in accord with the hypothesis of myotypic respecification. Eccles *et al.* (1962) therefore undertook an extended analysis of these earlier results, together with an extra series of experiments.

The hypothesis of myotypic respecification requires the growth of new monosynaptic connections which are appropriate to the newly-acquired function that derives from the nerve cross-union; this is "growth specificity". The hypothesis would also suggest regression of those monosynaptic connections that have been rendered inappropriate by the nerve cross-union; this is "regression specificity". The experimental arrangement used to analyse these two aspects of the respecification hypothesis are shown in Fig. 2.21. As may be seen in (b), the cross-union was effected between the

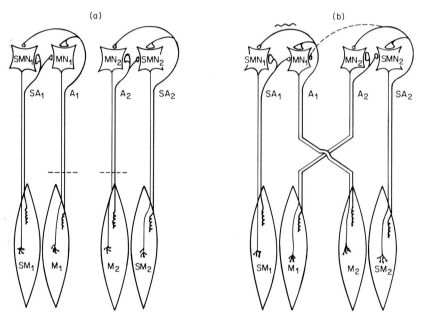

FIG. 2.21. Nerve cross-union. (a) Diagrammatic representation of monosynaptic pathways for two pairs of synergic muscles: M_1 and SM_1; M_2 and SM_2. The afferent fibres, A_1, SA_1, A_2, SA_2, respectively, from the annulospiral endings are seen to make monosynaptic connections to motoneurones of their own muscle (homonymous endings) and of the synergic muscle (heteronymous endings). The larger synaptic knobs for the homonymous endings symbolize the more powerful excitatory action. The broken lines drawn across the nerves to M_1 and M_2 muscles indicate the site of section and self-union in the control experiments: (b) Diagrammatic representation of cross-union of the nerves to M_1 and M_2 muscles with regeneration such as occurred for the two types of cross-union, $LGS \times Pl$ and $DP \times MG$. Broken line from SA_2 to MN_1 represents the new connections which appear to occur under certain conditions and which would be due to growth specificity. The wavy line above the connection from A_1 to SMN_1 symbolizes the decreased synaptic excitatory action which appears to occur under certain conditions and which would be due to regression specificity. From Eccles *et al.*, 1962.

nerves of two muscles, M_1 and M_2, leaving one member of each synergic pair (SM_1 and SM_2) undisturbed. Cross-union was effected between lateral gastrocnemius soleus and plantaris nerves in one series of experiments, and between deep peroneal and medial gastrocnemius in another. In relation to each cross-union situation it is possible to consider the

Table II

The statistical results of a series of nerve cross-union
experiments in the kitten

	Regression specificity		Growth specificity	
	1	2	3	4
	$SA_1 \to MN_1$ $SA_2 \to MN_2$	$A_1 \to SMN_1$ $A_2 \to SMN_2$	$SA_2 \to MN_1$ $SA_1 \to MN_2$	$A_1 \to SMN_2$ $A_2 \to SMN_1$
LGS × Pl	$MG \to LGS$ 0·20 $FDB \to Pl$ $\boxed{0·035}$ $FDHL \to Pl$ 0·001	$LGS \to MG$ $\boxed{0·017}$ $Pl \to FDB$ 0·18 $Pl \to FDHL$ $\boxed{0·5}$	$FDB \to LGS$ 0·062:0·042 $MG \to Pl$ $\boxed{0·09:0·25}$	$LGS \to FDB$ ~1·0 $Pl \to MG$ ~1·0 $LGS \to FDHL$ 1·0
DP × MG	$Per \to DP$ 0·59 $LGS \to MG$ 0·19	$DP \to Per$ 0·0035 $MG \to LGS$ $\boxed{0·18}$	$LGS \to DP$ ~1·0 $Per \to MG$ ~1·0	$DP \to LGS$ ~1·0 $MG \to Per$ 0·50
Per × MG	$DP \to PerL$ 0·60 $DP \to PerB$ $\boxed{0·054}$ $LGS \to MG$ ~1·0	$Per \to DP$ 0·001 $MG \to LGS$ 0·17	$LGS \to PerL$ 0·020:0·0001 $LGS \to PerB$ 0·25:0·0002 $Pl \to PerL$ 0·14:0·0007 $Pl \to PerB$ 0·10:0·010 $DP \to MG$ ~1·0	$Per \to LGS$ ~1·0 $MG \to DP$ ~1·0

The cross-unions were: lateral gastrocnemius soleus (LGS) and plantaris (Pl); deep peroneal (DP) and medial gastrocnemius (MG); and medial gastrocnemius and peroneus (Per).

The table gives the probability values that the observations on the specified afferent nerve to motoneurone actions could be due to random chance.

The results are arranged under the various subdivisions of the hypothesis of myotypic specification; there are two main column headings, regression specificity and growth specificity; and each of these is subdivided into two compartments which can be identified by the symbols that are shown diagrammatically in Fig. 2.21. Results that are contrary to predictions from the hypothesis of myotypic specification are boxed in.

FDB, flexor digitorum brevis; FDHL, flexor digitorum and hallucis longus; PerL, peroneus longus; PerB, peroneus brevis.

Where the tests were obviously of such low statistical significance that no calculations were attempted, the P values have been shown as approximately 1·0 (~1·0). The double values given in several entries in the third column are: first, for the self-union series as controls and second, for the pooled values of the self-union and normals as controls. From Eccles, Eccles, Shealy and Willis, 1962.

monosynaptic innervation of the motoneurones with changed function and also the monosynaptic action exerted by afferent fibres with changed function; both these aspects of the experiment can again be considered from the point of view of growth specificity and of regression specificity.

The results of these experiments by Eccles *et al.* (1962) were somewhat inconclusive. The general results for the three cross-union experiments (two from the 1962 experiments; one from the 1960 experiments) are shown in Table II. In this table there are two main headings of regression specificity and growth specificity; and each of these is subdivided into two components which can be identified by the symbols shown diagrammatically in Fig. 2.21. The results are given as probability values that the observations on the specified afferent nerve to motoneurone actions could be due to random chance; those results contrary to predictions from the hypothesis are boxed in.

In column 1 of this table some of the tests were against and some supported the hypothesis that changed motoneurone function would give loss of inappropriate monosynaptic connections; there were two results contrary to prediction (P = 0·035 and 0·054) and one very strongly in agreement with prediction (P = 0·001). The authors concluded that the hypothesis of regression specificity was not supported by these experimental tests. In column 2, four out of the six tests were in accord with the hypothesis that muscle afferent fibres with changed function suffered a regression of their monosynaptic connections to functionally inappropriate motoneurones; and two of these tests (DP to Per and Per to DP) were highly significant (P = 0·0035 and 0·001 respectively). There were two tests contrary to prediction, but neither was significant. It was concluded that in this situation the hypothesis of regression specificity had received significant support. In column 3 of the table there are listed the tests of the hypothesis that changed motoneuronal function resulted in growth of new monosynaptic connections that were appropriate to the new function. Five of the nine tests supported the hypothesis in a statistically significant fashion. The only test contrary to hypothesis was not significant. The results listed in column 4 of the table show that there was no experimental support for the hypothesis that muscle afferent fibres with changed function following cross-union grew new monosynaptic connections to functionally appropriate motoneurones.

These experiments of Eccles *et al.* (1962) have, in a very elegant fashion, made precise and specific some of the questions that can usefully be asked about the phenomenon of myotypic respecification. Unfortunately the answers given by the experiments are somewhat messy and conflicting. The dotted line in Fig. 2.21 shows one variety of growth specificity that occurred with a high degree of statistical significance and the wavy line in the figure indicates one type of regression specificity that also had considerable statistical significance. These statistically significant changes occurred with some nerve cross-unions and not with others. Moreover, not all the observed growth of new connections was what would be predicted on the basis of myotypic respecification. With one variety of nerve cross-union (DP to MG) there were statistically significant mono-synaptic connections that had no apparent functional meaning in terms of the new anatomical situation. Perhaps the only really remarkable result to emerge from these experiments is the fact that any changes were demon-strable at all; myotypic respecification, if it occurs, does so in amphibians, fishes and birds. There is no evidence that it can occur, or any comparable phenomenon, in mammals. It is rather a pity therefore, that this immense barrage of sophisticated tests should have been applied in the first place to kittens. What we would really like to know is whether it is possible to do comparable experiments in the lower vertebrates; and if so, what are the results in these animals where there is at least some evidence in favour of modulation.

PATHWAY SELECTION BY MOTOR FIBRES

In considering alternative explanations for the phenomenon of homo-logous response in reinnervated muscles we have two main possibilities which are not mutually exclusive: either [the regenerating motor fibres innervate the various muscles they encounter, in a random fashion, and thereafter myotypic respecification occurs and the modulated neurones achieve new central connections appropriate to their new effector organ; or else the regenerating fibres somehow manage to get back to their original muscles, thus automatically restoring the proper timing-sequence for coordinated movement.] If we recall some of the earlier work of Weiss which was quoted on previous pages (Weiss, 1931) it will be immediately obvious that the eventual answer is unlikely to lie in such a simple dicho-tomy. There is *some* evidence (Eccles *et al.*, 1962) for modulation influences on motoneurones and there is *some* evidence in favour of selective regrowth of neuromuscular connections, under suitable conditions (Feng *et al.*, 1965; Hnik *et al.*, 1965). It seems then, what is rather unsatisfactory for a simple idealist, that both mechanisms may be in action—an example of the "belt and braces" habit of the body. It is, however, worthwhile to consider the question of neuromuscular reinnervation in relation to the development of neuromuscular connections during embryogenesis, since it is at least conceivable that mechanisms operating in the embryonic state may have something useful to tell us about later regeneration.

The question we now ask is, therefore, what means does the developing embryo use to achieve the pattern of neuromuscular connection that is usually seen in the normal adult? The problem is complicated by the fact that neurogenesis leads not only to properly coordinated function, but also to a standard innervation structure. The occurrence of coordinated function could well be accounted for by a mechanism of the modulation type; the existence of a standard pattern of innervation cannot be so explained. Therefore, quite apart from the possible evidence of myotypic specification of developing neurones, we have to find a mechanism which will permit nerve fibres not merely to reach the correct destination but also to get there by the proper pathway. These intriguing questions of innervation have been extensively discussed by Cajal (1929) and more recently by Hughes (1968).

A transplanted limb in a larval amphibian becomes reinnervated and, provided that the innervation comes from limb-moving regions, the general pattern of the reinnervation resembles that of a normally innervated limb (Weiss, 1937b). This raises the question of how the pattern is reproduced. One possibility to be considered is that the existence, along the normal nerve pathways, of the debris of neural degeneration could perhaps exercise a form of chemical guidance on the newly growing fibres. Such an explanation, even if it were valid (which it is not, as will be seen later), could tell us nothing useful about the guidance of fibres growing into the embryonic limb, since in this situation there is no previously innervated path for them to follow.

In a developing amphibian limb-bud the ingrowing nerve fibres have only minute distances to travel. The fibres in a frog embryo grow into the bud at an early stage (stage L4 of Taylor), some considerable time before the muscles of the limb have developed. Figure 2.22 shows the innervation of such a stage L4 limb bud; the future nerve branches of the limb are already foreshadowed by a splitting up of the peripheral parts of the nerve mass; the forking distal to the plexus into the cruralis and sciatic (c and s), the division of the sciatic into peroneus and tibialis (p and t), the separation of the peroneus into medial and lateral branches and the division of the tibialis into profundus and superficialis (suralis) branches, may be seen. These characteristics of the adult innervation pattern have thus all developed in the absence of the target muscles. If the fibres present at this larval stage are the same fibres as are later present in the various branches, then the adult nerve pattern may thus develop in relation to cues laid down all along the pathway followed by the fibres.

Nerve fibres innervating a developing limb bud will be able to make first contact with their developing target muscles at a fairly early stage and thereafter the movements of the nerve are linked to those of the muscle— a process described by Weiss (1955) as "towing". However fibres growing into a transplanted limb do not have the benefit of this towing process; the muscles are already in their near-final positions and the fibres have to make their way over considerably greater distances than in the first development of limb connections. How is it that anything resembling a normal innervation pattern occurs under these circumstances?

This question was tackled by Piatt in a series of ingenious experiments on aneurogenic limbs. In order to present the ingrowing fibres with a task

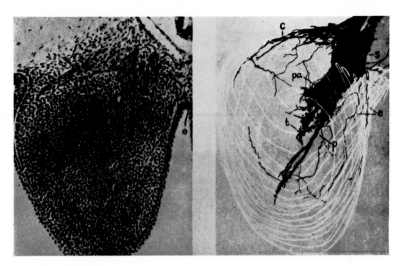

FIG. 2.22. Limb bud of a stage L4 *Rana pipiens* larva. Left: photomicrograph of an 8-micron section impregnated with silver. Right: photograph of glass plate reconstruction to show extent of development of the innervation pattern (white lines indicate the outlines of the limb bud). c, cruralis division. e, fibres of the epidermal primary innervation. p, peroneus branch. pa, profundus anterior branch. t, tibialis branch. From Fig. 5, Taylor, 1943, *Anat. Rec.* **87**, 390.

of maximal difficulty, Piatt (1942) observed the effects of innervation of transplanted larval urodele limbs, which, while they were well-formed limbs, with individual muscles identifiable, had never at any time previously been innervated. Such aneurogenic limbs were produced by removal of spinal segments 2–6 from embryos of *Amblystoma punctatum* at stages 23–25; this operation removes the source of forelimb nerve supply (segments 3–5) at a stage before the outgrowth of the limb nerve fibres. Operated animals were unable to feed themselves and were reared in parabiosis with a normal embryo (Fig. 2.23). Later the aneurogenic forelimbs from the operated member of the parabiotic pair was transplanted in place of the forelimb of a normal larva of similar age, 10–14 days after the onset of feeding (Fig. 2.24). The general result of innervation of these aneurogenic transplants was that the pattern of nerve distribution in the formerly nerve-free limbs was essentially normal as opposed to chaotic or abnormal (Fig. 2.25). In these experiments, as Piatt points out, the nerves had to find their way through a labyrinth of already differentiated tissues and yet they arrived at the toes in a close to normal fashion, without the "help" of any pre-established degenerating nerve pathways. Piatt also showed that the nerves were not merely following the path of least resistance—growing along the most readily available tissue planes; nor were the nerves merely following blood vessels. In two cases a nerve which had been accompanying an artery, left the artery and penetrated a

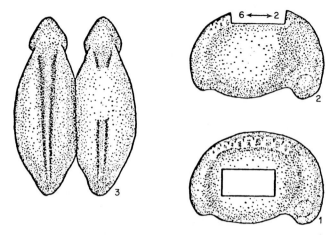

FIG. 2.23.   The formation of aneurogenic limbs. (1) Embryo showing region from which flank ectoderm and mesoderm was taken to cover the wound made by extirpation of cord segments. Stage 23: (2) Embryo showing extent of spinal cord removed. Stage 23: (3) Parabiotics representing operation, step two. Right embryo with brachial region of cord removed; left embryo normal. Stage 30. From Figs 1, 2, 3, Piatt, 1942, *J. exp. Zool.* **91**, 81.

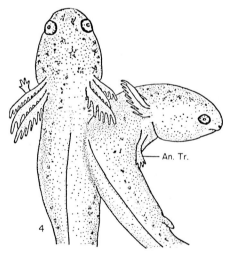

FIG. 2.24.   Aneurogenic limbs: drawing of parabiotics at the time the aneurogenic right forelimb was removed from the operated larva and grafted to a normal animal of the same age. Fourteen days post feeding. From Fig. 4, Piatt, 1942, *J. exp. Zool.* **91**, 81.

mass of cartilage to gain its region of normal distribution. Characteristic branchings of certain nerves were fairly frequently not accompanied by branching of the blood vessel, and vice-versa. In ten experimental animals, as may quite often be found in normal ones, the ulnaris nerve pierced the belly of the ulno-carpalis muscle instead of running superficial to it. From these observations, Piatt (1942) came to the conclusion that the role of the nerve fibre in establishing its characteristic distribution pathway may not be an entirely passive one.

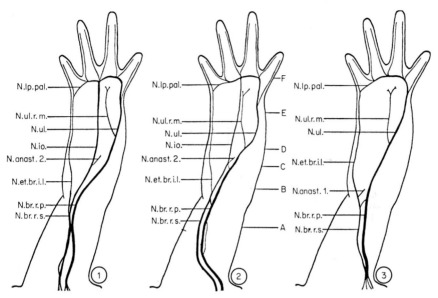

Fig. 2.25. Comparison of nerve patterns in aneurogenic transplants and normal limb: (1) Reconstruction of flexor nerves in experimental forelimb no. 9 to show comparative normalcy of nerve pattern: (2) Reconstruction of flexor nerves in a normal control forelimb: (3) Reconstruction of flexor nerves in experimental forelimb no. 1 to illustrate complete absence of N. interosseus and comparative normalcy of remainder of nerve pattern. From Figs 5, 6, 7, Piatt, 1942, v. *exp. Zool.* **91**, 91.

In a further series of experiments, Piatt (1952) extended his observations on the innervation of aneurogenic forelimbs by transplanting them in place of the hindlimb in a normal animal. In this situation, although innervated by limb-moving segments of the cord, the nerve patterns which developed in the aneurogenic limbs were, in general, very abnormal. In his 1952 paper, Piatt was unwilling to accept the idea that the difference in nerve source in the case of the heterotopic transplants was the cause of the abnormality of the nerve pattern in those limbs. Later, however, he (1956) performed a series of experiments involving the transplantation of forelimb primordia to various ectopic sites in *Amblystoma*. An entirely normal nerve pattern developed only when the transplanted primordium was placed in the orthotopic site and innervated by the proper forelimb nerves; not one instance was found in which a completely normal pattern resulted from innervation by foreign nerves.

One difficulty in attempting to disentangle the relative contributions made to the formation of nerve pattern by the geometry of the limb and

3*

by the source of the innervation, is that most transplanted limbs are less than perfect; and even when such a transplant is well-formed, the very fact that it is ectopically situated must mean that the region of junction with the trunk is wildly abnormal, which in turn will automatically introduce abnormalities, deviations of one sort or another in the course of nerve fibres entering the limb. One way round this difficulty is to leave the limb in its normal position, in normal relationship to its surroundings and to the spinal column, and to transplant the spinal cord instead. Experiments of this sort, where in particular the functional result was studied, have been discussed earlier in this chapter (pp. 47 *et. seq.*). This approach was used in an anatomical study of pathways, by Piatt (1957a), who transplanted medullary, thoracic or hindlimb segments in place of the brachial segments in *Amblystoma*, as well as transplanting, in other animals, brachial segments from donors as orthotopic controls. The orthotopic grafts were the only ones which gave a normal limb nerve pattern (nine out of 18). Seven of the remaining nine orthotopic grafts, though classified as abnormal, were described as being distinctly less abnormal than almost any limb in the three heterotopic series. The heterotopic cord grafts, even the hindlimb series, gave abnormal innervation patterns in the forelimb. The author concluded that, since under the same experimental conditions the normal nerve source is the only one which gives rise to an entirely normal pattern, the uniform presence of abnormalities in limbs with a foreign nerve supply must be, in part at least, the result of differences in the response of the nerve fibres themselves. The possibility that, during development, the matching specificities which presumably enable fibres to follow preneural pathways may be time-dependent, is suggested by some experiments (Piatt, 1957b) in which nerve pattern was studied in "reconstituted limbs"—limbs formed following extirpation of the forelimb bud at various stages. Following amputation of the limb bud at stage 27 in *Amblystoma* there developed limbs with normal innervation pattern; amputation at stage 29 (still before the limb bud becomes innervated) gave limbs showing some abnormalities of nerve pattern; while amputation at the much later stage 38 (after innervation had occurred) gave abnormal patterns in all cases. The observations of Piatt just described, taken together with those of Mark (1965) and Hnik *et al.* (1967) suggest that pathway selection by growing nerve fibres may play a very important role in the genesis of appropriate neuromuscular connections.

EFFECTS OF LIMB OPERATIONS DURING DEVELOPMENT ON VENTRAL HORN CELLS

Our discussion so far has been concerned mainly with the limb itself and the nature of the spinal segment innervating it. With the exception of the work of Eccles and his collaborators, discussed previously, we have not

considered the motoneurone itself except by inference. Yet the motoneurone, as originator of the fibre that eventually innervates the muscle,
is central to any consideration of homologous response. Unfortunately,
there is no adequate work dealing in detail with changes in the motoneurones in urodeles during normal development and following limb
transplantations. Detwiler (1924) described experiments on *Amblystoma*
which failed to reveal any diminution in ventral (motor) cell numbers
following limb ablation during larval life. This matter deserves to be
looked into again, with study of cell degeneration rather than total counts,
in view of the importance of the urodeles in the sum total of experimental
work on neuromuscular connection. As I have indicated earlier, the
organization of the urodele spinal cord is quite different from that of other
tetrapods; the most obvious difference from our present point of view is
the absence of ventral horns at limb levels of the cord. As Hughes (1968,
p. 196) remarks, the difference between the urodeles and the other
tetrapods are such as to warrant caution in extrapolating results obtained
in urodeles.

Since the phenomena with which we are concerned (homologous
response and neuromuscular specificity) are encountered also among anura,
fishes and birds however, we have to consider also the characteristics of
ventral horn cell responses in animals other than the urodeles.

Hughes and his collaborators have extensively studied the composition
of the ventral horns in relation to the development of limb behaviour, in
anura. In *Xenopus* Hughes (1961) found that each ventral horn, at the time
of its first appearance, contained some 5000–6000 cells, whereas by the
time of metamorphosis (some 60 days later) this number had become
reduced to 1200, which number thereafter remained fairly constant
(Fig. 2.26). Hughes calculated that the rate of cell degeneration was
greater than required simply to account for the overall reduction in cell
numbers; the total number of cells disappearing during development was
of the order of 10,000; so for each mature ventral horn cell surviving, eight
or nine had degenerated. There was thus evidence for a turnover of cells
in the ventral horn during development; and most of the overall decrease
in cell numbers occurred during the period of the development of limb
movements, from stages 54–59. The meaning of this extensive cell death
in the ventral horn, and the continued recruitment of new cells to replace
some of those lost, is problematical. It is tempting to think of cellular
overproduction as part of a "belt and braces" programme, whereby many
more cells (and perhaps fibres—see Prestige) are produced than are
necessary at any one time; and those fibres that fail to achieve a successful
termination, in the general fight for survival as they proceed down the
limb, degenerate (see Prestige, 1967b).

During larval development in *Xenopus* there are fibres present in the
ventral roots from about stage 53; at this stage the proportion of ventral

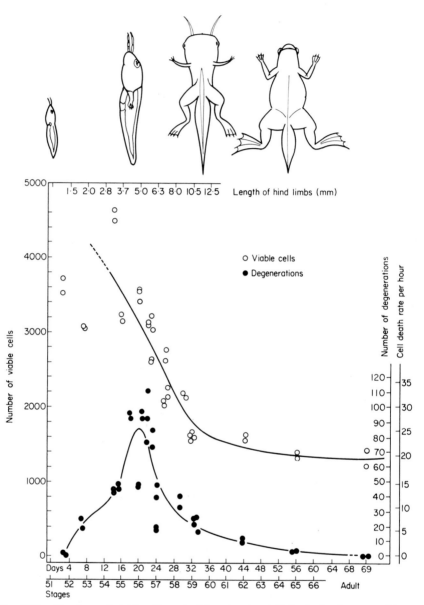

FIG. 2.26.   Numbers of viable cells and of degenerating cells in the lumbar ventral horn of *Xenopus laevis* during larval life. To the scale for numbers of degenerations is added a scale for cell deaths per hour, based on a duration of degeneration of 3·2 hours. From Hughes and Fozzard, 1961.

horn cells that send an axon into the lumbar ventral root is only 1 in 5 or 6 (Fig. 2.27). This proportion could be subject to revision upwards if electron microscopy were to reveal the presence in the root of fibres too small to be counted by light microscopy. During further development this proportion rises, presumably due to a combination of cell degeneration and new axon production (old axon enlargement?) so that at metamorphosis the number of ventral horn cells approximately equals the number of ventral root fibres.

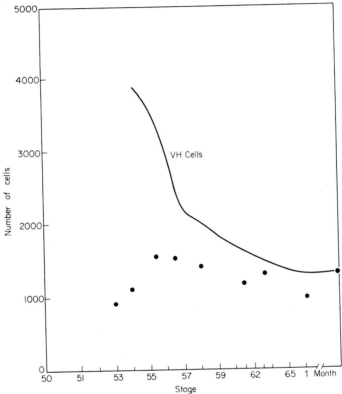

FIG. 2.27. Numbers of cells in one lumbar ventral horn of *Xenopus laevis* during development (continuous curve), together with the corresponding counts of the numbers of fibres in lumbar ventral roots. Ordinate: stages of development. From Prestige, 1966.

Amputation of the developing limb in *Xenopus* affects the course of development of the related ventral horn cells (Prestige, 1967b). Removal of the limb before the palette stage has no effect; from stage 53 histogenetic degeneration occurs in the normally developing limb and degeneration is also brought about by amputation of the limb. In either case, Prestige (1967b) argues that the explanation is likely to be the same, i.e. lack of a certain "maintenance factor" from the limb which would be required to permit the neurone to continue its development. This author has found that ventral roots and limb nerves are present at all times when amputation causes degeneration of ventral horn cells.

From these results we may make a tentative formulation of the course of events during limb development in *Xenopus*. Large numbers of ventral horn cells appear at the onset of limb innervation but only a small proportion of these cells have axons passing out yet in the ventral root; although it is possible that many more axons exist than have yet been counted. These axons pursue a course down the limb bud, following as best they may the preneural trails laid down under genetic control. Many more fibres are involved than can be used in the limb—perhaps as part of a developmental policy of survival of the most effective. Some of the fibres which have most accurately interpreted their directional cues will succeed in innervating the appropriate target organ. Most will not, and these are the fibres that come from ventral horn cells that will degenerate. As the limb grows, so more fibres are required to innervate the structure adequately and this requirement is met by the continued addition of new ventral horn cells during this stage of development.

SUMMARY AND CONCLUSIONS

The main theme of this chapter has been the myotypic response in transplanted limbs; the reason for this is that these experiments, whether or not the earlier interpretations of their results were right or wrong, have forced us to reconsider much of our classical neurophysiological dogma. We are required to ask some very basic questions about the meaning of coordination and the intimate nature of neuromuscular connection and nerve-to-nerve contact.

When an amphibian larval limb is transplanted it will become re-innervated and may then show homologous response with the normal limb. Various restrictions have become obvious in this response: the limb must be reinnervated by limb-moving segments, thus revealing a significant difference between these segments and non-limb-moving segments of the cord. This requirement for brachial or lumbosacral segments exists in relation to coordinated homologous movement, to maintenance of the limb musculature and to the establishment of a normal pattern of limb innervation.

Before any great attempt is made to explain the phenomenon of homologous response it is advisable to determine whether, and if so, to what extent, the phenomenon exists. All early work on myotypic respecification was done either using cinephotography of the moving parts, or smoked-drum kymography, to analyse the time relations of the various muscular contractions. These methods are inherently inadequate to the task and most recently appropriate electrophysiological recording has been used for this purpose (Székely, 1968). Early results with this technique suggest a certain caution in accepting all the previous assertions about the synchronicity of the timing of contraction in normal and transplanted limbs.

There is no doubt, however, that reinnervated transplants may function in a coordinated fashion with the rest of the body; and this fact also requires explanation. Székely (1965) has shown that the basic pattern of efferent impulses controlling urodele limb movement is organized within the spinal cord and moreover, since adequate limb movement may be maintained by one spinal segment only, we have to say that the elements of this basic "limb-moving apparatus" are replicated in each limb segment of the cord. After mid-thoracic spinal transection the hindlimbs are paralysed; however, when the animal starts to drag itself over the ground by its forelimbs, the hindlimbs start to move in a coordinated fashion, but independently of the forelimbs. Rhythmic afferent impulses from the moving limb are apparently not necessary for coordinated limb movements, since excision of the spinal ganglia at limb level does not impair the coordinated movement of the limbs. Furthermore, the motor response to a mechanical stimulus applied to a limb is determined by the position of that limb at the time of the stimulus, and consists of the movement that would normally follow from this position in the course of a normal step.

It has been customary, since the early work of Weiss, to represent the walking movements of a salamander limb by a simplification into comparatively few phases, each controlled by a group of muscles. Székely (1965) adopted this approach and was able then to simulate the limb-moving functions of the urodele cord by a logical network which delivers rhythmic outputs on non-rhythmic inputs, and in which the discharge sequence of the output elements is determined (Fig. 2.28). When this network was tested electronically, using the artificial neurones of Jenik (1962) a rhythmical discharge (Fig. 2.29) was obtained which resembled fairly closely the type of activity seen in a urodele limb. Various networks with different properties have since been described by Székely (1968) and Kling and Székely (1968).

It is not possible to say, at the present time, whether such networks have biological as well as logical and electronic validity. The networks of Kling and Székely (1968) have recurrent cyclic inhibition as a basic structural principle; however, as the authors point out, biological networks with this property have never been demonstrated in the central nervous system. And even if these networks represent any form of biological reality, this would hardly simplify our biological problem very much; for we would still have to arrange for the outputs of each of the neurones A, B, C, D, to reach appropriate muscle for the system to provide the coordinated activity actually seen.

We must maintain a certain scepticism about the synchronicity of homologous response until a sufficient number of normal animals and

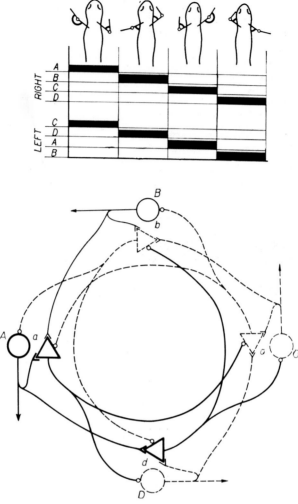

Fig. 2.28. Top: Simplified myochronogram illustrating the contraction sequence of limb muscles during stepping. A: extensory of the elbow, B: adductors of the shoulder, C: flexors of the elbow, D: abductors of the shoulder. The movement of the wrist and the overlap actually existing between neighbouring muscle groups has been disregarded. Bottom: Diagram illustrating the connections of four motoneurones (circles) and four inhibitory neurones (triangles) in a network capable of delivering rhythmic outputs to non-rhythmic inputs. Fork-shaped endings (⤙) denote excitatory synapses, circle endings (–o) inhibitory synapses. Nerve cells drawn with heavy line (A, a, d) are excited, B with thin line is in "responsive state", and those drawn with broken line are inhibited. From Székely, 1965.

animals with transplanted limbs have had electromyographic recording performed on them. Even so, while the precision of muscular timing is open to question, the general existence of the phenomenon of homologous

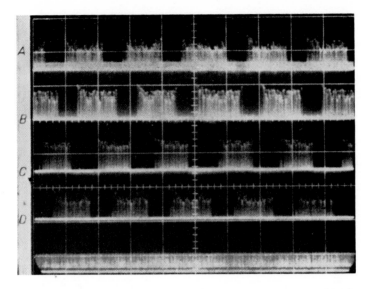

FIG. 2.29.   Action potentials of the four output elements of a network of artificial neurones evoked by a series of random inputs at a frequency of 500 pulses per sec (lowermost trace). Time calibration; one division, 200 msec. Note the prolonged discharges of the artificial neurones and the big overlap. From Székely, 1965.

response is not. Two main mechanisms may be put forward to account for this. The first is the modulation or respecification of nerves by their target organs and the second is selective reinnervation of the muscles by their original motoneurones. Weiss has maintained consistently that selective reinnervation could not account for his findings; however, as will be apparent from the discussion earlier in this chapter, much of Weiss' interpretation is open to serious question. I would also argue, in this neuromuscular context, as I shall argue in the next chapter, on skin innervation, that the whole problem of homologous response has been very considerably over-interpreted by most of the early investigators. There is a difference between saying that a few major groups of limb muscles reaquire an adequate timing, and saying that all 40 or so limb muscles each reaquire their proper phasing. There is evidence in favour of the former statement but none in favour of the latter.

There are only two of Weiss' experimental arrangements where it would be very difficult to conceive of selective reinnervation occurring: these are the experiments (Weiss, 1937b) in which a distal limb nerve was shown to be capable of adequately reinnervating an entire limb; and the experiments (Weiss, 1930a,b; 1931) involving homologous response in individually transplanted muscles supplied with a predetermined innervation.

The experiments which must compel most attention are those of Mark (1965) and Sperry and Arora (1965) on fishes. In this work the recovery of coordinated muscle function was shown unequivocally to be due to selective reinnervation of individual muscles by their appropriate fibres. In these situations myotypic respecification did not occur. We must ask, therefore, whether a form of selective reinnervation might not account for *all* the observations of homologous response, including those in transplanted limbs and transplanted individual muscles.

In the case of whole-limb-replacing grafts, it is quite possible and seems to me to be quite likely that selective reinnervation may account for the motor recovery found. The nerves entering the limb show massive branching even under light microscopy and the tendency for a normal nerve pattern to be restored in the graft suggests a form of intimate chemical guidance; the fibres appear to be able to sniff their way along a previously laid down pathway. This form of pathway-selection would be manifested with greater or lesser efficiency according to circumstances. Fibres growing on the "wrong" substrate would grow randomly, their direction determined only by the steric configuration of the ground; however, given a choice, the fibres will tend to follow the appropriate paths.

Depending partly on the age of the animal, we may also have to consider the effect of amputation of a limb on the number of ventral horn cells, or motor cells in urodeles. In anura, chicks (Hamburger, 1934) and possibly in urodeles, limb amputation results in increased degeneration of motor cells. This may be accompanied by recruitment of new motor cells and new motor axons, which could aid the appropriate reinnervation of the limb muscles. There is evidence suggesting that such degeneration and replacement is part of the normal course of limb innervation in anura (Hughes, 1968) and it would seem reasonable to involve this mechanism in the case of limb transplantation.

With supernumary limb grafts it has been customary to sever one of the host's limb nerves and lead it into the graft. In this case, since each root in urodeles contains fibres adequate for all limb muscles, the problem is essentially similar to that in the case of replacement grafts, except that we now have an expanded peripheral field of action for the limb fibres.

In the experiments of Weiss (1937b; 1930a,b; 1931) involving reinnervation of a transplanted limb by a distal limb nerve, and those involving muscle transplantation, it is difficult to avoid the requirement for modulation to account for the findings. In these experiments in particular, since they are crucial to the case for modulation, it would be most useful to have reliable electrophysiological evidence. Since this is not available we have to say that selective innervation involving merely choice of peripheral pathway by the nerve fibres would not explain the results. For the muscles in these experiments to become reinnervated by their appropriate fibres would require the fibres actually innervating the muscle to be replaced, at cord or plexus level, with appropriate fibres. This would in turn require passage back up the nerve of a message to the effect that the muscle was "wrong", together with selective regrowth of the proper nerve fibres. Such a mechanism, apart from being difficult to conceive of, is perhaps even more unlikely than modulation in this situation. The experiments on muscle transplantation (Weiss, 1930a,b; 1931) have never been successfully repeated and this is really necessary if we are to attempt a useful reassessment of their meaning. The time-factors involved in these experiments, where animals examined after longer intervals showed more evidence of homologous response than animals examined sooner after operation, could suggest that either a time-related modulation process was occurring or perhaps that time was required for nerve fibre regeneration after degeneration of inappropriate fibres.

Apart from the experiments just mentioned, the only evidence in favour of modulation is that of Eccles and his collaborators (Eccles *et al.*, 1960; Eccles *et al.*, 1962) and here the results are, firstly, conflicting and secondly, from the wrong animal. We have to conclude therefore that the phenomenon of myoneural modulation is unproven in most cases where it has been invoked and that selective reinnervation is more likely to be the mechanism at work. There are, however, certain observations that cannot, at present, be explained adequately on this basis.

3. SOMATIC SENSORY CONNECTIONS

Sensory nerves from the skin transmit to the central nervous system information on the nature, intensity and position of peripheral stimuli. During adult life the sensory innervation of the skin is derived from the dorsal root ganglia of the spinal cord. In the lower vertebrates the initial afferent innervation of the skin during development is provided by various forms of extra-ganglionic sensory neurones (Hughes, 1957) of which one variety, the Rohon-Beard cells, is found in the larval cord of fishes and amphibians. In both urodele and anuran amphibians the Rohon-Beard cells provide the first sensory system for the skin. These cells and their processes are unlike any other neuronal variety commonly found in the vertebrates; they send their peripheral fibres out between the myotomes to innervate both skin and muscle. As larval life proceeds this primary afferent system is gradually replaced by the developing system of dorsal root ganglia, until at the approach of metamorphosis the Rohon-Beard cells begin to degenerate. The role these cells may play in sensory activities or in the further development of the secondary sensory system, is unknown.

In the present context we are concerned with how the cutaneous sensory fibres achieve their eventual pattern of connections during development; and with the nature of the connections formed during nerve regeneration. As with the neuromuscular system, much of the experimental work to be discussed in this chapter deals with inferences about neural connections derived from studies of neural functions. Again, as with neuromuscular connections, it will (I suspect) become obvious as we go on that some of the conclusions that have been reached are unwarranted. Since, however, so much investigation has been done on the functional aspects of sensory innervation, it is necessary to consider briefly the nature of the sensory message. We may here treat the information content of the sensory message separately, in terms of the three components mentioned above, and our concern will be particularly with positional information.

At the present time it is rather generally accepted that the strength of a sensory stimulus is signalled to the CNS by a combination of the number of fibres excited and the frequency of the impulses in each fibre. If we accept this approximation to the truth, we have no need to consider this aspect of sensory information further in the present context.

As concerns the *nature* of the sensory response to a peripheral stimulus, the specificity of the pathway for the mode of sensory response, as predicated by Müller (1840) in his doctrine of specific nerve energies, is still the subject of vigorous controversy. The discussion, somewhat crudely summarized, relates to whether one type of sensation reflects the activity particularly of one corresponding class of peripheral nerve fibres; or whether one type of sensation results from the central analysis of a certain spatiotemporal pattern or patterns of impulses in many varied types of peripheral nerve fibres.

The specificity of many afferent nerve fibres for one particular type of *stimulus* is well established, by many investigations from the early work of Adrian and his collaborators (Adrian, 1926; Adrian and Zotterman, 1926) up to the present time; this does not, unfortunately, tell us much about the specificity of such fibres for a particular sensation. The arguments in favour of an "impulse pattern" type of interpretation of sense modality signalling have been put forward at length by members of the Oxford neuroanatomical school (Lele and Weddell, 1956; Sinclair, 1955) and by Melzack and Wall (1962). Discussion continues and at present shows no sign of reaching a conclusion. In so far as the experiments to be described in this chapter involve the responses of animals to different forms of sensory stimulation, our present uncertainty about the nature of the mechanism of modality signalling is highly relevant to any conclusions that may be drawn from the experiments.

THE NATURE OF POSITIONAL INFORMATION

Most of the work to be discussed here, however, deals principally with positional information in cutaneous afferent messages. And here we are (perhaps) on firmer ground. The ability of an animal to distinguish the positions of two stimuli applied to widely separated regions of the body surface, must reflect an ability to distinguish the inputs from different sets of nerve fibres and not merely a different pattern of impulses in the same set. It will, however, emerge from the discussion of the experiments about to be described, that even spatial sensory resolution of this sort does not provide us with conclusive evidence about the nature of the peripheral sensory mechanism.

The identification by the CNS of the *position* of a stimulus applied to the skin could be made in several ways. (1) The most obvious mechanism could utilize the known differential distribution of sensory nerve fibres across the skin. Thus with non-overlapping receptive fields in the skin, activity passing centrally along fibre A automatically transmits topographical information to the CNS differentiating this stimulus position from any other by virtue of the fact that fibre A and not fibres B or C has been activated; and for this to happen, the stimulus must lie within the receptive field of A. For this to be a useful mode of identification, the central terminals of fibre A must also be separate, in a spatial or a functional sense, from those of other fibres. (2) With partially overlapping cutaneous receptive fields, a situation corresponding more closely with what we know of cutaneous innervation than the previous one, stimulation at one position on the skin will result in activation of more than one afferent fibre. And since the stimulus will lie in the centre of one field and towards the periphery of another, the various fibres involved will be differentially excited by the one stimulus. Consequently, in this case, sensory localization could be achieved through central recognition that a certain *pattern* of impulses in several adjacent fibres was different in topographical import from another pattern in another group of fibres. In this situation, importance still attaches to the topographical distribution of the fibres, but the central analysis has to involve a more statistical approach. This arrangement represents what is probably the most widely held view of the nature of sensory localization at the present time. (3) With totally overlapping cutaneous receptive fields, if the fibres are identical in sensitivity, the presence of impulses in one fibre rather than another cannot be used as the basis of sensory localization since any stimulus within the common receptive field, if it excites one fibre, should excite them all; and to the same extent. In this situation (which may not correspond to any biological reality) positional information could not be signalled along the peripheral-central link indicated. However, if the overlap of receptive fields is less than 100%, then sensory localization could be achieved by an extension of the process of central statistical analysis mentioned previously. In this case, if the field overlap were very extensive, information from any one fibre would carry relatively little positional information; and the accuracy of localization might be expected to increase with the number of neurones (each of slightly different peripheral distribution) included in the central analysis. In this situation also, the precise spatial distribution of the central terminals of any one fibre may perhaps come to be of less significance than in situation 1. A further possibility, relevant to the case of totally overlapping receptive fields, would be that positional information might be signalled within the field of any one fibre, by characteristic differences in the temporal pattern of impulses in that fibre. Our knowledge of the relationships found in single-fibre discharges between stimulus intensity and impulse frequency however, makes it difficult to see how this mode of signalling position could be other than highly ambiguous.

While it is so that changes in stimulus strength are indicated by alterations in impulse frequency, we now know that sensory signalling may be more subtle than this; how much more subtle remains to be discovered.

In one particular *central* system, the spinocervical tract of the cat, for instance, pulse-interval distributions in a single fibre may be characteristically different for different modes of peripheral stimulation (Brown and Franz, 1970); and, of course, analysis of post-stimulus-time histograms of the responses from various cells in the occipital cortex reveals, in many cases, quite different temporal patterns of activity, from the same cell, to different modalities of sensory stimulation (Morrell, 1967). If this can be done with the aid of a simple laboratory computer, it is hard to believe that the central nervous system cannot do comparable analyses even better. It would therefore perhaps be unwise for us to abandon "impulse-pattern" hypotheses as impossible; for whereas we know that the pattern of discharge in single sensory nerve fibres tends to be regular following the carefully graded stimuli used in such electrophysiological analyses, the form of stimulation used in the embryological studies here being discussed is seldom if ever so rigorously controlled. And furthermore, since a detailed analysis of the properties of receptors over a wide area of the skin surface has never been undertaken, we are not in a position to say whether small graded differences of the sort being considered exist or not.

In normal neurological or neurophysiological investigations the various possible mechanisms considered here (and there are presumably others) are mostly not considered, it being fairly generally accepted that stimulus localization is a function of fibre localization in the periphery and synaptic localization in the appropriate centres. But in the present discussion we are not dealing with ordinary neurophysiology. We are dealing with a nervous system in the process of *becoming*, and any experimental procedure adopted in these circumstances may possibly alter the mode of becoming and certainly alters the eventual structure. We are not entitled to assume that the modes of signalling apparently appropriate to a normal nervous system are necessarily so to the distorted nervous system produced by operation on the embryo—some of the abnormalities of which have undoubtedly never been encountered by these animals in the absence of human intervention.

LOCAL SIGN IN THE AMPHIBIAN BLINK REFLEX

The mechanisms underlying the signalling of cutaneous positional information, and their development, were studied by Weiss (1942) in urodeles. The question he posed was that, if the correct identification of a peripheral stimulus is dependent on constant topographical relations between periphery and centres, thus requiring correct connections between receptor and central unit of corresponding specificity, how could the presumed stereotypism of central-peripheral connections be assured during development? Weiss (1942) then adapted the arguments from his previous work on neuromuscular connectivity to this situation and maintained that it would be difficult to account for sensory specificity without conceding specificity to the nerve fibres themselves: fibre specificity, presumably of some unknown biochemical nature, could provide a mechanism for bringing about orderly central-peripheral connections during development⟩

If such fibre specificity exists, the next question is whether the bio-chemical diversification of the fibres is of central or peripheral origin. It is conceivable (and, as mentioned in the previous chapter, there is some evidence for this) that the differentiating neural centre could impose its specificity on the outgrowing nerve fibres, which would then make selective connection with the periphery which was also specified appro-priately by the process of differentiation. Alternatively, and in agreement with Weiss' concept of neuromuscular modulation, sensory nerve fibres could grow out with a greater or lesser degree of randomness, and have their specificity imprinted on them by contact with the terminal organ of a particular biochemical character. In this latter case, as with neuro-muscular modulation, the central connections of the afferent fibres would then become adjusted to provide an adequate sensory-motor linkage.

⟨One way of investigating the mode of formation of sensory connections would be to connect, in a developing animal, a sense organ with a nerve originally serving a different sensory function; it should then be possible to see whether the central response to stimulation of the end organ con-tinued to conform with the type of function originally manifested by that nerve, or whether instead the function now conformed with the new type of end organ.⟩ Information of this sort may be obtained by transplantation experiments; either by transplantation of a given sensory area of the periphery into the domain of a strange nerve, or by deflection of a given sensory nerve into a foreign peripheral area.

Weiss (1942) adopted the former alternative in his experiments on the reflex responses obtainable from transplanted urodele eyes. In amphibia, a localized mechanical stimulus applied to the surface of the cornea evokes a localized motor response—lid closure and eye retraction. This reflex response to corneal stimulation only develops at about the time of meta-morphosis (Kollros, 1942a) even though the afferent and efferent paths involved in the reflex apparently become functional separately some time before this. Maturation of the central part of this reflex arc is thus related to the changes of metamorphosis; and in keeping with this, the reflex may be induced to appear prematurely by treatment with thyroid. Indeed, localized implantation of thyroid hormone into the hindbrain may result, if the implant is asymmetrically located, in the unilateral appearance of the reflex (Kollros, 1942b).

⟨The cornea is innervated by part of the ophthalmic division of the trigemi-nal nerve. Parts of the rest of the face area are also supplied by sensory fibres from the trigeminal. Yet stimulation of the cornea or skin immediately surrounding the eye results in the corneal, or blink reflex, while stimulation on the top of the snout gives reflex depression of the head and stimulation under the chin causes head elevation, and so forth (Sperry and Miner, 1949). Different afferent nerve fibres are associated with these different responses.⟩

The reflexogenic area for lid-closure in a normal *Triturus* is fairly narrow (Fig. 3.1). To investigate the relative effectiveness of central versus peripheral factors in the setting up of the reflex arcs involved in

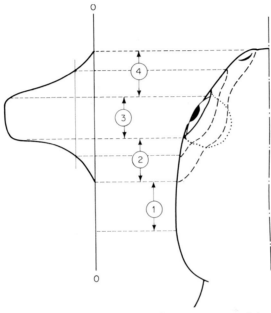

FIG. 3.1. Sensitivity distribution within the reflexogenous area of the lid-closure reflex in a normal animal several months after metamorphosis. Area 1 is the ear region; area 2 is the skin between area 1 and the eye; area 3 is the corneal region; area 4 extends from the anterior edge of the eye to the nose. The left half of the diagram represents a profile of the sensitivity distribution along the anteroposterior diameter of the reflexogenous area; elevation of the curve above the zero level indicates in a qualitative fashion the reciprocal threshold values in arbitrary units. From Fig. 8, Weiss, 1942, *J. comp. Neurol.* **77**, 148.

these responses, Weiss (1942) transplanted an eye to the region of the ear or the nose in *Triturus torosus* at mid-larval stages of development. The eventual results of his experiments can be summarized by saying that touching an eye transplanted to the ear or nose region is just as effective in producing a blink reflex of the normal eye on the same side as is touching the cornea of the latter (Fig. 3.2).

Thus in these experiments, stimulation of areas of skin well outside the normal reflexogenic zone gives rise to the blink reflex. Furthermore, the thresholds of the intermediate region, between graft and normal eye, were higher than those of either cornea but lower than those of the same area on the normal side; and the intensity (duration) of the reflex response to corneal stimulation was greater on the operated side. Thus the increase in sensitivity following the grafting of an extra eye extends beyond the confines of the graft itself. This overexcitability of the affected region was apparently not due to the immediate effects of injury, since the reflex testing was performed at metamorphosis, several months after the operation. The hypothesis offered by Weiss, to account for these findings, is that outgrowing sensory neurones become modulated by the specific biochemical character of their end organs; and that the modulation so acquired determines the central interrelations of the fibres, thus explaining the conformance between the reflex response and the type of end organ stimulated. We may note that this hypothesis has nothing helpful to say about the fact that skin between graft and normal eye has a lower threshold than normal.

gradient?
or dispersion of nerve through area because of biochemical attraction of supernumerary eye.

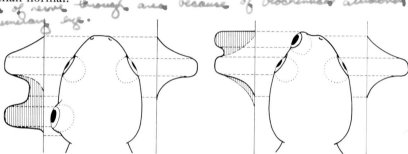

FIG. 3.2. Sensitivity profiles for lid-closure reflex in animals with eye-to-ear grafts (left side of figure) and eye-to-nose grafts (right side of figure). The mode of plotting is the same as that in Fig. 3.1. From Figs 9, 10, Weiss, 1942, *J. comp. Neurol.* **77**, 161.

In the normal development of the corneal reflex in *Triturus torosus* (Weiss, 1942), the first trace of a response appears as a weak retraction following strong mechanical stimulation of the centre of the cornea. As development continues, the reflex threshold decreases, the reflexogenic area spreads and the motor response increases in strength. Several weeks after metamorphosis the reflexogenic area shrinks again and becomes confined to the eye and its immediate vicinity. Thus, while in the early stages of the appearance of the reflex it could be elicited from the ear zone, during the normal course of development the reflexogenic zone would shrink away from this area. In the presence of a transplanted eye in this region however, its reflexogenic character persists.

It is conceivable (Weiss, 1942) that the widespread nature of the early reflexogenic zone reflects the functional equivalence of the immature sensory fibres. As more specialized end organs develop in the metamorphosing skin, their neurones would become correspondingly modulated. All trigeminal fibres would evoke the reflex in the early stages, but those with cutaneous endings would gradually become modulated so as to render them increasingly unfit to release the lid-closure mechanism, while at the same time linking them more firmly to the mechanism of the head-jerk

Does reflex occur in super-numerary eye as well as normal eye. In absence of normal musculature would there be any evidence for relatively normal efferent activity.

reflex (Weiss, 1942). Whether the apparent change in function that normally occurs during development in the trigeminal fibres reflects an increasing *corneal* modulation, or merely that the corneal fibres have remained in a primitive condition, unmodulated by skin, Weiss was unable to say. In one or other of these directions, however, the results of the experiments were interpreted as indicating the existence of peripheral modulation of the trigeminal fibres. And whereas in Weiss' (1942) experiments all the nerve fibres involved belonged to the trigeminal nerve, making it possible to argue that all these fibres may have some general property which enables them, under appropriate circumstances, to form blink reflex connections, Kollros (1943) has shown that eyes implanted between the ear capsule and the base of the gill, a region innervated by the vagus nerve, will also yield a corneal reflex from the normal eye. Similar results from eyes transplanted to the base of the gills have been described by Székely (1959b) in *Pleurodeles* and *Triturus vulgaris*.

The argument for modulation as the mechanism at work in these experiments depends on (1) the specific character of the motor effect, which is normally only elicited by localized stimulation of the eye; (2) the assumption that the specific reflex effect reflects the topographical distribution of fibres rather than some configuration of impulse pattern; (3) the assumption that selective outgrowth of nerve fibres does not occur; and (4) the assumption that the abnormal reflex, elicitable after corneal transplantation, is uniquely related to the particular character of the transplanted tissue. Point (1) is valid; point (2) is unproven; point (3) is quite possibly untrue (similar arguments to those presented in the previous chapter will apply here); and point (4) is invalid, as shown by Székely (1959b).

While studying, for other purposes, the limbs of urodele larvae, transplanted to the base of the gill, Székely (1959b) observed that the distal part of an implanted limb had been bitten off by another animal. A regeneration blastema developed at the site of amputation and mechanical stimulation of the regeneration blastema evoked a corneal reflex from the ipsilateral eye. This effect was never seen on stimulation of an intact implanted limb. Since this observation was inconsistent with the assumption that "corneal specificity" was the cause of the abnormal blink reflex obtainable from transplanted eyes, Székely (1959b) performed a further series of operations to test this point. Limbs were transplanted to the base of the gill in young larvae of *Pleurodeles waltlii* and *Triturus vulgaris*; a few days before the onset of metamorphosis the foot of the limb graft was cut off and the animals frequently tested for reflex effects of stimulation of the resulting blastema and regenerated limb. In control experiments an eye was transplanted to the same place.

At the onset of metamorphosis, stimulation of the transplanted eye evoked a corneal reflex from the ipsilateral normal eye; however, during the first half of larval life, stimulation of the transplanted eye evoked the gill depression reflex, which in this period is normally elicited exclusively from the vagal sensory area (Székely, 1959a). Thus reflex connections from the transplanted eye existed both before and after metamorphosis but the functional connections changed at the time of metamorphosis. Similarly with transplanted limbs: stimulation of the intact limb during larval life evoked gill depression. Shortly before the onset of gill reduction during metamorphosis, the foot was cut off and within a week a blastema developed at the site of amputation. Weak mechanical stimulation of the blastema evoked the blink reflex. Stimulation of the skin immediately next to the blastema was completely ineffective in evoking this reflex. The further the regeneration of the foot proceeded, the higher became the threshold of the blastema for the blink reflex. When the foot had completely regenerated the reflex was no longer elicitable. Reamputation of the foot one month after metamorphosis enabled a blink reflex to be elicited again from the resulting new blastema.

This experiment of Székely shows conclusively that, while the presence of corneal tissue may be a sufficient condition for the establishment of the blink reflex, it is not a necessary one. Cornea and limb blastema evidently cannot have any common biochemical properties which could be called cornea-specific. The ability of a regeneration blastema to evoke the blink reflex immediately removes the necessity to invoke "corneal modulation" as the explanation for the earlier results of Weiss. There is a sense, however, in which Weiss' original interpretation might retain some relevance; and this relates to his suggestion (1942) that the corneal tissue may be such as to cause the innervating fibres to remain in some "primitive" state while the fibres innervating the surrounding skin become progressively modulated in the direction appropriate for other reflexes. This suggestion would require the "primitive", non-specified fibres to be generally effective in eliciting the corneal reflex. As Székely (1959b) points out, there is some similarity between the mode of terminal innervation in the cornea and in a blastema; both form an extensively arborizing plexus with free and apparently unspecialized naked terminals. This author suggested that the fibres supplying a limb regeneration blastema retain their ability to evoke a corneal reflex for as long as they remain in a low state of differentiation; this ability is lost when, as the foot regenerates, the character of the innervation changes to that characteristic of a fully differentiated limb.

We must agree that there is a certain similarity between the innervation of a cornea and that of a limb blastema; but without further experiments this similarity does not take us very far. It will be recalled that in both Székely's (1959b) and Kollros' (1943) eye transplantations, and Székely's limb transplantations, the innervating fibres came from the *vagus* nerve, which never normally gives rise to the blink reflex. Székely (1959b) has put forward the suggestion that the different forms of peripheral innervation may give rise to different forms of afferent messages, in terms of spike height, duration, frequency and so forth, and that the central nervous system possesses the ability to disentangle these differing incoming messages and distribute them appropriately to the various motor systems. An alternative mechanism was suggested by Kornacker (1963), who investigated the spatial and temporal patterns of synaptic activity in the frog's medulla, following localized peripheral stimulation of the head region, in an attempt to obtain direct evidence concerning the neurological basis of stimulus specificity. His electrophysiological results suggested that small diameter myelinated sensory fibres of the trigeminal terminate laterally in the medulla while the larger diameter fibres terminate medially. Most corneal nerve fibres are of small diameter and in keeping with this the response to corneal stimulation was almost entirely confined to the lateral medullary locus, whereas the greater part of the response to snout stimulation (fast fibres, 20–30 m/sec) occurred medially. This distribution is in keeping with the known localization of trigeminal afferent terminals in the gelatinous part of the spinal tract nucleus of the cat, as shown by Szentágothai and Kiss (1949); these authors found that the ophthalmic branch of the trigeminal gave endings ventrolaterally while the mandibular division ended dorsomedially in the nucleus. Szentágothai and Kiss also described the larger fibres terminating in the spongy medial part of this region while the finer fibres mostly ended more peripherally. This suggests that the basic anatomy of this region is similar in cat and frog. Kornacker (1963) found that activity occurring in the lateral locus alone appeared to be sufficient to elicit an eye blink.

On the basis of this result, Kornacker (1963) suggested that the factor underlying the abnormal corneal reflex from a transplanted limb blastema might be the diameter of the fibres innervating it. If the tissue character of the blastema was such as to lead to a reduction in the diameter of the nerve fibres innervating it, and this change were associated with a shift of fibre terminations within the brain towards the more lateral of the medullary sites, the blastema could perhaps take on some of the reflexogenic capabilities of the cornea. This suggestion, while doing away with the requirement for tissue-specificity, is hardly an advance over previous suggestions, since we have no reason to expect that nerve terminations, already functionally established in one part of the brain, should get up and go elsewhere when the peripheral fibres are decreased in diameter. On the other hand, since the periphery *has* been surgically disturbed, we have to do with regenerating peripheral fibres; and if we postulate that small fibres have a tendency selectively to innervate "undifferentiated" tissues, then perhaps we could account for the findings on the basis of a low-grade form of selective reinnervation. Note: it sure is difficult to evaluate what is going on when you don't know what else happens with stimulation in question in regard to the patterns of activity obtainable at any one time.

TRANSPLANTATION OF SENSORY GANGLIA

As mentioned earlier, the two most commonly used approaches to the problem of the specificity of sensory nerves are the transplantation of the sensory nerve or the sensory target area, each into the territory of the other. A third, highly ingenious, variant on these procedures was devised by Székely (1959a), who transplanted the anlage of one sensory ganglion into the place of another in urodele embryos. Thus in some animals the anlage of the V ganglion was removed and replaced by a vagal ganglion anlage; and in other embryos the vagal ganglion anlage was replaced by a trigeminal ganglion anlage in the same way. These animals were then tested for the presence of the various reflexes normally characteristic of the vagal or trigeminal sensory areas (Fig. 3.3).

In a normal *Triturus* or *Pleurodeles* tactile stimulation of the gill or the skin posterior to the ear evokes, in early larval life, a reflex depression of the gills. Both the afferent and efferent fibres concerned in this reflex are furnished by the vagus nerve and up to the mid-larval stage this is the only local reflex that can be elicited by tactile stimulation of the head. Light touch applied to the skin elsewhere on the head, even on the cornea itself, is ineffective in producing the reflex. Another reflex, specific for the trigeminal nerve, normally appears only around the time of metamorphosis; this is the corneal or blink reflex and its motor pathway is via the 6th nerve to the eye retractor muscles.

Animals with two vagal ganglia and no trigeminal ganglion on one side differed from normal animals in their response to light touch on the cornea in early larval life. In these larvae, stimulation of the cornea resulted in a gill depression reflex (Fig. 3.3 row 2, column 1). Thus the afferent fibres of the transplanted vagal ganglion could establish effective functional connections with the motor vagal nuclei, in spite of the trigeminal location of the ganglion. Furthermore, at the onset of metamorphosis, the corneal reflex appeared on the operated side as well as on the normal side (Fig. 3.3 row 3, column 1), suggesting that the afferent fibres of the transplanted vagus could also establish orderly connections with the 6th nerve nucleus.

This experiment would suggest that, in larval life, the character of the reflex connections formed by the fibres concerned corresponds to the nature of the nerve and not to its locality. Yet at metamorphosis these fibres appear to establish functional connections with the abducens nucleus, a connection not normally revealed by reflex activity. The difficulties of interpretation inherent in these results may be emphasized by two further observations: Székely (1959a) noted that, in some of these animals after metamorphosis, stimulation at the site of the resorbed gill on the side of the operation would elicit a corneal reflex; and Kollros (1942a) had observed that, in underfed animals the reflexogenic area for the corneal reflex could extend to the base of the gill. In both of these cases, stimulation within what is normally the vagal area evoked the typical

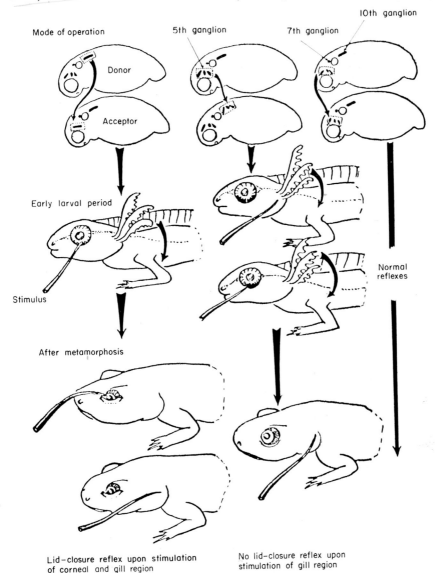

FIG. 3.3. Diagram summarizing the functional result of transplantation experiments replacing trigeminal by vagal ganglia and the reverse. The third column with orthotopic transplantation of trigeminal ganglia serves as control. Normal reflexes were observed in this group during all stages of development. From Székely, 1959a.

trigeminal reflex of eye retraction. This suggests that, even in unoperated animals, either the peripheral distribution of sensory fibres from the trigeminal is more extensive than is revealed by normal testing; or that the central synaptic connections of vagal fibres may extend to embrace the abducens centre, even though such connections are not normally activated.

In his second type of transplantation Székely (1959a) produced animals with two trigeminal and no vagal ganglia on one side. During the first half of larval life such animals produced a normal gill depression reflex in response to stimulation of the skin posterior to the ear (Fig. 3.3 row 2, column 2). Thus in this situation fibres from the transplanted trigeminal ganglion, which innervated this region, were able to form central reflex connections appropriate to their new location and not to their original character. Moreover, on stimulation of the cornea in many of these animals a gill reflex occurred during the first half of larval life (Fig. 3.3 row 3 column 2). This indicates that the fibres of the normal trigeminal ganglion, which innervates the eye, can form functionally effective connections with the vagal motor nuclei when there are two trigeminal ganglia present on the one side. At the onset of metamorphosis the corneal reflex developed in the normal fashion but no corneal reflex was ever seen following stimulation of the skin posterior to the ear (Fig. 3.3 row 4, column 2). Thus the fibres of the transplanted trigeminal ganglion seem unable here to form functional reflex connections appropriate to their character.

Székely (1959a) interpreted these observations as indicating that the sensory neuroblasts of the cranial ganglia show signs of functional specificity; that is, there is a qualitative difference between the neuroblasts of the 10th and 5th ganglia which becomes manifest before the outgrowth of their axons. The difference between the existence of an extra vagal ganglion, which enabled the animal to give a gill reflex on corneal stimulation, and the existence of an extra trigeminal ganglion, which did not yield corneal reflexes on gill stimulation, was thought by Székely to be due, perhaps, to the differences in the two anatomical situations. Fibres from a transplanted vagal ganglion grow back into the brain stem and follow the normal descending course of the trigeminal tract, thus having ample opportunity to achieve connection with the secondary neurones of the vagal system; whereas trigeminal ganglionic neurones transplanted to the site of the vagus ganglion suffer from the disadvantage that there is no preformed tract for them to follow, to direct them to the region of the 6th nerve nucleus. These and other relevant experiments are described in an excellent review by Székely (1966).

There are too many undetermined factors in these experimental situations, involving the innervation of limbs and eyes transplanted to the head, to permit us to make any definitive statement about what is actually happening. It is not known, for instance, how the trigeminal and vagal innervation develops; less is known about the course of the outgrowth of these fibres than about the innervation of the normal limb. It would be interesting and relevant to know whether, at the time of metamorphosis, any new wave of sensory fibres grows out to the periphery. Also, whether the normally restricted reflexogenic fields represent fibre distributions or restrictions of functional activity brought about by some means within considerably greater peripheral fields of fibre distribution. So much interpretation of neurophysiological experiment involves the implicit assumption that where impulses are not to be found, there fibres do not go; in everyday human terms the analogy would be that, on a map of the countryside, only those roads with people on them actually exist. The doubtful nature of this proposition is evident; there may be gates on some roads. Indeed, the probable existence of such "gates" in a neurological situation is indicated by recent work of Wickelgren and Sterling (1969) on cortico-collicular interactions in visually deprived kittens. Even when we take into consideration the inadequacies of these transplant experiments, however, we may still say that the work just discussed, on eye and limb transplants to the head region, provides no compelling evidence in favour of the hypothesis of peripheral modulation in sensory fibres.

LOCAL SIGN IN AMPHIBIAN HEAD-WITHDRAWAL REFLEXES

Stimulation of different regions within the area of trigeminal innervation on the head of a newt evokes reflexes appropriate to the point stimulated. It is likely that the different reflex effects of such stimulations reflect the different peripheral distribution of trigeminal fibres to the face region; in which case the central functional connections of these fibres must, during development, become adjusted to match the cutaneous distributions of the fibres. This would be necessary to account for the local-sign properties of the various reflexes. An investigation of the mode of formation of these orderly relations between sensory cutaneous field and brain centres was carried out by Sperry and Miner (1949), using urodeles and anurans. They considered three possibilities: (1) The sensory-motor organization might be the outcome of some form of functional adaptation; i.e. the central associations might be adjusted through activity in accordance with the adaptiveness of their functional effects. (2) The central organization might be developed during growth as a result of an orderly spatiotemporal sequence of events during neurogenesis; an "accident of development" hypothesis, where the formation of specific connections would automatically follow the phased arrival of certain fibres at a certain place at a certain time. (3) Proper sensory-motor associations might be formed on the basis of selective physicochemical affinities between central and sensory neurones. These hypotheses were tested by a variety of experimental approaches involving sections and cross-unions of parts of the trigeminal nerve in post-larval urodeles and anuran tadpoles.

4

In the first place (Sperry and Miner, 1949) the central root of the nerve V was cut intracranially and then allowed to regenerate in efts and aquatic newts. After two months the roots had re-established central connections and the reflex responses of the animals to stimulation of the various parts of the trigeminal area were then normal. Similar results were obtained when the same operation was performed in late larval tadpoles of *Rana catesbiana* and testing was performed after metamorphosis. When adult frogs were used, the recovery of function (and the fibre regeneration) were too poor to provide useful analysis. Sperry and Miner argued that the disorganization which they found histologically to occur at the site of the scar ruled out the possibility that mechanical and timing factors were responsible for the orderly restoration of functional connections during regeneration. If the positional accuracy of the reflex reflects an orderly arrangement of central synapses, then these results indicate that the regenerating central fibres of the nerve V had succeeded in getting back to their proper sites of termination. The authors noted occasionally an interesting abnormal crossed response in the adult frogs following stimulation on the operated side and sometimes in the opposite direction. This observation, so far unexplained, may indicate that the restoration of fibre connections can occur to either side in the centres, as is the case in the anuran visual system (see chapter 4); the occurrence of the reciprocal crossed response cannot be accounted for in this way however and remains very perplexing.

In a variation on this experiment, the authors cross-united the peripheral end of the cut root of N V to the central end of the cut root of N VII, thus causing the fibres regenerating centrally from the trigeminal ganglion to enter the brain via root VII (Fig. 3.4a). The operation was performed in efts and aquatic newts and reflex responses from the affected trigeminal sensory area returned within 2–4 months. These reflexes were normal in character and histological examination confirmed that the trigeminal root had regenerated via the root of N VII. This experiment merely extends the result of the previous one by placing yet more obstacles in the way of the regenerating fibres. The results were essentially the same in both cases and neither experiment ruled out a functional adjustment to altered central connections during regeneration.

This point was specifically investigated in the other two experimental situations devised by Sperry and Miner (1949). In efts and newts the peripheral ophthalmic division of the trigeminal nerve to the dorsal surface of the snout was cut and its central end cross-united to the peripheral end of the cut mandibular division, which supplies the lower jaw and chin (Fig. 3.4b). The central root of the trigeminal was then cut, between 13 and 20 days after the nerve-cross operation. The central stump of the mandibular nerve was excised far centrally to impede its regeneration into its own stump. After regeneration of the ophthalmic nerve along the

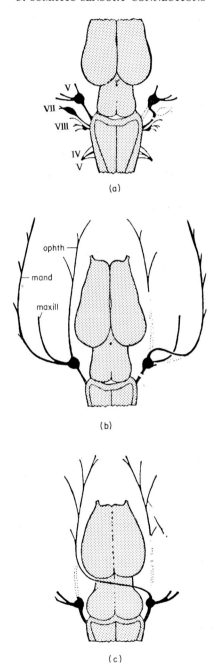

FIG. 3.4. Experiments involving cross-union of trigeminal fibres: (a) Cross-union of nerve roots V and VII; (b) Cross-union of ophthalmic and mandibular nerves with transection of root V; (c) Contralateral cross-union of ophthalmic nerves. From Figs 2, 4, 5, Sperry and Miner, 1949, *J. comp. Neurol.* **90**, 403.

peripheral path of the mandibular nerve, stimulation of the under side of the rostral third of the mandible between the chin and the eye led to depression of the head instead of the normal elevation. The animal thus responded by pressing its head more strongly against the stimulus rather than withdrawing from it. Some animals were kept for as long as 137 days after the initial signs of reflex recovery and these showed no evidence of correction of the reversed responses. The maladaptive nature of these inverted reflexes rules out any form of functional adaptation as the effective mechanism during regeneration. Similarly, when the central end of the ophthalmic division on the right side was cross-united to the distal end of the left ophthalmic nerve in anuran tadpoles prior to the emergence of the forelimbs (Fig. 3.4c), stimulation of the left ophthalmic region after metamorphosis resulted in wiping responses of the contralateral limb aimed at the right ophthalmic area. These laterally reversed reactions also remained unchanged for periods of up to 4½ months.

These experiments of Sperry and Miner show that, in this situation, cutaneous modulation of outgrowing sensory fibres did not occur. It could be argued, however, that the animals used were already too old at the time of operation for this process to take place; the specification of cutaneous sensory neurones might have already reached an irreversible state in postlarval *Triturus*. If the existence of localized reflexes from different parts of the head reflects the existence of distinct fibre pathways and central synaptic associations from these cutaneous regions, then the experiments indicate that the appropriate synaptic connections were restored during regeneration, to an extent at least sufficient to permit normal reflex activity.

THE GENESIS OF CUTANEOUS LOCAL-SIGN IN THE SENSORY INNERVATION OF LIMBS AND BODY

The local sign properties of cutaneous innervation have been further investigated by Miner (1956) using limb-specific, and by Miner (1956) and Jacobson and Baker (1968; 1969) using body-specific, reflexes in frogs. The problem in these experiments is the same as in the ones just described: how does the CNS locate the position of a peripheral stimulus? The interpretation to be put on the results of any such investigation will depend to a large extent on the ideas held by the interpreter on what mode of signalling is being used by the animal. On any hypothesis of local sign generation, the CNS has to be able to recognize the stimulated point on the body surface. If recognition depends on central analysis of which *fibres* are activated by the periphery, and the peripheral distribution of these fibres is then changed, local sign information should be wrongly interpreted and the animal make misdirected reflex responses to cutaneous stimulation. This is what actually happens in amphibia if the nerve or skin is misplaced sufficiently late in life, as was discussed previously (Sperry and Miner, 1949). Moreover, if a skin flap with much of its innervation intact is swung across the midline of a metamorphosing frog tadpole (Fig. 3.5), after metamorphosis the frog shows localizing reflexes that are misdirected across the midline when the flap is stimulated (Sperry, 1951a).

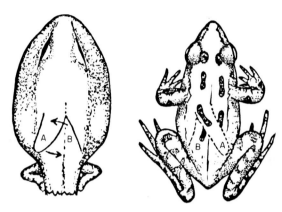

Fig. 3.5. Contralateral translocation of skin flaps. Skin translocation across the midline of the back in frog tadpoles results in contralateral misdirection of localizing reactions after metamorphosis. From Sperry, 1951a.

Similarly if, in a frog tadpole, the central ends of the cut dorsal roots supplying the leg are cross-united to the peripheral ends of the cut dorsal roots on the other side of the cord (Fig. 3.6), then, again after metamorphosis, cutaneous stimuli applied to the cross-innervated foot result in characteristic reflexes from the other leg, while the foot stimulated remains motionless (Sperry, 1951a).

Miner (1956) accepted the view, put forward by Sperry (1945a), that the local sign properties of cutaneous fibres are determined by their central relations and that for accurate localization, the peripheral terminations must match precisely the pattern of central synapses. ". . . the map of the body surface must be reflected in the central circuits" (Sperry, 1951a). Since earlier work (Sperry and Miner, 1949) had shown that the organization of cutaneous connections, considered in this fashion, was not brought about by any form of functional adjustment or mechanical guidance of sensory root fibres to their proper central destinations, it seemed reasonable to assume that the cutaneous sensory fibres supplying different areas of the skin differ chemically from one another and that appropriate central reflex patterning is achieved through selective termination of the root fibres, regulated by specific chemical affinities between the sensory fibres and the central neurones.

Several different ways of misinforming the nervous system were devised

(Miner, 1956): the normal sensory innervation of the developing hind-limbs was destroyed; a hindlimb bud was transplanted to the back, where it could become innervated by thoracic fibres; and pieces of skin were excised, rotated and reimplanted to investigate the effects of the altered central-peripheral relationships.

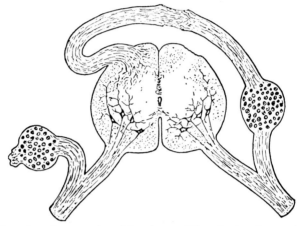

FIG. 3.6.   Contralateral cross-union of dorsal roots. When the dorsal roots of the hindlimb nerves are crossed in the manner indicated, the regenerating sensory root fibres establish functional relations with the spinal centres of the contralateral limb similar to those that they establish with the ipsilateral limb centres. This selective formation of the central reflex connections cannot be attributed to mechanical guidance or to functional adjust-ment. From Sperry, 1951a.

In tadpoles of *Rana clamitans* at late paddle and early foot stages, the sensory spinal ganglia 8, 9 and 10 were removed on the left side. This destroyed the innervation source that would normally supply the hindlimb. Later histological examination showed that the operations were successful, and Miner noted that the dorsal roots immediately above and below the excised ones were 2–4 times the size of the corresponding roots on the normal side. After metamorphosis the animals were tested by stimulation of the skin at various positions on the leg, to determine the nature of any reflex responses brought about by the abnormal innervation caused by the operation. Seven out of thirteen frogs showed good localizing reactions (wiping or kicking reactions specific for the point stimulated) correctly aimed and at approximately normal threshold. The other animals gave either poor responses of high threshold or no clear responses at all.

If these results may be accepted at their face value, they suggest some rather surprising conclusions. The normally located reflex responses were obtained from a leg which received its sensory innervation from non-limb segments, segments which normally have nothing to do with the limb. And in this situation it is not possible for us to urge selective reinnervation as an explanation of the normality of the results, since the cells of origin of the normal fibres had been removed. If fibre and synaptic connections were of importance in achieving these results, either the thoracic fibres that innervated the limb had become modulated by their terminal connections in the skin, or the new fibres formed in the adjacent roots may have come from newly differentiated ganglion cells which were able somehow to form the proper central as well as peripheral connections. Alternatively, the fibres were comparatively unimportant in obtaining the result and the pattern of impulses in the abnormal fibres, set up by leg receptors, led to appropriate leg reflexes.

The next type of operation (Miner, 1956) involved transplantation of the left hindlimb bud to the dorsal trunk region, to the right of the midline, in tadpoles of *Rana pipiens* at stages IV–VII of Taylor and Kollros. Again, in these experiments, the innervation of the transplanted limbs came from cord levels rostral to the hindlimb segments. And in these animals both motor and sensory innervations were from this abnormal source. These transplanted limbs, innervated by non-limb segments, showed no intrinsic movements and became muscularly atrophic and ankylosed, as is generally the case with transplants with such innervation (Székely and Szentágothai, 1962; Straznicky, 1963). However, the limbs were sensitive via the thoracic innervation and in 10 of the 47 cases tested after metamorphosis, stimulation of the transplant elicited responses in the normal ipsilateral hindlimb that were specific for the region stimulated. These responses, in a normal animal, are such that toe stimulation leads to a backward kick of the foot; heel stimulation leads to a sideward kick; stimulation of various points on the dorsal aspect of the leg leads to brushing responses of the foot aimed differentially at the point stimulated.

If this had been the only result achieved, we could make the same statements about these experiments as about the former ones: that is, the nature of the reflex response obtained suggests that either the thoracic fibres had become modulated to suit their abnormal hindlimb terminations, or the results indicated a "pattern" mechanism. However there were other results as well. In a larger number of cases (18), the responses were effected by the ipsilateral forelimb, not the hindlimb. In general, these forelimb responses appeared to be properly directed, according to the homologous point stimulated. In 19 animals a combination of forelimb and hindlimb responses was obtained. Histological analysis showed that in those animals in which forelimb responses were predominant, the transplant tended to be innervated by more rostral segments while those which showed the best hindlimb reactions were innervated by more caudal segments.

The thoracic innervation area in *Rana pipiens*, when mechanically stimulated, normally evokes wiping reactions of the limbs aimed at the site of stimulation. Stimulation of the rostral half of the belly elicits reflexes from the ipsilateral forelimb while the back and sides, as well as the caudal half of the belly, elicit reflexes from the hindlimbs (Jacobson and Baker, 1969). There is normally a small area of overlap of the forelimb and hindlimb reflexogenic areas on the trunk. Responses directed *at* the hindlimb are normally effected *by* the hindlimb. In the experimental situation being discussed, responses elicited from a *hindlimb* situated on the dorsum of the body are aimed appropriately at the right *part* of the (a?) limb and may be exerted by the forelimb.

These peculiar results are indeed very useful from our present point of view in that they emphasize the inadequacy of our conception of what we call "normal function." These forelimb motor responses evoked by stimulation of a heterotopic hindlimb are "normal" in the sense that they are apparently aimed at the appropriate part of the limb. But it is the wrong limb—in a double sense; not merely is it not the limb stimulated, it is not even the homologous normal limb. Such responses can only be called normal when considered from a very high plane of conceptual abstraction.

Certainly, as in the limb denervation experiments, we may not argue that selective reinnervation of the ectopic limb has occurred; innervation is by the "wrong" ganglion cells. Similarly we may not talk, in this case, of modulation proper; for this should lead to appropriately-directed responses of the ipsilateral *hindlimb*. There is no meaningful sense in which modulation could lead to appropriate responses of the *wrong* limb.

We are fortunate indeed that these interesting results of Miner do not stand alone. In essence, similar results have been obtained by Székely and Szentágothai (1962) in chicks. They observed that, irrespective of whether a wing or a leg had been grafted into the body wall, limb-specific reflexes on stimulation of the graft were always effected by the limb nearest the graft. Székely and Szentágothai suggest, as an alternative to the modulation concept, which appears to be inadequate in view of these results, that the CNS may have the ability to recognize incoming information on the basis of certain cues (for example spatiotemporal impulse patterns) independently of the channels through which they have been received, and to direct them to more or less adequate "addresses". The work of these authors is further of interest in that it shows that these phenomena are obtainable in vertebrates other than the amphibians.

The third and final variety of operation reported by Miner (1956) involved the excision, rotation and reimplantation of pieces of larval skin in *Rana pipiens* at stages X–XIII of Taylor and Kollros. A rectangular piece of skin 7–10 mm wide, on the left side, extending from the dorsal midline to the ventral midline, was cut free from the surrounding tissues, removed completely, rotated 180° and grafted onto the body again in this reversed position. The animals were then tested for localizing reactions to skin stimulation after metamorphosis (Fig. 3.7). Stimulation of the belly skin on the back evoked wiping responses directed at the belly while stimulation of the dorsal skin over the belly led to reflexes directed at the back. The reversed responses were most marked from the central parts of the dorsal and ventral skin of the graft and from near the edges of the graft the responses were frequently normal. A cut through the skin and extending completely round the graft reduced the normal responses and gave reversed responses from right up to the edge of the graft, whereas normal responses could be elicited from the other side of the cut. These results of Miner were interpreted by her as indicating that the pattern of central synapses formed by cutaneous fibres is determined in part by the nature of the skin with which the fibres connect in the periphery: that is, by modulation.

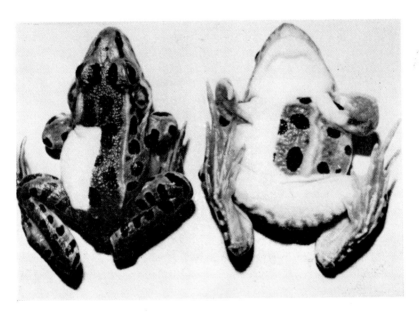

Fig. 3.7.   Frogs with back-to-belly rotated skin flaps. From Fig. 2, Miner, 1956, *J. comp. Neurol.* **105**, 166.

These various experiments by Miner demonstrate the difficulties in the way of any attempt to make a coherent hypothesis about what connections are actually formed and how these are achieved. However the situation gets really confusing in view of the more recent work of Jacobson and Baker (1968, 1969), who repeated and extended the observations on rotation of larval skin in *Rana pipiens*. These authors confirmed that reversed reflexes are obtained from back to belly skin reversals; they also showed, however, that reflex reversal was not obtained in the rostrocaudal axis of the body. Long, narrow strips of skin taken running rostrocaudally along the dorsum of the body did not, after rotation, result in anteroposterior reversal of wiping reflexes. The developmental stages over which back to belly reversal led to reversed reflexes were shown to extend from stage I

4*

to XV of Taylor and Kollros. Animals with skin rotations performed after stage XV gave normal localizing reactions.

Jacobson and Baker (1969) found that the reflex responses from rotated skin grafts were normal on first appearance. Seventeen out of 34 animals showed the full complement of normal and reversed reactions simultaneously from the first time of testing; the other 17 showed first the normal reactions which then gradually reversed over a period of 3–8 days. When the reversed responses did appear, they were initially confined to stimulation of a small region within the graft, on back and belly, and the reflexogenic area giving reversed responses then gradually spread, over the following weeks, until most of the graft gave reversed reactions (Fig. 3.8). The rate of spread of the area eliciting abnormal reactions was 0·5–1·0 mm per day. In animals with reversed responses, the skin graft was re-rotated to its original position, in adult life; four out of nine animals thereafter gave normally directed reflexes from the graft, while five gave reversed reactions; in these latter animals, stimulation of the back skin replaced on the animal's back gave responses misdirected towards the belly and vice-versa.

Jacobson and Baker (1969) also recorded electrophysiologically the extent of the multiunit receptive fields of various skin nerves from inside and outside the grafts. As in normal animals, receptive fields on the dorsal surface were circular or oval, with the long axis running rostrocaudally and were smaller than ventral fields. Fields on the ventral skin were oblong, with long axis running mediolaterally, and were larger than dorsal fields. In animals with back-to-belly reversed grafts, the receptive fields of single units were occasionally seen to cover an area within the graft including parts of both the normal reflexogenic region and the reversed reflexogenic region. In these back-to-belly grafts, multiunit receptive fields usually ended precisely at the graft margins, with the receptive field assuming the contours of the graft (Fig. 3.9). This was not so in rostrocaudally inverted grafts, where receptive fields frequently overlapped the edge of the graft.

INTERPRETATIONS OF THE SKIN-ROTATION EXPERIMENTS

Jacobson and Baker (1969) held that their results indicated that the central connections of the cutaneous fibres were altered by the process of cutaneous modulation of the fibres. There are however, certain observations that appear to conflict with this interpretation. Firstly, there is the fact that in many cases the first responses obtained from the grafts were normal, with the reversed responses only developing over a period of days (Fig. 3.10). As these authors have themselves shown, normal cutaneous receptive fields exist and may be mapped electrophysiologically as early as stage XIV. The rotations were performed not later than stage XV.

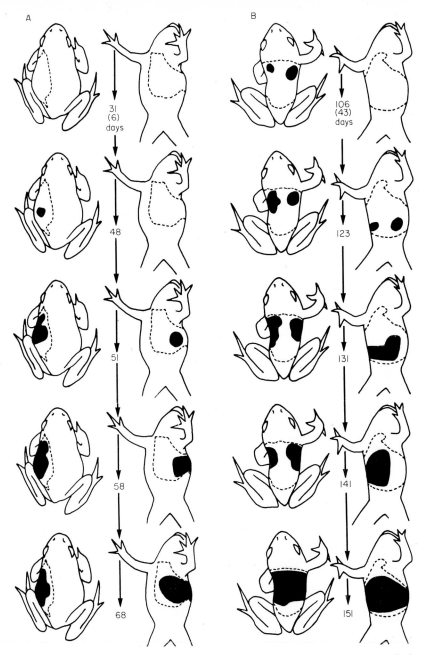

FIG. 3.8. Spread of area of skin graft from which misdirected reflexes were evoked at progressively later postoperative times. The graft is outlined by a dashed line. Misdirected reflexes were evoked from the black area, normal reflexes from the rest of the graft. A shows dorsal and ventral views of a frog with a back-to-belly inverted skin graft made at larval stage VI and tested 31 days postoperatively (6 days after metamorphosis) and 48, 51, 58 and 68 days postoperatively. B shows dorsal and ventral views of a frog with back-to-belly reversal of the skin of the trunk made at larval stage V and tested 106 days postoperatively (43 days after metamorphosis) and 123, 131, 141 and 151 days postoperatively. From Fig. 2, Jacobson and Baker, 1969, *J. comp. Neurol* **137**, 129.

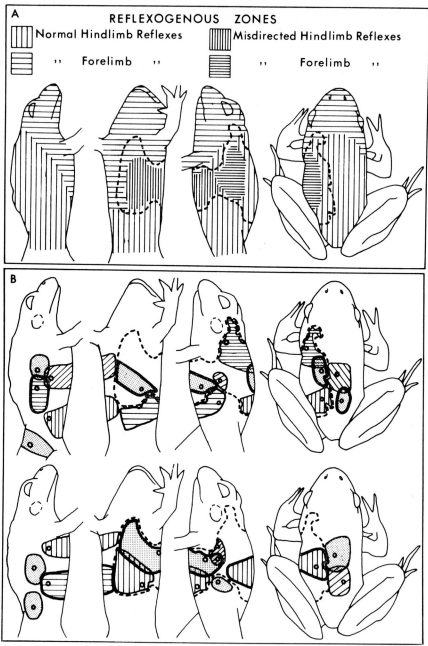

FIG. 3.9. A. Reflexogenous zones of the skin are shown in four views of the same frog with a back-to-belly inverted skin graft (dashed outlines) made at larval stage XIV. The reflexogenous zones remained as shown during frequent tests from 31 to 280 days after the grafting operation. Stimulation of the normal reflexogenous zones evoked a movement of a limb to the point of stimulation. Stimulation of the zones for misdirected reflexes resulted in movement of the fore- or hindlimb, as indicated, to the original position of the grafted skin: B. Receptive fields of cutaneous sensory nerves of the frog shown in fig. A, mapped 280 days after skin grafting. The area of skin within which a stimulus evoked action potentials in each cutaneous nerve is shown. Each cutaneous nerve enters the skin at the position shown by a small circle in its receptive field. From Fig. 4, Jacobson and Baker, 1969, *J. comp. Neurol.* **137**, 131

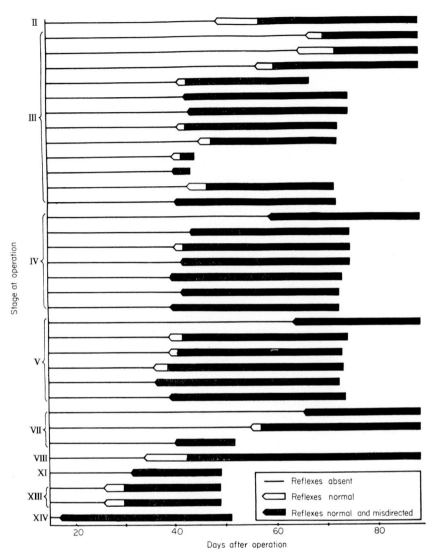

FIG. 3.10. Time of onset of normal and misdirected reflexes in 34 frogs with back-to-belly inverted skin grafts made at larval stages shown on the ordinate. Reflexes were tested daily during the postoperative period shown on the abscissa. From Fig. 1, Jacobson and Baker, 1969, *J. comp. Neurol.* **137**, 126.

The cutaneous fibres were therefore probably in effective contact with the rotated skin for a considerable period of time, several days at least, before the reflexes could be tested at metamorphosis. Yet the initial reflexes were *normal.* If the character of the skin modulates the fibres, why are the responses not reversed from the start? The operated animals developed wiping reflexes at the same time as normals, that is, about stage XXII.

why should modulation not take time

The next observation of Jacobson and Baker (1969) that is difficult to fit with the mechanism of modulation, is the result of re-rotation of the graft in the young adult, back to its original position. In this case, if modulation of the fibres innervating the skin has occurred as the authors suggest, we must assume that ventral fibres innervating dorsal skin have become modulated so as to produce reflex effects appropriate for the back, while dorsal fibres innervating ventral skin have become specified to give responses appropriate for the belly. The reversal of reflexes only occurs if the larval skin is rotated prior to stage XV; we must therefore assume that whatever "modulation" is going to occur has already taken place at this stage. If so, then rotation back of the skin after metamorphosis should result in reversed responses, since ventral fibres, although now reinnervating ventral skin, have previously been specified for dorsal skin and the process is irreversible. No matter what skin the fibres now innervate, they should give rise to dorsal reflexes. But the experimental result indicates differently: four out of nine animals gave normal reflexes after the skin had been rotated back to its original position. Jacobson and Baker (1969) argue that this indicates that the neuronal connections are still modifiable at this time. If this is so however, one would expect an initial skin rotation performed at these late stages to produce (even if only in half the cases) reversed reflexes; and this apparently does not occur. "Modulation" only takes place if the skin is rotated before stage XV. Unfortunately, this observation that, after re-rotation, half the animals gave reversed responses and half gave normal reflexes is equally difficult for any of the hypotheses yet mentioned. We may be reduced to admitting that the real trouble is that we do not yet know enough about the normal mode of working (and wiring) of these responses.

Some aspects of these experimental results could suggest that selective reinnervation of the graft eventually occurs, shortly after metamorphosis:

(1) The initial responses occurring at about stage XXII were normal and were replaced by the first sign of reversed responses within 3–8 days. This might suggest either that, at this time, some signal was sent back to the ganglion from the reversed skin, indicating that the connections were inappropriate; or that such a signal, given previously, now became effective with the onset of metamorphic climax. The delay between the onset of normal reflex responses and the first reversal could then perhaps be attributed to the time required for the message to give rise to the regeneration of new fibres from the ganglion cells and for these fibres to get to the periphery.

(2) A slow evolution of the abnormal reflexogenic area would be expected if reflex reversal was due to fibre regeneration in the periphery. The rate at which the reflexogenic area was found to spread, about 1 mm per day, could perhaps fit this idea.

(3) Since thoracic nerve fibres normally grow more or less dorsoventrally

in the frog, the presence of reflex reversal along the dorsoventral axis and its absence along the rostrocaudal axis could be attributable to an inability of the fibres to grow in the rostrocaudal direction, as Jacobson and Baker themselves suggest.

(4) The moulding of the receptive fields to the contours of the graft in dorsoventral inversions would agree with selective reinnervation by specified fibres. The observation that, in rostrocaudally inverted grafts the receptive fields *did* overlap the graft edges could be related to the fact that the mediolateral reversal which these grafts also showed was of minor extent; the grafts were long, narrow strips with the long axis lying rostro-caudally. In terms of a possibly graded distribution of "dorsoventral character" across the skin, the differences between the dorsal and ventral edges of the graft would be rather small and perhaps not sufficient to stop the fibres from growing across the border of the graft.

In these experiments, the factor immediately responsible for the changes involved in reflex reversal would appear to be some effect associated with metamorphosis. We may not suppose that initial, or even extended, contact of the nerves with their end organs has, by itself, resulted in any change in the central organization of the reflexes; in fact, since the reflexes, when first they can be evoked, are normal, it obviously has not. Thus if modulation in the classical sense has occurred it must be (at least) a two-stage phenomenon: the neurone has to be considered as modifiable by the specified skin up to stage XV and yet the modulation of the neurone must remain latent, not affecting the initial reflex pathways, which are put together on the basis of the anatomical *position* of the nerves. Later, with metamorphosis, we would have to consider that the second stage of the modulation process occurred; the reflex connections begin to change in consonance with the original nature of the skin, which had been impressed on the axon before stage XV. It would be interesting to know what would happen if the skin, rotated before stage XV, were re-rotated back to its original position just before metamorphosis, since on the modulation hypothesis the ventral nerve fibres would already carry an irreversible latent specificity for dorsal skin.

Whatever the mechanism of reflex reversal, it obviously depends on the orientation of the skin by stage XV. Thus some message from the skin to the nerve fibres is a necessary postulate no matter what mechanism is favoured. Furthermore, on the evidence available we must accept that the mechanism is a two-stage one and leaves us with no useful answer to the question of what led to the formation of the localized *correct* reflex con-nections that were found before the reflex reversal. It is worth emphasizing, however, that the results of these experiments are interpretable (or, rather, equally uninterpretable) *either* on the basis of modulation *or* on the basis of selective reinnervation; that is, if we ignore for the present the possibility of a "pattern" mechanism.

might it be that a necessary condition for modulation is functioning innervation

These experiments were designed to throw light on the mode of forma-tion of the central connections of certain cutaneous reflexes. This the results and their interpretation by Jacobson and Baker (1969) indeed do, but only at the expense of ignoring half the problem. If modulation leads to the reversal of the skin reflexes, such that these become appropriate to the original nature of the transplanted skin, what mechanism are we to invoke in regard to the (equally complex) formation of the *normal* reflex connections found before the reflexes reverse? It seems that to fill in this logical gap we would have to assume that modulation in fact occurs *twice*; once when the first outgrowth of cutaneous fibres reaches the end organ and again later, following skin reversal. We would in this case also need to assume that the original, early modulation was immediately effective, in contradistinction to the second modulation which remained latent until metamorphosis.

It seems, however, unlikely that the original innervation of the skin involves a process of modulation. We may first note that, in anurans, differences exist between some cells in the ganglia of the limb region and those elsewhere, even *before* the limb bud appears (Taylor, 1943; Hughes and Tschumi, 1958). These characteristics are thus independent of any influence exerted by the limbs and presumably indicate certain cellular differences inherent in the developing nervous system. Moreover, as Taylor (1943) points out, in the anurans all the major branches of the limb innervation are already recognizable when the limb bud is less than a millimetre long; and at these early stages the histogenesis of the muscles and limb skeleton has not progressed beyond local condensations of mesenchyme. The pattern of the limb nerves is thus shaped by factors other than the end organs of the limbs themselves. And since, in this situation, the pattern of innervation is fairly constant from one animal to another, the pattern of innervation cannot simply be due to random out-growth of fibres followed by peripheral modulation to achieve adequate central connections. A further argument pointing in the same direction may be obtained from the work of Straznicky and Székely (1967) who found that, when brachial cord segments were replaced by thoracic segments at progressively older embryonic stages of *Pleurodeles*, neuromuscular in-nervation failed in a proximo-distal sequence along the limb. With the later operations, the only muscles to be innervated were those of the distal forearm. This means that the innervating fibres had grown through the upper arm musculature to reach their destinations. There is no reason why this should happen if neuromuscular innervation were based on a more or less random outgrowth of fibres, followed by modulation by the muscles which happened to get in the way of the fibres These experiments therefore suggest that modulation plays no major part in the development of normal peripheral innervation.

It seems to be an a priori assumption that effects should be strictly decomposable and that implies the causes to be also decomposable. Why exclude the possibility of coalitions or non-decomposable interactions. Without evidence that such an exclusion is justified.

THE DEVELOPMENT OF THE DORSAL ROOT
SENSORY SYSTEM

The development of the lumbar spinal ganglia has been investigated in *Xenopus* by Prestige (1965), who studied cell turnover in the ganglia of tadpoles. He found that, as in the ventral horn, extensive cell degeneration takes place during development. This histogenetic degeneration occurs between stages 53 and 59, starting when the development of the hindlimb has reached the stage of toe differentiation. On the assumption that the degeneration of spinal ganglion cells, like that of ventral horn cells (Hughes, 1961), takes 3 hours, Prestige (1965) estimated the rate at which ganglion cells were degenerating. This turned out to be between 400 and 1000 per day (Fig. 3.11); with the effect that, between stages 53 and 59 some 20,000

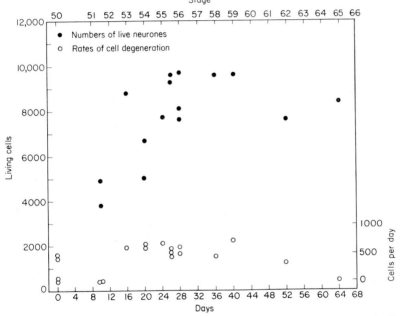

FIG. 3.11.   The number of live neurones and the rates of cell degeneration in the limb ganglia S 8+9+10 in *Xenopus*. From Prestige, 1965.

to 24,000 cells in the hindlimb ganglia degenerate. The number of cells in these ganglia at stage 52 was found to be 1500, whereas at stage 59 it was 9000–10,000. These figures indicate that, in *Xenopus* hindlimb dorsal root ganglia, two out of every three neurones degenerate during differentiation. The same applies to the trunk ganglia (Prestige, 1965), as shown in Fig. 3.12.

In another paper Prestige (1967a) investigated the control of cell numbers in the dorsal root ganglia during development. This he did by observing the effects, on the numbers of living and degenerating cells present, of amputation of the leg at various developmental stages. Before cell turnover starts, at stage 53, leg amputation merely results in a decreased rate of cell production (Hughes and Tschumi, 1958); during the period of cell turn-over amputation decreases both the rate of cell degeneration and the rate

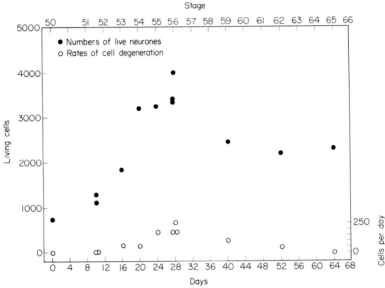

Fig. 3.12. The numbers of live neurones and rates of cell degeneration in the trunk ganglia S 5+6+7 in *Xenopus*. From Prestige, 1965.

of production of new cells. The overall effect of amputation after stage 53 is an irreversible fall in the number of ganglion cells (Prestige, 1967a). The rate at which ganglion cells degenerate during normal development must be maintained in some way by the limb itself, since amputation leads to a fall in the absolute rate of histogenetic degeneration; Hughes and Tschumi proposed (1958), and Prestige (1967a) supports this, that some factor produced by the developing limb effects this control over cell numbers.

The question next to be asked is, *why* do so many dorsal root ganglion cells degenerate during development? According to Prestige (1967a), the initial production of cells is independent of the limb; the limb itself controls the rate at which further cells are produced; the differentiated limb controls the number of cells, and the excess degenerate. In this connection it is relevant to ask what is meant by "excess". Does excess simply mean that too great a number of cells is produced in relation to an ideal number layed down in the plan of the limb? It seems more likely to me that, as previously argued for neuromuscular connections (Chapter 2), the degenerating cells in the ganglia represent mostly those that have failed to make adequate connections in the periphery. If some form of neural pathway selection exists, and this is less than completely effective, then it is reasonable to argue that the centre must produce more cells than will eventually be required, in order to allow for those fibres that make inadequate connections and have to be abandoned. Such a postulate of central-peripheral matching would also allow leg amputation to decrease the number of cell degenerations since the actual basis for fibre-periphery incompatibility would be removed by this operation. We would still require the developing limb to induce the formation of ganglion cells, so that after amputation the eventual cell numbers would decline; the cells that remain could then either be those that innervate proximal, non-amputated structures, or cells that have not yet produced an axon (Prestige, 1967a).

If this concept of the nature of the developing dorsal root system is valid, it would suggest that a fundamental characteristic of the growth of peripheral connections is a specific matching between the ganglion cells and their appropriate terminations. This would indicate that the individual sensory or motor neurones become specified during development such that, after specification, each neurone is labelled as belonging to, or due to innervate, a particular muscle or sensory region. Obviously, for such a system to work, the prespecified neurone would have to make contact with its appropriate region of termination. The hypothesis would suggest that this selective innervation is achieved in two mutually facilitatory ways: first, the entire neural periphery is considered to undergo, during development, a refined field-like differentiation such that each region (e.g. skin or muscle) is biochemically distinguishable from the others (Sperry, 1951); secondly, nerve fibres growing out to the periphery are aided in reaching their appropriate terminations by means of guidance by various factors, including preneural pathways, probably laid down under genetic control.

Evidence for the existence of such preneural pathways is available from the work of Piatt discussed in the previous chapter (Piatt, 1942; 1952; 1956), and the masterly analysis by Hamburger (1961) of the dual origin of the trigeminal nerve. This author managed to separate the placodal and neural crest components of the trigeminal ganglion by operative removal, early in embryonic life, of either the placode or the rostral medulla. He showed that the ophthalmic and maxillary rami are produced by the large cells of placodal origin and that in the formation of their peripheral distribution the trigeminal fibres showed in high degree the ability to form a normal pattern, no matter how the cells of origin had been displaced by the original operation. Steric features of the tissue being traversed were obviously helping to guide the fibres in the correct nerve pathways, but these preneural paths could not be entered indiscriminately; the small cells of neural crest origin never formed ophthalmic or maxillary nerves. And the specifications seemed to extend even to subgroups within the large placodal cells. Opposing the conclusion that preneural specific pathways exist for nerve fibres is the view of Narayanan (1964), who found essentially normal nerve patterns in variously transplanted chick limbs. Narayanan concedes the need for a certain specificity of fibres for their appropriate endings but concludes that the formation of nerve primary pathways is essentially by random outgrowth; however Narayanan did not identify the cells of origin of the nerves and in any case the limbs were all innervated in great part by the normal limb segments. His observations thus appear to support the conclusions of Hamburger.

Also relevant to the question of the control of limb innervation are the observations of Weiss and Litwiller (1937) who found that the mass:innervation ratio was approximately constant for all levels of a regenerating limb at one stage of regeneration. This suggested to them that the tissues of the limb exert a control over the admission of new fibres, establishing a "saturation point" for the number of possible terminations in a given volume of tissue. A similar conclusion, qualitatively, was reached by Cajal (1929, p. 103). It would be of interest to know if this control which the target organ exerts over the number of incoming fibres extends to the *nature* of the fibres; for instance, sensory versus muscular.

SELECTIVE INNERVATION AS THE BASIC MECHANISM IN PERIPHERAL INNERVATION AND REINNERVATION IN LOWER VERTEBRATES

A useful hypothesis accounts for the observations from which it was derived and predicts others accurately. To the extent that the predictions accord with reality, the hypothesis gains support. But a hypothesis can never be *proved*, it merely becomes more probable when it is adequately supported; the only logically certain thing one can do with a hypothesis is to prove it wrong in that it does not accord with the deductions made from it. A hypothesis is useful to the extent that it exposes itself to the possibility of refutation. Unfortunately the hypothesis of modulation is, in practice, remarkably difficult to disprove. This is largely because those animals that display the phenomena that are classed as modulation, have also a very great ability to sprout collateral nerve fibres on the slightest provocation.

The idea of modulation was based on the study of neuromuscular connectivity; from the analysis in the previous chapter I hope it will be clear that much of the original interpretation of the evidence from this field is now suspect in view of the recent work of Mark (1965) and Sperry and Arora (1965). It appears that when a critical experiment (in this case, properly controlled nerve crossing) can be done, the result is to exclude modulation. Similarly, the first demonstration of modulation on the somatic sensory side of the nervous system came from the work of Weiss (1942) on the lid-closure reflex; and in this situation also the attribution of the result to modulation is most probably invalid, as I argued earlier (Székely, 1959b). The only outstanding experimental situation where modulation may yet be invoked is that of the skin innervation experiments of Miner (1956) and Jacobson and Baker (1969). Some criticism of the attempt to explain these results in terms of modulation has already been made; the crucial experiment in this situation has yet to be done however; this would involve the controlled misregeneration of dorsal cutaneous nerves into ventral skin and vice-versa. And even this experiment is likely to turn out less crucial than one would hope, as will be shown later. On previous evidence from an analogous neuromuscular situation, however, we might expect (Mark, 1965; Sperry and Arora, 1965) the result of such an experiment to tell against the hypothesis of modulation.

In view of the unsatisfactory state of modulation as a neural mechanism it is worth while putting forward the arguments for an alternative which could account for the known facts of peripheral neurogenesis and regeneration, or most of them. The suggested mechanism is based on neuronal specificity with selective innervation and reinnervation of target organs. In this respect it is essentially similar to the ideas of Sperry before the experiments of Miner in 1956.

(1) The initial innervation of the skin is effected by pioneering fibres, some of which find the right pathway and the right end organ. Those that do not, atrophy. The finding, by Prestige (1965; 1967a), that two out of every three dorsal root ganglion cells degenerate during development in *Xenopus* could well fit with this mechanism. Some guidance appears to be offered to the initially outgrowing fibres, and those that follow, by a system of preneural pathways which presumably carry directional information for specific fibre groups. It is hard to avoid this conclusion in view of the work of Piatt (1942; 1952; 1956) and Hamburger (1961). The fact that fibres tend to produce typical distribution patterns does not, of course, tell us whether this is because they are being selectively guided by some biochemical characteristics of the substrate or are merely receiving "contact guidance" in the sense of Weiss (1955). It seems highly unlikely, however, that mere guidance by the steric configuration of tissue planes, etc., could account for the degree of pathway selectivity observed in Hamburger's (1961) experiments on the trigeminal fibres; or, for that matter, for the cases described by Piatt (1942) where a nerve penetrated a muscle, or mass of cartilage, to reach its normal area of distribution. The likelihood that contact guidance does play a major part in many cases is indicated by further observations of Piatt (1952), who showed that when older, previously innervated forelimbs were transplanted to the site of the hindlimb in *Amblystoma*, they developed a nearly normal nerve pattern; whereas aneurogenic forelimb transplants to the same site did not. Thus if previous nerve pathways exist, they may be followed by regenerating fibres. The essence of Hamburger's (1961) observations, and Piatt's (1942) orthotopic

aneurogenic transplants, however, is that a normal nerve pattern develops when the operation is performed *before* there are any previously innervated pathways for the fibres to follow. The requirement that the particular nerve fibres innervating a limb should be properly matched to the limb tissues for a normal innervation to develop, was emphasized by Piatt (1957a) in experiments where he left the limbs alone and merely altered their innervation by transplanting segments of the cord anlage. Piatt found that the normal (i.e. brachial) segments were the only ones to give an entirely normal pattern in the forelimbs; from which he concluded that the uniform presence of abnormalities in limbs with a foreign nerve supply must be, at least in part, the result of differences in the response of the nerve fibres themselves. The possible role of differences in the timing of innervation by the various spinal segments was discussed in a further paper (Piatt, 1957b) and this point requires further investigation.

(2) On arrival at the periphery, aided by the mechanisms just discussed, a proportion of the fibres find the "right" target and make effective and permanent contact. Those that do not may degenerate. At this point it is conceivable that information is transmitted back to the centre indicating that appropriate contact has been made; thereafter further fibres of the same type follow the paths of the correctly-lodged fibres. In this fashion a "normal" distribution is set up.

(3) The basis for normal central interconnections may be laid down at this time (Cajal, 1952). Barron (1943; 1946) found that the development of dendrites tended to occur at about the time the axon reached its target organ. It may be that the general pattern of dendritic-axonic spatial relationships are formed at this time, but the formation of effective synapses waits for the metamorphic stimuli. The relevance of metamorphosis in this context follows from the fact that skin innervation exists, and is functional (in that it gives rise to action potentials in cutaneous nerves on peripheral stimulation) some considerable time before metamorphosis (Jacobson and Baker, 1969); also, the limb motor apparatus is fairly well developed before metamorphosis; yet the specific cutaneous reflexes only appear *at* metamorphosis.

The significance of metamorphosis for the maturation of certain neural connections is also well demonstrated in the case of the blink reflex. Here again, while both motor and sensory sides of the arc are present some time previously, the reflex only appears at or near metamorphosis. This suggests that it is the central connections that are induced to appear, or become functional, at this time. Another case in which metamorphosis appears to play a role in the formation of intracentral connections is the development of the anuran ipsilateral visual projection, to be discussed in another chapter.

The reflex changes and new neural connections that presumably develop at metamorphosis are part of the structural alterations that fit the animal for its new post-metamorphic mode of life. At metamorphosis the gross structure of the anuran body changes dramatically; it could almost be said that at this time the frog develops a body for the first time, since the tadpole consists largely of head and tail. Obviously, such major changes in external morphology must involve comparably drastic changes in the relationship between the nervous system and the periphery.

The aquatic tadpole does not show localized reflexes on stimulation of the skin innervated by thoracic nerves. It is possible to argue that cutaneous local sign only becomes of major importance to the animal when it undergoes metamorphosis and changes its mode of life. Indeed, cutaneous localization can have no meaning for the animal until the development of the appropriate central connections at metamorphosis. At this time we know that new functional central connections appear and we may expect that, in view of the major changes in body configuration, the animal makes final adjustments to the relationship between centre and periphery. It would be reasonable to expect that, at metamorphosis, a considerable growth of new sensory fibres take place to innervate the new areas of skin become available.

(4) It is now relevant for us to consider the nature of cutaneous innervation at the time of metamorphosis. In urodeles the spinal ganglia are capable of responding to a peripheral overload by producing new ganglion cells up to the time of metamorphosis (Carpenter, 1932). And in *Xenopus* there is a continued turnover of dorsal root ganglion cells during larval development up to stage 59, which is near metamorphic climax (Prestige, 1965). Cell turnover in the ganglia ceases after metamorphosis, since no degenerating cells are then visible and cell numbers are constant. However, amputation of the leg even 1–2 months after metamorphosis in these animals can initiate cell turnover in the ganglia again for a brief period (Prestige, 1967a). Thus in *Xenopus*, in the immediately post-metamorphic stages, the ganglia are still capable of producing new cells.

In *Xenopus* and in *Eleutherodactylus* (Hughes, 1968) the number of cells in the *ventral* horn at metamorphosis is about equal to the number of fibres in the ventral root; thus it may be assumed that there are at this time no more ventral horn cells that have not yet produced an axon. The situation in the dorsal root ganglia however, is quite different. Here (Fig. 3.13) the proportion of cells which have sent fibres into the central processes of the lumbar ganglia is still only one in four in the early juvenile as determined by light microscopy. If a similar situation exists in the thoracic ganglia, and if *Xenopus* and *Eleutherodactylus* are in this respect comparable to *Rana pipiens*, then at the time that Jacobson and Baker (1969) report reflex reversal following skin rotation, three out of four dorsal root ganglion cells may still be undifferentiated and without connections.

(5) When tadpole skin is rotated, misregeneration occurs into the rotated skin. The cut fibres regenerate from close to their injured ends, into the

(now inappropriate) skin of the transplant. We may perhaps surmise that the animal is not particularly concerned about this misregeneration during larval life; and in any case it has no central connections functional yet which would allow it to manifest reflexes of any sort. We must accept, however, that the neurones are "informed" of the change in peripheral distribution if the operation is performed before stage XV of larval life.

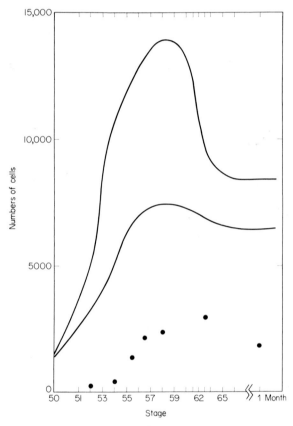

FIG. 3.13. Total numbers of cells in lumbar ganglia of *Xenopus laevis* during development (limits shown by continuous curves), together with light-microscopic counts of the corresponding numbers of fibres in lumbar dorsal roots to same scale. Ordinate: stages of development. From Prestige, 1966.

(6) At metamorphosis several things happen:

(*a*) New functional connections develop within the nervous system. In an animal with rotated skin, these first connections are normal, as foreshadowed by the original innervation pattern. The metamorphic stimulus at this stage would appear to induce the formation or maturation of synapses on endings that are already in close proximity to cells and dendrites.

(*b*) The metamorphic stimulus leads the nervous system to produce new neurones to innervate the newly available areas of skin. New fibres grow out from newly differentiating dorsal root ganglion cells.

(*c*) In animals with rotated skin these connections with the periphery are found to be inadequate. The fibres present when the skin was rotated prior to stage XV, remember the inadequacy of their terminal connections and inform the centre of the existence and nature of the abnormality. These fibres then gradually degenerate and are replaced by new fibres, either grown from existing ganglion cells or from newly differentiated ganglion cells. The newly-formed central-peripheral connections then result in the development of reversed reflexes in accordance with the nature of the reversed skin.

In the experiments of Jacobson and Baker (1969) the reversal of reflexes only occurred in the larval skin that had been rotated prior to stage XV; yet the first reflexes to develop were normal and were only replaced by reversed reflexes later. We must argue, therefore, that the factor immediately responsible for the changes in response was *not* the skin contact; it was rather some effect associated with metamorphosis. It is metamorphosis that is the common factor in these experimental results and those on the blink reflex (Weiss, 1942; Székely, 1959b). In each case the analytical reflexes only appear at metamorphosis, indicating the occurrence of major changes in the nervous system at this time. It is, indeed, possible to argue that skin contact by the nerve fibres at about stage XV or earlier leads to a latent change in the neurone soma, which is then triggered by some metamorphic stimulus to produce the required synaptic alterations; it is equally possible to argue that the metamorphic stimulus, which is required in either case, leads to an increase of cutaneous nerve fibres in accord with the extended areas of body surface.

Since some form of information transfer from the inappropriate skin to the nerve is required on either interpretation, the discussion reduces to whether the neural alteration induced by the skin leads eventually to alteration in preformed central synaptic connections, or to the outgrowth of new, appropriate peripheral fibres. It is of interest to attempt to decide whether one or the other, or both, of these mechanisms actually exist. Further information about this could be obtained by looking for degenerating fibres in the cutaneous nerves at the time the reflex reversal was occurring; and also by estimations of the numbers of fibres (and ganglion cells) for each of the affected dorsal roots in the period of development extending from immediately premetamorphosis to several months afterwards.

A developmental scheme involving selective innervation could also perhaps enable us to account, at least partially, for the differences between the sensory and motor results of ectopic limb transplantations. When limbs are transplanted into the thoracic region in urodeles (Detwiler, 1936), frogs (Miner, 1956), or chicks (Székely and Szentágothai, 1962; Straznicky, 1963) they do not show motor function and the muscles eventually degenerate. On the other hand, in frogs and chicks, their sensory innervation (by thoracic roots) *is* functional and even shows some signs of "proper" local sign characteristics. The failure of the motor innervation could then be related to the absence of any cellular response showing increase in ventral horn numbers associated with such a peripheral overload. The existing motor fibres which initially innervate the limb are inappropriate; it is noteworthy that they do *not* show modulation which would lead to coordinated motor function and proper maintenance of limb muscles. On the other hand, on the sensory side, the dorsal root ganglia can probably respond to overload by producing new cells up to metamorphosis in urodeles; and the evidence from *Xenopus* suggests that there may be a pool of unconnected dorsal root ganglion cells in anura at this time. If these cells were induced to differentiate in the appropriate direction by information coming from degenerating *inappropriate* fibres, this could be related to the occurrence of "limb specific" sensory behaviour in such ectopically transplanted limbs. In this context it is worth noting that the first reflexes elicited by stimulation of an ectopically-sited chick limb (Székely and Szentágothai, 1962) were non-specific, i.e. general escape movements indicative of pain; the limb-specific responses in these animals following stimulation of the transplanted limb only emerged gradually, within the first three days, and more complex behavioural responses even later.

Most of the evidence that has been adduced in favour of modulation is indirect, by inference from the functional results of reflex testing. It becomes increasingly obvious that this form of evidence is highly unreliable. Indeed we may now say that it is not possible, in most cases, to make meaningful statements about specific neural connections, solely on the basis of behavioural observations. There are always too many alternative hypotheses that could account for the observations. The only methods available to us which may indicate, without ambiguity, the nature of nerve connections, are those of experimental morphology: anatomical and electrophysiological analysis; and even with these methods, positive results only are of real value.

The electrophysiological and anatomical evidence for modulation is slender and unconvincing. The work of Eccles and his collaborators has already been discussed in the previous chapter; in the sphere of neuromuscular innervation their results suggest that *some* changes may occur in synaptic connectivity after central-peripheral alterations in kittens, but the direction of the changes was not particularly illuminating from our present point of view. Unfortunately no other useful electrophysiological investigations of modulation have yet been undertaken. What one would like to see would be an Eccles-type experiment performed on an animal in which "modulation" was known to occur: that is, on newt, frog or fish.

More direct modes of investigation of modulation, using classical anatomical techniques, are also completely lacking. [This undoubtedly reflects partly the inherent difficulty of devising an unambiguous experiment. The need would be to demonstrate that a particular fibre, or fibres, changed its function following peripheral contact.] The difficulty lies in being sure that the fibre investigated after the modulation has occurred is the same fibre as that investigated before. One experimental approach which seems promising and could perhaps be applied to the investigation of modulation, is that used by Illis (1964), who examined the synaptic boutons on motoneurones in the cord of the cat, following experimental dorsal root section. He found that, within 24 hours of root section, there is a widespread disorganization of synaptic terminals on the motoneurone surface; the normal mosaic appearance is lost, which must imply the disorganization, at least temporarily, of terminals belonging to fibres other than those cut. Some 15 days later only those terminals presumably belonging to the cut fibres were still obviously degenerated; the other terminals had become reorganized, leading to a partial restoration of the normal mosaic appearance.

This result is of great interest in that it indicates a widespread effect of root section, one not confined to the injured fibres. Unfortunately the time scale of the effects, as reported, is of the wrong order to be immediately relevant to the problem of modulation. Modulation following section and regeneration of a peripheral nerve could only occur after contact with the end organ had been re-established, which would undoubtedly take more than 24 hours. Furthermore the synaptic results of section of a peripheral nerve have not yet been examined; they may differ considerably from those following section of the dorsal root. Another observation that may be relevant to the question of spinal cord plasticity is that of Liu and Chambers (1958) who severed unilaterally an extensive series of dorsal roots in a mammal, leaving one in the middle intact. Then, more than 200 days later, when all Nauta-Gygax stainable material had disappeared, they cut the intact root on the normal side. They found, using Nauta staining, that the distribution of degeneration was much wider on the previously operated side than on the other; this they interpreted as evidence that the previous section of adjacent fibres had led to the sprouting of collaterals in the remaining intact root. Such results can be no more than pointers for future work; they do suggest, however, that the conditions for the modification of synaptic connections may exist in the adult mammalian spinal cord and, according to recent work by Raisman (1969), in the mammalian brain. Further experimentation along these lines is highly desirable and much needed.

SUMMARY AND CONCLUSIONS

Doubt has been cast on the existence of modulation as the mechanism accounting for the development of normal sensorimotor coordination in embryogenesis and in neural regeneration in the lower vertebrates. In particular, in the only experiment on cutaneous innervation which can be put forward as a serious candidate for this mechanism, that is, the skin-rotation experiments of Miner (1956) and Jacobson and Baker (1969), the reversal effect observed involved, essentially a two-choice situation; either the animal wiped at his back or at his front. Indeed, this particular mechanism of testing, carried to the limits of its accuracy, could probably subdivide the dorsoventral strip of skin into no more than three or four areas. The actual number of functionally-differentiable positions on such a skin strip is unknown; the experimental evidence, however, reveals only a simple back-belly choice. No evidence exists to suggest that the system can provide any further resolution than this.

(1) When the hypothesis of modulation is submitted to a critical test, the results of experiment do not support it (Székely, 1959b; Mark, 1965; Sperry and Arora, 1965).

(2) Certain observations on development of neuromuscular connections do not support, and indeed contraindicate, modulation (Straznicky and Székely, 1967).

(3) The reversed responses that may follow skin rotation in frogs (Jacobson and Baker, 1969) only develop some time after initially *normal* responses have appeared. There is likewise a time-lag of some days before limb-specific reflexes appear from ectopically transplanted chick limbs. The delays in these cases could suggest a mechanism involving growth of fibres. The modulation hypothesis indicates the growth to be central; it could equally well be peripheral.

Extensive consideration of the material presented in this and the previous chapter, leads me to think that the most obvious deficiency in all these studies is the almost complete lack of adequate anatomical knowledge of the systems being dealt with. The experimental analyses I have discussed have, many of them, been of very considerable ingenuity; the concepts being argued are of high sophistication; yet the almost universal ability of the experimenters to ignore the possible existence of unknown premises, and to argue as if they were dealing with a logically closed system, suggests a lack of respect for the complexities of the nervous system that is rather surprising.

I suggest that the modulation hypothesis is unconvincing and difficult to test; the major alternative mechanism, involving selective innervation, would have the merit that it could be refuted more easily—by adequate search for degenerating fibres in "modulating" nerves. There can be no doubt, however, that new central nerve connections do develop at metamorphosis. This occurs in the cutaneous innervation system, in the maturation of the blink-reflex mechanism and also in the development of the anuran ipsilateral visual projection (see Chapter 5). Our discussion is thus mainly about what controls the establishment of these new central connections, and whether new peripheral connections are important also. While the weight of my arguments has been against the existence of the phenomenon of modulation, yet I would point out that most of the evidence so far presented, *even that arguing against modulation*, is behavioural. And the criticisms I have already made of this form of evidence will apply also to my own arguments. Furthermore, modulation, as a concept, is so neat and could be so useful biologically that we could argue, as did Voltaire on a different topic, though one that also raises passions, that if modulation did not exist it would be necessary to invent it.

4. RETINOTECTAL CONNECTIONS

In considering the specificity with which nerve fibres form and reform connections on the sensory side of the nervous system we have so far been concerned mainly with cutaneous sensibility and in particular localization. Comparable questions can however be asked of the visual system, where the geometrical arrangement of the sensory surface is more favourable for our purposes. The study of cutaneous localization mechanisms is bedevilled by the irregular geometry of the body surface; and while the cutaneous sensory surface is topologically equivalent to that of the retina, the existence of continuously and irregularly varying curvatures on the body surface, together with the projections of the limbs, make this sensory surface difficult to investigate. Further, the segmental nature of cutaneous innervation introduces complexity into the analysis of the neural input: output relationships. The retina, on the other hand, represents, for all practical purposes, a simple, regular, two-dimensional sheet of sensory epithelium on which the visual world is optically projected.

The vertebrate retina sends its optic nerve fibres to various neural centres, in particular the lateral geniculate nucleus and the optic tectum or superior colliculus. In lower vertebrates such as amphibians, fishes and birds the main visual projection area within the brain is the optic tectum, which presents a receiving surface over which the incoming fibres are distributed. Anatomical and histological studies have revealed, in all vertebrates so far studied, that there is a continuous mapping of the retinal surface on to the tectal surface by means of the optic nerve fibres. Thus one place (point; region; district) on the retinal surface projects fibres to one corresponding place (point; region; district) on the tectal surface; and a different retinal locus to another, corresponding, tectal locus. The comparative simplicity of this mapping enables the experimenter to investigate, in a fairly straightforward and meaningful way, the mode of formation and reformation of the retinotectal connections.

The general comments I have made, in previous chapters, on the difficulties inherent in the attempt to analyse form from the study of function will apply also to the visual system. Thus by far the greatest number of experiments on visual connections rely on alterations in visuomotor behaviour, induced by crude surgical alterations in the visual pathway; from these changes in visual behaviour the experimenter attempts to determine the intimate alterations in connectivity that may have resulted from his operative interference. Since (as will emerge from the discussion as we go on) we do not know the basic rules by which the visual system processes positional information, obviously the premises for discussion are inadequately established and such attempts are likely to be less than completely successful.

The most widely-held view on the mechanism of selective connection between nerve fibres is, at the present time, Sperry's hypothesis of neuronal specificity. This states that different neurones develop, during embryonic differentiation, different (and in certain cases, matching) cytochemical specificities; and that those neurones with like or matching specificities become linked up. This is the hypothesis with which I shall be most concerned in the present chapter; and since the hypothesis derived mainly from observations on the growth and regrowth of fibre connections in the amphibian visual system, it will be useful to consider the experimental evidence in roughly chronological order. The order of discussion may seem somewhat odd, in that I deal with various experiments on adult animals before considering the development of the system. This back-to-front method is necessary because the adult experiments indicate what has to be explained, and the experiments on developing systems are the most complex.

HISTORICAL: STUDIES ON THE RESTORATION OF THE VISUAL PROJECTION

The present era in the study of regeneration of fibre connections within the CNS may be considered to start with the work of Matthey in 1925. A good discussion of earlier experiments in this field is given in a later paper by the same author (Matthey, 1927). Matthey reported (1925) the results of observations on two animals (*Triturus cristatus*), in one of which he resected both optic nerves and in the other he resected a short length of one nerve and cut the other. Both animals showed incontrovertible evidence of restoration of vision when tested four and a half months after operation. Surprisingly, anatomical investigation of the animals revealed that the regenerated optic nerves had each entered the brain on its own side, with no sign of restoration of the optic chiasma. In view of the later experiments of Sperry (1945b) one would have expected Matthey's animals to show lateral inversion of their visuomotor prey-catching reflexes; presumably the testing situation used by Matthey was not sufficiently refined to allow this point to be cleared up. A similar recovery of visual function was demonstrated when an eye was homografted into another animal (Matthey, 1926).

These observations were repeated and extended by Stone and his collaborators (Stone, 1930; Stone, Ussher and Beers, 1937; Stone and

Zaur, 1940), who showed that *normal* visually controlled behaviour occurred after optic nerve regeneration; but no major advance occurred in the field until 1943, when Sperry observed the results of optic nerve regeneration in urodeles and thought about what this visual recovery must mean (Sperry, 1943b). Normal newts can accurately identify the position of a lure in the visual field and this indicates that excitation of one part of the retinal surface is distinguishable by the centres from excitation of other parts. Simple rotation of a newt eye by 180° results in inverted visual behaviour (Sperry, 1943a) and this back-to-front and upside-down response to visual stimulation persists indefinitely without any sign of functional modification. The restoration of normal visually-controlled behaviour after regeneration of the optic nerve indicates that the unique localization properties of each part of the retina, the local sign properties, are appropriately restored when the eye reconnects with the brain. Functionally each part of the retina regains its behavioural effect.

Since the publication of Sperry's formulation of the problem (Sperry, 1943b; 1944) discussion has continued, and still continues, on the implications of these observations. Restoration of normal visual behaviour could mean (1) that the regenerating optic nerve fibres each get back to their proper destinations, thus restoring the *status quo ante* and so automatically allowing a normal visual function; or (2) that the regenerating fibres grow back randomly to the tectum, all mixed up (as they certainly are at the site of the nerve lesion) and thereafter terminate at the "wrong" sites in the tectum. In this case, a readjustment of central connections in the tectum could enable proper motor results to follow excitation of individual retinal regions; another possibility (with which we will now be familiar, after our discussion of cutaneous sensibility) is (3) that it is immaterial *where* the retinal fibres end up—conceivably retinal positional information is transmitted in the form of an impulse code which can be decoded at the tectal end and the individual messages then passed on to the appropriate motor mechanisms.

The first two of these three mechanisms imply that connections are important in determining behaviour; the third implies that they are not. The fact that it is possible to propose such conflicting hypotheses is an indication of the extent of our lack of knowledge about how the nervous system actually functions; and it again adds point to my earlier comments that argument from function to form is unwise.

Sperry (1943b; 1944) considered all three of these mechanisms; selective reconnection of the optic nerve fibres, random regeneration with subsequent central "adjustment" and impulse-pattern specificity. Regeneration of the optic nerve in urodeles was followed by restoration of good visual localization and of perception of direction of movement of a visual stimulus. Since rotation of the eye by 180° and section and regeneration of the nerve resulted in reversed visual responses, obviously functional adaptation of any sort was not influential in determining the character of the recovered visual perception. After recovery of vision the animals' responses were persistently incorrect and maladaptive. These animals, relying on the operated eye, are worse off than totally blind animals; a blind animal may come across prey by accident, whereas an animal with reversed vision sees the prey and consistently jumps away from it.

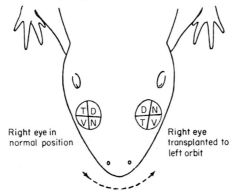

Right eye in normal position

Right eye transplanted to left orbit

Right-left transplant with inversion of naso-temporal axis

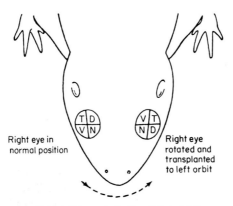

Right eye in normal position

Right eye rotated and transplanted to left orbit

Right-left transplant with rotation of eye and thus inversion of dorso-ventral axis

Fig. 4.1.   Transplantation of right eye to left orbit. The right eye is divided into quadrants in order to show the inversion of the axes. D, dorsal; V, ventral; T, temporal; N, nasal. From Gaze, 1960.

Rotation of the eye by 180° around the optic axis results in inversion of both nasotemporal and dorsoventral axes of the retina. It is possible to transplant an adult urodele eye from one orbit to the other (Stone, 1944; Sperry, 1945b) and obtain visual recovery. The same may be done in the frog tadpole (Sperry, 1945b). If the eye is transplanted so, with dorso-dorsal orientation, only the nasotemporal axis is reversed (Fig. 4.1); in this case the animals later show visual behaviour that is correctly directed dorsoventrally but reversed in the nasotemporal field axis. If the eye is transplanted to the other orbit and also rotated 180° (Fig. 4.1) the result is an eye which is inverted in the dorsoventral axis and normally oriented

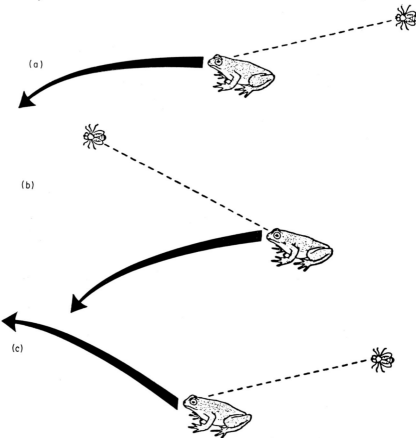

Fig. 4.2.   Sample types of error in spatial localization of small objects following rotation and inversion of the eye. (a): with eye rotated 180°, frog strikes at a point in the visual field diametrically opposite that at which the lure is actually located. (b): after dorsoventral inversion of the eye, frog strikes correctly with reference to the nasotemporal dimensions of the visual field, but inversely with reference to the dorsoventral dimensions. (c): after nasotemporal inversion of the eye, frog strikes correctly with reference to the dorsoventral dimensions of the visual field, but inversely with reference to the nasotemporal dimensions. From Sperry, 1951a.

in the nasotemporal axis; such an animal later shows visual behaviour reversed in the dorsoventral axis and correct in the nasotemporal axis (Fig. 4.2).

In amphibia the retinotectal connection is completely crossed and each eye sends tectal fibres only to the contralateral tectum (Wlassak, 1893; Cajal, 1898; Knapp *et al.*, 1965; Scalia *et al.*, 1968). This situation provided

Sperry with yet a further opportunity to interfere in an elegant fashion with the normal spatial relationships between eye and brain. In various adult anurans he uncrossed the optic chiasma (Sperry, 1945b) and allowed each optic nerve to regenerate back to its ipsilateral tectum. The functional result was that the animals erroneously localized a visual stimulus at a corresponding position on the opposite side of the midsagittal plane. Only if the stimulus was actually in the midsagittal plane was it localized correctly (Fig. 4.3). This erroneous localization following uncrossing the

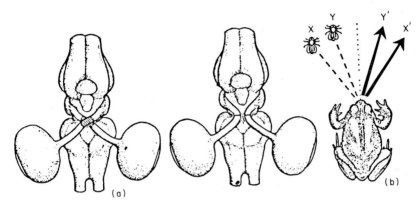

Fig. 4.3. Contralateral transfer of retinal projection on the brain. (a): by excising the optic chiasma and crossuniting the four optic nerve stumps as diagrammed, the central projection of the two retinas can be interchanged. (b): after optic-nerve regeneration the animals respond as if everything viewed through either eye were being seen through the opposite eye. For example, when a lure is presented at X or Y, the animal strikes at X' or at Y' respectively. From Sperry, 1951a.

optic chiasma is what would be expected to occur if the optic nerve fibres grow back to their correct locus on the tectum, irrespective of laterality (Fig. 4.4).

Following these experiments involving eye rotations, transplantation and uncrossing of the chiasma, Sperry was able unequivocally to rule out functional adjustment as the cause of the (abnormal) visual recovery (Sperry, 1943b; 1944; 1945b). No form of "relearning" of the visual field, or adjustment of connections according to the principle of the achievement of optimal functional results, could lead to the consistent abnormalities found in these experiments. The results showed with certainty that the restoration of function proceeded according to some predetermined plan irrespective of the usefulness of the result to the animal.

In a normal amphibian, since stimulation of different retinal areas evokes different responses, each retinal locus must possess *functional* connections with the brain centres differing from those of all other retinal loci. After optic nerve regeneration these differential *functional* relations between retina and visual centres are systematically restored in their

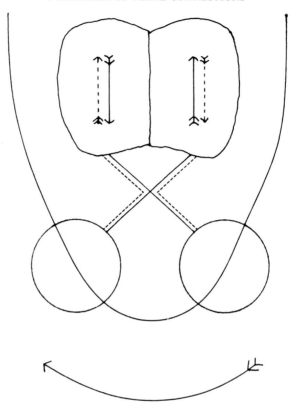

FIG. 4.4. This diagram illustrates the reason for the lateral misdirection of visual pursuit reflexes after uncrossing the optic chiasma in a frog. Each eye connects normally with the contralateral tectum (full lines connecting each eye with opposite tectum, and crossing at the chiasma). Each eye connects with its contralateral tectum such that nasal field for that eye is represented rostrally on the tectum (solid arrow on each tectum). Thus the arrow representing the visual field points in a different direction on each tectum.

When the chiasma is uncrossed, each eye connects with its ipsilateral tectum (dashed lines connecting eye to tectum). However, in these circumstances, as well as in a normal animal, temporal retina (nasal field) still projects to rostral tectum; thus the orientation of the field arrow as it projects directly to the ipsilateral tectum (dashed arrow) is appropriate to the normal contralateral projection and is so interpreted by the animal.

Thus if we assume a stimulus to lie at the head of the field arrow, the normal contralateral projection of this stimulus via the right eye would be to the caudal part of the left tectum; after uncrossing the chiasma, the projection of the stimulus would be to the caudal part of the right tectum. But in a *normal* animal, this tectal position is associated with a stimulus at the tail of the field arrow; and this is the direction in which the animal jumps.

original form, as shown by tests of visual localization. As Sperry points out (1943b), the different functional results of stimulation of different parts of the retina, both in normal animals and in those with regenerated optic nerves, must imply that fibres arising from different retinal loci must be distinguished in the centres by some differential property. Ganglion cells in the retina must differ intrinsically from each other according to their position on the retinal surface. The eventual result of these differences is that the animal responds appropriately in terms of visual localization; the *mechanism* of this appropriate response could be either that the differentiated optic fibres, by virtue of their characteristics acquired from their cells of origin, terminate selectively at appropriate positions in the optic tectum; or that the differentiated ganglion cells each emit characteristic, position-related, messages which are then suitably decoded at the tectum and transmitted into the appropriate motor channels.

Since studies on optic nerve regeneration in adult amphibians show restoration of visual function according to the retinal position stimulated, we have to consider two aspects of retinal differentiation; first, there is the continuing existence in the adult of the distinguishing factors which identify individual ganglion cells in the retina; and second there is the problem of how the system got that way during embryonic development. We can agree with Sperry (1943b) that

"it is easiest to conceive of this retinal cell differentiation (i.e. the differences between cells existing in the adult—RMG) as being orderly and continuous so that the differences between cells located far apart across the retina is greater than that between cells which are nearer together. The development of such a condition is readily interpreted embryologically in terms of a polarized, field differentiation of the optic cup. The retinal field would thus become, in respect to cellular differentiation of the ganglion cell layer, a true 'field' in the physical sense of the term."

Furthermore,

"To attain a complete differential specificity of all retinal loci the retinal field must undergo differentiation on at least two separate axes. Possibly, as in the developing limb bud (Harrison, 1921) the anteroposterior and dorsoventral axes are determined separately in the order given. If so, one would expect that contralateral eye transplantation carried out at increasingly early embryonic stages would begin at a certain point to yield normal vision after dorsoventral inversion while continuing to yield inverted vision after nasotemporal inversion" (Sperry, 1945b).

This prediction about the separate times of nasotemporal and dorsoventral axial determination has been borne out by later work of Székely (1954b) and Jacobson (1968a).

The experimental results so far discussed are fairly straightforward and merely tell us that, whatever the nature of the functional relationship between retina and visual centre, it (or something similar) is restored after regeneration. From these experiments we do not know whether the visual recovery indicates a selective restoration of fibre connections or restitution of an impulse-pattern mechanism for signalling retinal position. Unfortunately this distinction, which is of major importance both to our ideas on neural function and to our understanding of the developmental problems, has tended to get blurred as the experimental analysis continued. Thus in 1943 Sperry carefully restricts himself to statements concerning the restoration of *functional relations* between eye and brain, while later (1945b) he talks about precise patterning of central synaptic associations in optic nerve regeneration.

In normal amphibians the phenomenon of visual localization, or retinal local sign, is associated with an orderly fibre projection from the retina to the optic tectum (Stroer, 1940; Sperry, 1944; Gaze, 1958a). And it is reasonable to assume (although it cannot be proven) that visual local sign is dependent, in normal animals, on this simple mechanism. Since fibres from different parts of the retina normally go to different parts of the optic tectum, we have here a built-in mechanism for allowing the centre to distinguish between excitation of different retinal areas. Why look further? When presented with such an essentially simple explanation for the local sign properties of the normal visual system, what is the point of speculation about possible functional coding systems that might inform the tectum of retinal position—which the tectum knows already by virtue of the maplike distribution of retinal fibres across its surface? The tentative answer to these questions is that, while in a normal animal such speculations seem excessive, the visual results of experiments on animals with regenerated optic nerves have such startling implications that *no* possibility must be ignored merely because it seems to us initially to be unlikely. I will consider the question of impulse-specificity in the visual system further on.

Sperry (1944) attempted to provide evidence on the nature of the fibre distribution after optic nerve regeneration by observation of the effects of localized lesions in the tectum. Animals (*Rana* and *Bufo*), otherwise normal, in which the caudal part of the tectum had been removed, made no response when the lure was presented in the back part of the visual field, but struck vigorously and accurately when the lure was presented in the front part of the field. Animals in which the rostral part of the tectum had been removed, turned rapidly when the lure was presented behind, so as to face the lure in preparation for a strike; but when they had turned and the lure was directly in front of them they made no further response until the lure was again moved into the back part of the field. These animals could thus be caused to turn round in circles, by moving the lure, without their ever striking at it, although they reached a good striking position with each turn. Thus rostral tectal lesions result in the appearance of a scotoma in the anterior field. The behaviour of these animals with rostral tectal lesions also demonstrates that the normal striking behaviour is continuously controlled visually. The animals were unable to complete the strike on the basis of information from the back of the field, although this information told them where the lure was. This supports the observation of Gaze (1960) that the strike reaction is a two-stage phenomenon involving first an orienting reflex and then the strike itself.

These experiments of Sperry thus demonstrated the existence, in normal frogs, of an orderly quadrantic functional projection from retina to tectum, and confirmed the earlier observations of Stroer (1940) on urodeles. Similar lesions made in animals with regenerated optic nerves gave comparable results. Sperry therefore concluded that the regenerating optic nerve fibres had re-established functional associations in the same regions of the tectum with which they were originally associated. These observations however do not tell us anything directly about the sites of termination of the fibres themselves, for two reasons: firstly, a localization mechanism based on impulse-pattern specificity would give the same answer even in the presence of random regeneration; and secondly, the tectal lesions, of course, not only destroy the terminations of incoming sensory fibres, but also a considerable part of the tectal efferent system as well.

Before we discuss the factors that may underly the various phenomena of optic nerve regeneration it will be as well to take a brief survey of the field, to establish what it is that has to be explained. Since the early experiments of Matthey (1925) and Sperry (1943b) on urodeles, visual recovery (localization) has been demonstrated after section of the optic nerves in frog tadpole (Sperry, 1944), adult anurans (Sperry, 1944) and teleost fishes (Sperry, 1948). Apart from localization of a target in the visual field, after regeneration of the optic nerve perception of direction of movement may be restored in frogs (Sperry, 1944) and colour vision in fishes (Arora and Sperry, 1963). Weiler (1966) has also shown that goldfish may recover their visual acuity to approximately 80% of normal.

To account for the apparent restoration of orderly central connections during regeneration of the optic nerve, Sperry put forward the hypothesis of neuronal specificity (Sperry, 1943b; 1944, 1945b; reviewed in Sperry, 1951a; 1963). Briefly, this hypothesis states that, during embryonic development, there occurs a field-like differentiation of the retina such that each ganglion cell becomes cytochemically distinguished from all the others; a comparable and matching specification of tectal neurones also occurs; and on ingrowth of the optic nerve fibres, axons and tectal cells with matching specificities link up selectively. The original specification of the retina (and tectum) is to be considered as occurring separately across two axes.

Sperry's hypothesis thus suggests that differentiation within the developing nervous system leads to the appearance of differences between retinal ganglion cells, and likewise between tectal cells, such that, by means of some intercellular recognition phenomenon, cells with matching specificities connect with each other. The degree of specificity demanded of the hypothesis is very high indeed—"so refined as to approach the level of the individual nerve cell and its axon fiber" (Sperry, 1965). In order to examine this hypothesis in detail I shall discuss, in the following sections, the following topics: the structure of the normal visual projection; the structure of the regenerated visual projection; the mode of development of the visual system; and various analytical experiments that have been performed and which illuminate the question of specificity.

STRUCTURAL OBSERVATIONS ON THE NORMAL VISUAL SYSTEM

The optic nerve

Amphibian optic nerves differ from those of most other vertebrates in that they contain a greater preponderance of unmyelinated fibres. Early counts of the numbers of fibres in the anuran optic nerve (Bruesch and Arey, 1942) gave figures of approximately 15,000 for *Bufo* and 30,000 for *Rana*. However, Bruesch and Arey used light microscopy, which is inadequate to reveal the fine, close-packed unmyelinated fibres. When Maturana (1959) examined the optic nerve of the frog with the electron microscope he found some 470,000 fibres, and the unmyelinated fibres outnumbered the myelinated ones by 30:1. The unmyelinated fibres form compact bundles bounded by glial cells; within a bundle the unmyelinated fibres appear to be in direct contact with each other, with a gap of approximately 200 Å between membranes (Fig. 4.5). The great majority of these unmyelinated fibres are between 0·1 and 0·6 microns in diameter.

Maturana (1960) states that, in the anuran optic nerve, individual unmyelinated fibres follow a sinuous course and remain in contact with their neighbours for only a very short distance (a micron or so). It has also been claimed that fibres may frequently pass from one bundle to another (Maturana *et al.*, 1960) and that adjacency in the optic nerve does not correspond to adjacency in the retina. While this could well be the case in the frog, the situation may be rather different in the goldfish; for when one records with a microelectrode from the fish optic nerve, it is true that, at any one position in the nerve the electrode tip may pick up single-unit activity from widely separated retinal regions, yet it is also true that, along with the large single-units there may frequently be recorded a multi-unit "fuzz"; and this tends to come from a localized region of retina—usually the region from which one of the single units is coming (Gaze, unpublished data). This would suggest that, at the level of a fasciculus, most of the fibres do in fact come from a limited region of the retina. Light microscopy of the silver-stained frog optic nerve, close to the chiasma, shows a roughly parallel arrangement of fibres (Fig. 4.6).

In *Xenopus* the fibre-arrangement is similar to that in *Rana* (Gaze and Peters, 1961) but the number of fibres is smaller. Adult Xenopus optic nerve has approximately 50,000 fibres of which the great majority are unmyelinated. In the newt the visual system is altogether more primitive than in the anurans. Electron microscopic fibre counts in *Triturus vulgaris* give a figure of 29,000 fibres, of which 28,500 are unmyelinated (Gaze and

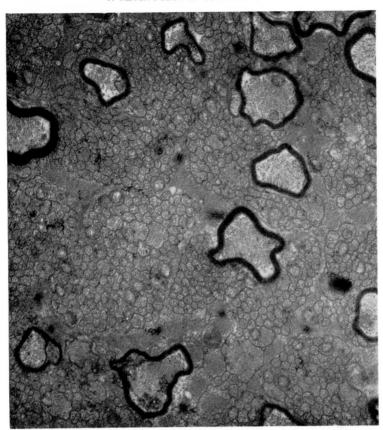

Fig. 4.5. Transverse section of frog optic nerve. ×5,000. (From photograph by Margaret Wilson.)

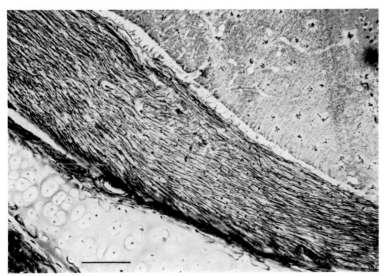

Fig. 4.6. Coronal section of normal frog nerve as it approaches the chiasma. The fibres appear to lie more-or-less parallel to each other. Holmes' silver stain. Calibration, 100 μ.

5*

Wilson unpublished) (Fig. 4.7). These fibre counts give the order of magnitude of the nerve populations in these animals, but since the eye continues to grow, by the addition of ganglion cells, into adult life, the total fibre counts will be expected to vary with the age of the animal, particularly in urodeles and *Xenopus*.

The optic nerve of the goldfish (*Carassius auratus*) is quite different in structure and composition from that of the amphibia. In goldfish almost all the optic nerve fibres are myelinated and 90% of those are $1\,\mu$ in

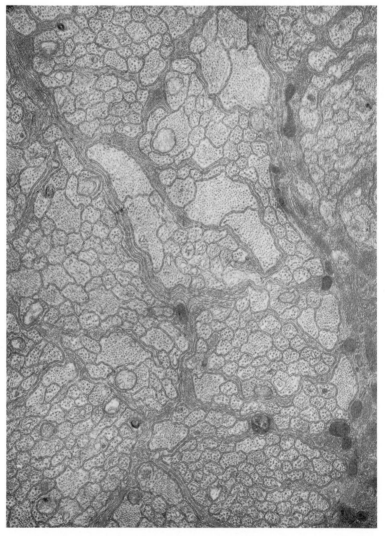

FIG. 4.7. Transverse section of newt optic nerve. $\times 15{,}000$. All the fibres in this section are unmyelinated. (From photograph by Margaret Wilson.)

diameter or less (Fig. 4.8). The number of myelinated fibres is approximately 68,000 and while the nerve does contain some unmyelinated fibres (Fig. 4.8), they tend to be restricted to one or two fascicles near the edge of the nerve; their number has not been counted, but most are 0·3–0·4 μ in diameter. The degree of fasciculation in the goldfish nerve is much greater than in *Rana*. Light microscopy in fact shows the goldfish nerve to be made up of numerous (80–100) almost separate fascicles. At the

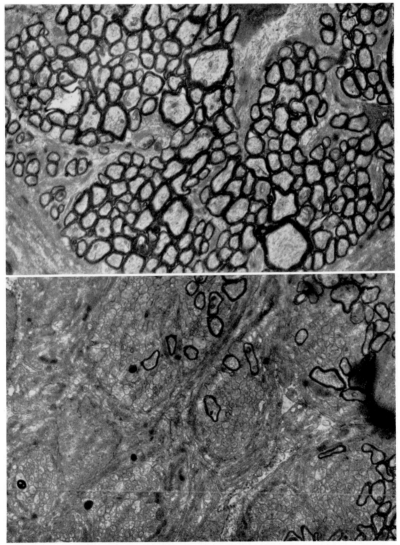

FIG. 4.8. Transverse section of goldfish optic nerve. ×5,000. Top: one of the fascicles of myelinated fibres. Bottom: some of the unmyelinated fibres. These tend to be concentrated in a few fascicles near the edge of the nerve.

chiasma the goldfish nerve also behaves differently to that of the frog. In the latter the fibres of the two nerves intermingle at the chiasma, whereas the goldfish nerves curl round each other, maintaining apparently complete separation on their way to the tracts running up the sides of the diencephalon.

The nature of the retinotectal fibre projection

The first demonstration that there was an orderly retinotectal fibre projection in a lower vertebrate was that of Stroer (1940) who showed, by analysis of fasciculation in a normal *Triturus* optic nerve, that the various quadrants of the retina projected in order upon the contralateral tectum. Similar conclusions were reached by Sperry (1944) about the quadrantic retinal projection as a result of experiments involving tectal lesions. Sperry showed that the anterior part of the visual field was functionally related to the rostral tectum, the posterior field to the caudal tectum and the dorsal field to the dorsal tectum. The same basic type of quadrantic projection was indicated for a teleost fish (carp) by the work of Buser and Dussardier (1953), who used local electrical stimulation of the retina and electrophysiological recording from the tectum. These last experiments would appear to rule out any mechanism dependent on impulse-pattern for the transmission of positional information in the normal animal. Investigation of the retinotectal projection by electrical stimulation of the retina is analogous to investigation of the function of a telephone exchange by throwing bombs through the windows; if, in either case, a meaningful answer is achieved, it is likely to reflect the existence of preset connections rather than specific codes of impulses.

The optic tectum of the lower vertebrates is a most precisely layered structure. The cellular architecture of the frog's optic tectum has been described by Cajal (1952) and, more recently, by Lázár and Székely (1967). According to the classification adopted by these latter authors, the various layers of the tectum are numbered from 1 to 9, going in the direction from ependyma to outer surface. Layers 1 to 6 comprise the deeper half of the tectum and contain most of the cells; whereas layers 7, 8, 9 make up the outer, mainly fibrous, half. Optic nerve fibres from the contralateral eye enter the tectum via the medial or lateral branch of the marginal optic tract and course through the outer half of the tectum in four distinct layers (Fig. 4.9). The tectal distribution of optic terminals has recently been investigated by Lázár and Székely (1969), using the Fink-Heimer technique, and it also shows a comparable arrangement into four more-or-less distinct layers (Fig. 4.10). This anatomical layering could well be the structural basis of the layered depth-distribution of unit types which is found electrophysiologically. The general arrangement of the tectal layering in Xenopus appears to be similar to that in the frog.

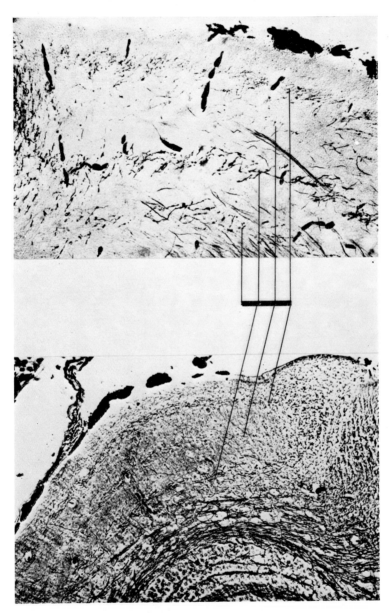

Fig. 4.9. Top: Degenerating optic nerve fibres entering the frog tectum from the lateral branch of the optic tract. Four layers of fibres may be seen, indicated by the markers. Nauta-Gygax. 14 days degeneration; Bottom: Comparable section of a normal tectum, silverstained. The three most superficial layers of fibres may also be seen in this preparation.

No one has so far used localized retinal lesions together with a selective stain for degenerating fibres (Nauta) to demonstrate the fine details of the retinotectal projection in the frog, newt or fish. In the absence of this sort of experimental approach no histological method is adequate to show details of the retinotectal projection finer than the quadrantic distribution already mentioned. By the use of electrophysiological recording from the optic tectum, together with physiological stimulation of the eye by small objects moved in the visual field, it is however possible to map the fibre

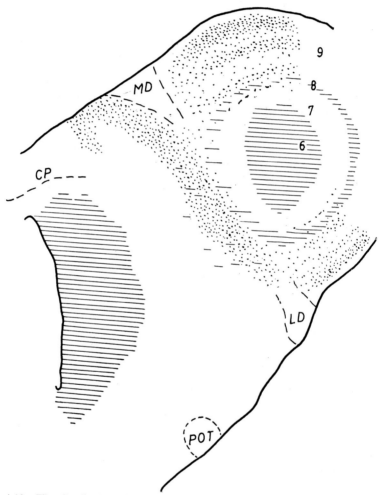

FIG. 4.10. The distribution of optic terminals in the tectum of the frog. Degeneration (Fink-Heimer technique) is indicated by dots. Hatched lines indicate the grey matter. CP, posterior commissure; MD and LD, medial and lateral divisions of the marginal optic tract; POT, posterior accessory optic tract. The numbers refer to the corresponding layers of the tectum. Four layers of terminal degeneration may be seen in the tectum, the deepest lying just below layer 8. From Lázár and Székely, 1969.

projection from retina to tectum with considerable accuracy in a normal animal.

The technique of electrophysiological mapping

Our method of electrophysiological mapping is performed in the following way. The animal is anaesthetized, the skull opened with a dental drill and the forebrain removed or destroyed. The animal is then curarized, the optic tecta are covered with mineral oil and the meninges removed. The tecta are then photographed and a print prepared at $50\times$ magnification, with a 1 cm grid superimposed (Fig. 4.11). The presence of a detailed melanophore pattern on the tectum of frog and *Xenopus*

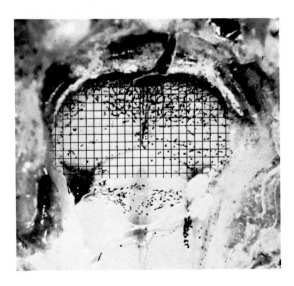

FIG. 4.11. Photograph of frog brain with 200 micron grid superimposed on the optic tecta.

facilitates the later placing of electrodes at predetermined surface positions. The animal is then set up at the centre of a perimeter of 33 cm radius with the eye under investigation centred on the fixation point of the perimeter (Fig. 4.12). The perimeter is so arranged that it can be tilted to provide for the optic axes of *Xenopus*, which look upwards and outwards. Centring of the animal's eye is performed by observing the reflection of a spot of light, projected to the cornea from a mirror at the fixation point of the perimeter, and observed from the same position. Tectal activity, consisting of either single-unit action potentials or grouped multi-unit potentials, is recorded by placing a microelectrode on the tectum at a position predetermined with reference to the grid on the tectal photograph. For each tectal position the corresponding optimal stimulus position in the visual field is found by moving the stimulus-objects, or spots of light, on the perimeter arc. The microelectrodes used are normally either sharpened tungsten wires, insulated except at the tip, which is about one micron in diameter, or glass micropipettes filled with low-melting-point metal and tipped with platinum; these latter have tips of 3–10 microns in diameter. Since we prefer working with action potentials rather than evoked slow-wave activity (which is more difficult to interpret), we normally use a short time-constant of amplification (0·002 msec) which selectively cuts out all

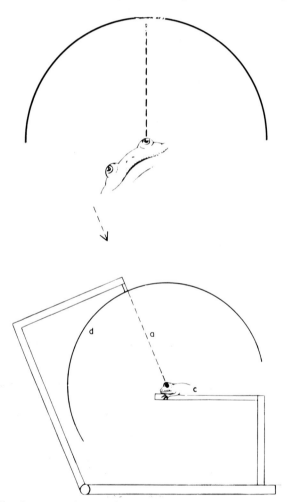

FIG. 4.12. Showing approximate relationship between animal and perimeter when a *Xenopus* is being recorded. In the lower diagram the arrow indicates the orientation of the charts of the visual field. The animal (which here seems to be a cross between a *Xenopus* and a newt) should be lying somewhat laterally, to permit the eye to look at the centre of the perimeter arc. The perimeter can be tilted as shown, or lowered to a horizontal position for work with frogs or fishes. a, optic axis of the eye; c, animal; d, perimeter arc.

slow potential changes and enables us to record unit spikes against a quiet electrical background.

This standard method of producing an electrophysiological map of the visual field (and thus, with camera-inversion, of the retina) produces results as shown in Fig. 4.13 for the frog (Gaze, 1958; Jacobson, 1962), Fig. 4.14 for *Xenopus* (Gaze *et al.*, 1963), Fig. 4.15 for the goldfish (Jacobson and Gaze, 1964) and Fig. 4.16 for the newt (Cronly-Dillon, 1968). In each case the optimal stimulus position in the visual field for a particular tectal recording position is represented as a *point* on the perimetric chart; it will be realized, however, that the "receptive field" for one recording position comprises in all cases an *area* of visual field. Thus when single units are being recorded the size of the unit receptive field may be 3° in frog, perhaps 5° in *Xenopus*, 10–15° in goldfish and 3–12° in newt; when multi-unit recording is used (as is usually the case in mapping experiments) the receptive fields tend to be somewhat larger and in this case the experimenter can determine subjectively the optimal position by listening to the responses over a loudspeaker.

The interpretation of electrophysiological maps

It may be seen from these maps of the retinotectal projection in various animals, that they are all remarkably similar. They confirm the previous histological observations already mentioned and they extend these into a further dimension of accuracy. For each small (of the order of 200 microns) step across the surface of the tectum, the most effective retinal position changes regularly. If these maps can be taken to represent *fibre distributions* across the tectum, then we have a powerful tool for the analysis of re-generated visual projections. If, on the other hand, the maps represent tectal postsynaptic activity, then the argument that they reveal fibre distributions becomes much less direct.

There are compelling reasons for believing that the technique of micro-electrode recording from the superficial layers of the optic tectum picks up selectively the activity of terminal arborizations of incoming optic nerve fibres. The question of the origin of the recorded potentials is so important for our further arguments that I shall present the evidence in some detail. These arguments have been presented previously by Maturana *et al.* (1960).

(1) A microelectrode on the surface of the optic tectum records activity (either single-unit, multi-unit or slow wave and spikes, depending on type of electrode and electrical characteristics of amplification) from a localized region of visual field (retina). Movement of the electrode tip across the tectal surface to a new position, even if only 100 microns away, results in an appropriate shift of the effective region of visual field. This means that the electrode cannot be picking up from fibres travelling past its tip. If an electrode could pick up from fibres of passage, then at tectal position

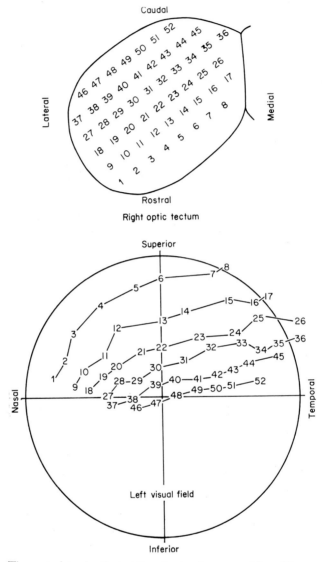

FIG. 4.13. The contralateral retinotectal projection in a normal frog. The upper diagram represents the outline of the optic tectum, seen from above. Each number on the tectum indicates an electrode position. It will be seen, that in this case, the orientation of the tectal grid is different from that shown in Fig. 4.11, which is the more usual arrangement. The lower diagram is a perimeter chart of the left visual field, as seen by the experimenter, looking towards the animal. The chart extends radially for 100° from the centre of the field, which is the "fixation point" of the frog's eye. The numbers on the chart represent the optimal stimulus positions which correspond to the numbered recording positions on the tectum. From Gaze and Jacobson, 1963c.

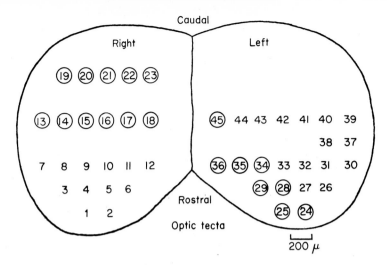

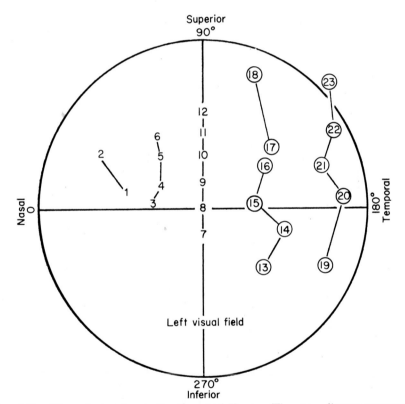

FIG. 4.14. The retinotectal projection in normal *Xenopus*. The upper diagram represents the optic tecta, seen from above; the numbers are electrode positions. The lower diagram is the left visual field showing the stimulus positions corresponding to the electrode positions on the right (contralateral) tectum. The visual field chart extends outwards for 100° from the centre of the field. Positions in the temporal field are indicated by ringed numbers.

The numbers on the left tectum refer to a different field chart, not shown in this figure. From Gaze, Jacobson and Székely, 1963.

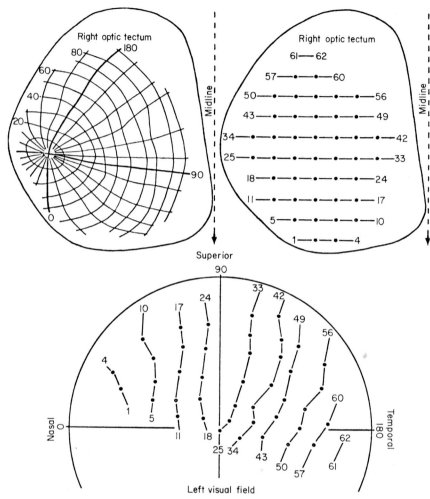

Fig. 4.15. Projection of the left visual field onto the right optic tectum in the goldfish. Upper right: dorsal surface of tectum showing rows of numbered electrode positions. The arrow along the midline points rostrally; Lower: chart of left visual field showing optimal stimulus positions, each corresponding to its appropriate electrode position. The chart covers 100° from the centre of the field; Upper left: map of the meridians and parallels of the visual field on the tectum, prepared from the information in the other two diagrams. From Jacobson and Gaze, 1964.

(a) (Fig. 4.17) it should record activity evoked from field positions (a, b, c). This does not occur. With the electrode at position (a) one records from one field position only, (a); movement of the electrode to (b) or (c) always results in appropriate movement of the field positions. We conclude that the electrode is either picking up postsynaptic activity or else it is recording from a particular point on the presynaptic fibre, e.g. the terminal arborization.

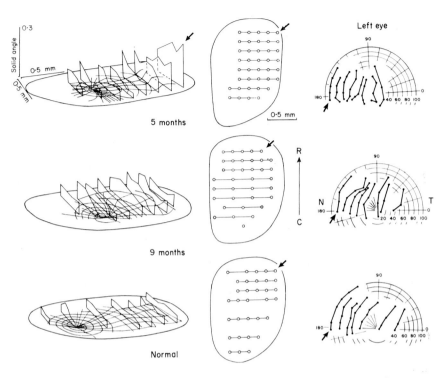

Fig. 4.16.   Newt visual projections: Normal animal and at intervals after retinal regeneration. Characteristics of the retinotectal projection recorded from individual animals
belonging to the 5 month group (top row); the 9 month group (middle row); and the normal
group (bottom row). In each row, the centre diagram shows the right optic tectum of the
animal, seen from above (open circles indicate electrode positions). Black dots in each
right-hand diagram indicate the stimulus positions within the visual field corresponding
to the electrode positions on the tectum. Thus each array of black dots linked by a line is
correlated with a particular row of electrode positions on the corresponding tectum.
Short black arrow indicates the relative position of the "first" row in each of the corresponding diagrams. On the extreme left, each diagram shows the dorsal surface of the
tectum, seen from an angle. Here, the "vertical" component indicates the size of the multi-
unit receptive field (measured in units of solid angle) found for each electrode position
on the tectum. N, nasal; T, temporal; R, rostral; C, caudal. From Cronly-Dillon, 1968.

(2) When mapping is performed using single-unit recording, the field
characteristics of the tectal units are the same as those recordable in the
optic nerve. In this latter situation there are no neurones, there are only
axons. The implication is thus very strong that the units recorded in the
tectum and showing identical receptive-field characteristics to optic nerve
axons, are also optic nerve axons.

(3) It is possible to record unitary activity, deep in the tectum, which
has receptive-field characteristics, and other characteristics, quite different
from those of optic nerve axons. These deeper tectal units are presumably
tectal cells and their processes.

(4) The electrical characteristics of the superficial tectal units are similar to those of optic axons, while those of the deeper units are not.

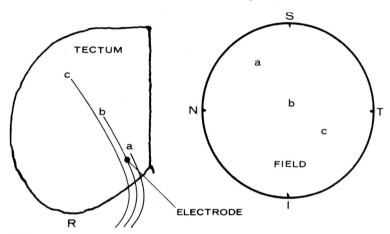

FIG. 4.17.   Diagram showing why the mapping electrode cannot normally pick up the activity of fibres of passage. See text.

For these various reasons it seems highly likely that the recordings made from the superficial tectal regions represent the distribution of the incoming optic nerve fibres. The probable site of origin of the signals is the terminal arborization of the fibre, since here the branching would be expected to increase the signal. It may be mentioned again that the fact that Buser and Dussardier (1953) were able to demonstrate a retinotectal localization using electrical stimulation of the retina, argues forcibly against positional information being transmitted by an impulse-code; an electrical shock applied to the retina is a most unphysiological stimulus and may be confidently expected to upset any finely-organized impulse signalling system heading for the tectum. Yet retinal position is adequately indicated at the tectum by this procedure.

STRUCTURAL OBSERVATIONS ON THE VISUAL SYSTEM AFTER REGENERATION OF THE OPTIC NERVE

The optic nerve

The simplest assumption one could make to account for the restored visual function after optic nerve regeneration is that the fibres grow back to their original destinations in the optic tectum; and the most obvious mechanism that might achieve this would be for the fibres to be straight-forwardly directed back along their normal channels—a form of mechanical guidance. Several observations show that this cannot be the case.

In the first place, at the site of an optic nerve section, there occurs an extensive scar formation; the result is that the fibres, growing in through the scar, are forced to form a complex tangle which, one must assume, successfully disrupts any spatial relationship existing in the normal nerve (Fig. 4.18). In the normal frog optic nerve bundles of unmyelinated fibres are each enclosed within a glial sheath (Maturana, 1960). And while

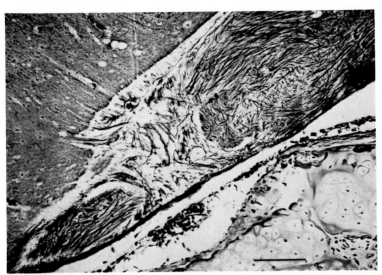

FIG. 4.18. Photomicrograph of the regenerated optic nerve of a frog at the site of section near the chiasma. Coronal section. Holmes' silver stain. Calibration 100 μ.

Maturana maintains that fibres frequently cross from one bundle to another, yet it may still be possible that within a bundle fibres tend to stay together and come from closely adjacent regions of retina. It would be reasonable to think that the relationship of a group of fibres to its sheath cells could be of great importance for the proper directing of the fibres. While a certain amount is known of the structure of the optic nerve itself, however, we have no information at all, at electron microscopic level, of the structure of the tracts between chiasma and tectum. The fact that it is fairly easy to record unit action potentials from the nerve distal to the chiasma, while it is very difficult to do so between chiasma and tectum, suggests that the arrangement of fibres with respect to each other and to the supporting cells may be different in the two situations. At the site of a nerve section, however, a massive tangle of fibres develops and if the fibres are to find their way back to "normal channels" beyond the lesion, something more than mere mechanical guidance is necessary.

A second factor arguing against any major role of mechanical guidance in the fine control of direction of regenerating fibres is that, after transplantation of an eye in *Amblystoma*, Stone (1930) found that the proximal stump of optic nerve had degenerated and disappeared completely by 10 days after the operation, whereas the new nerve growing out from the eye had only reached the optic foramen by the same time. In this situation therefore there is no possibility that the regenerating fibres could regain their original pathways—the pathways were no longer present.

A third type of observation, and one that is critical for the question of pathway following, is that an optic nerve may be caused to regenerate along a totally abnormal pathway (the oculomotor nerve) and may still re-establish appropriate functional (electrical or behavioural) connections in the tectum (Gaze, 1959; Hibbard, 1967). Since the oculomotor nerve obviously does not contain the "proper" channels for optic nerve fibres, these experiments prove that, while channel-selection (if it occurs) may be an adequate condition for ordered regeneration, it is not necessary. A functionally appropriate retinotectal connection may be established in the absence of a properly ordered optic nerve; and moreover this may occur even when the incoming fibres approach the tectum from an incorrect direction (Fig. 4.19).

The nature of the regenerated retinotectal projection

The behavioural experiments of Sperry had suggested that the normal retinotectal connections were reformed during optic nerve regeneration; and his observations on animals with localized tectal lesions (Sperry, 1944) indicated at least a quadrantic restoration of functional relationships between retina and tectum. However the detailed nature, and mode of establishment, of the regenerated projection had to await the application of electrophysiological recording methods. I have described above the electrophysiological map of the retinal projection in normal animals; the same technique has been used after section and regeneration of an optic nerve in Xenopus (Gaze, 1959), frog (Gaze and Jacobson, 1963c), goldfish (Jacobson and Gaze, 1965; Gaze and Sharma, 1970), newt (Cronly-Dillon, 1968), in each case with similar results: under certain circumstances, the regenerating nerve fibres may re-establish the electrophysiological retinotectal projection that previously existed, or a close approximation to it.

The restoration of the electrophysiological retinotectal projection under these circumstances may be taken as indicating that the fibre projection is appropriately restored; this we may claim because the arguments applied earlier to the projection in a normal animal also apply after full regeneration. Maturana et al., (1959) and Gaze and Keating (1969, 1970c) have shown that the various functional types of optic nerve fibre found in the normal tectal neuropil are also to be found after regeneration of the optic nerve. Gaze and Keating (1970c) have used a combination of single-unit analysis with retinotectal mapping; and in this case the arguments relating to the nature of the units recorded are directly applicable to the regenerated projection. Maturana et al. (1959) also showed that, during regeneration the normal differential depth distribution of the various classes of optic

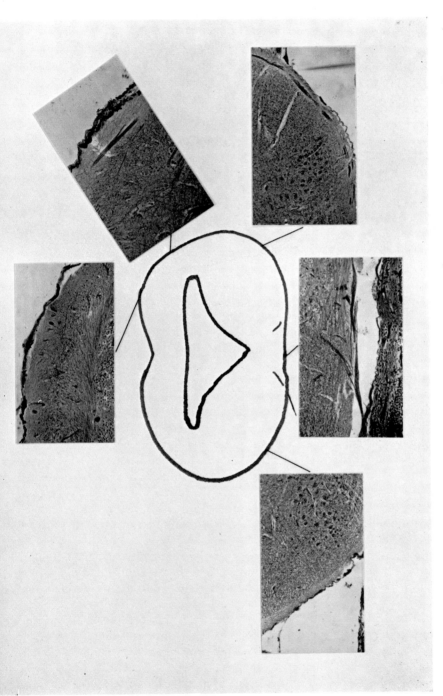

FIG. 4.19.   Regeneration of the optic nerve of a larval *Xenopus* via the oculomotor nerve. The central diagram shows, in outline, a section through the tecta at the level of the oculomotor nerves. The photomicrographs, taken from this and the adjacent sections of the series, show the abnormal bundles of regenerating fibres entering with the oculomotor nerve and running up to the contralateral tectum. (Animal from the series described in Gaze, 1959.)

nerve terminals was restored in the tectal neuropil. This observation adds a third dimension of localization to the previous findings that the retino-tectal map across the surface of the tectum was restored. The observations on tectal depth distribution of the unit types before and after regeneration of the nerve have been extended by Gaze and Keating (1969, 1970c), who found that, while the relative depths of the different classes of endings were approximately correct after nerve regeneration, the absolute depths after regeneration were somewhat less than normal. This finding agrees with the observation that, after nerve regeneration, the affected tectal neuropil is thinner than normal; thus regenerating fibres appear not to be following any instructions of the nature of "grow down into the tectum for x microns and there terminate"; rather they appear to grow down until they come upon certain structures, which, in the thinner tectum after nerve regenera-tion, will lie nearer the surface. Conceivably the distinct layers of incoming fibres are correspondingly displaced in the thinned tecta.

The electrophysiological experiments just described give us, therefore, strong evidence that, when fibres from an otherwise normal eye grow back to an otherwise normal tectum, they end up in the proper distribution across the tectum as well as in depth in the neuropil. Thus the original conclusions drawn by Sperry (1943b; 1944; 1945b) from his observations on the visual behaviour of animals after optic nerve regeneration have received dramatic confirmation.

The evidence that restoration of the fibre projection may occur is not only electrophysiological; histological observations point in the same direc-tion. As I mentioned previously, the only histological methods capable of giving resolution even approaching that of electrophysiological methods are those involving selective staining for degenerating fibres. Such methods have not yet been applied to the problem of optic nerve regeneration, but Attardi and Sperry (1960; 1963) devised a modification of the Bodian silver stain which enabled them to identify bundles of newly-regenerated fibres. In goldfish they removed part of the retina and cut the correspond-ing optic nerve; histological examination some 17–25 days later revealed that the fibres regenerating from the remaining part of the retina formed arborizing plexuses only in the appropriate part of the tectum. After re-moval of the dorsal or ventral hemiretina, fibres regenerated only to the dor-sal or ventral regions of tectum respectively (Fig. 4.20). This is the normal distribution of these fibres, for ventral retina (dorsal or superior visual field) projects to the dorsal surface of the tectum and vice-versa (see Fig. 4.15). After removal of the nasal or temporal hemiretina, fibres regenerated only to the rostral or caudal regions of the tectum respectively (Fig. 4.21); while after ablation of a peripheral ring of retina fibres were found distri-buted in the central region of the tectal neuropil (Fig. 4.22). In each case the distribution of the fibres from the residual retina appeared to be normal after nerve regeneration. Moreover those fibres which, normally,

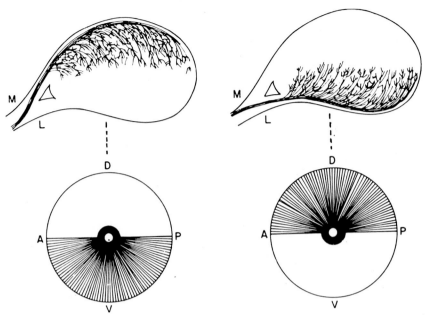

Fig. 4.20. Diagram of the regenerated fibre patterns obtained with nerve section and ablation of dorsal or ventral hemiretina respectively. Goldfish. From Attardi and Sperry, 1963.

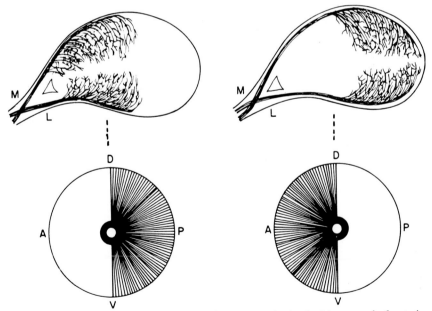

Fig. 4.21. Diagram of the regenerated fibre patterns obtained with removal of anterior (nasal) or posterior (temporal) hemiretina respectively. Goldfish. From Attardi and Sperry, (1963).

pass through the medial or lateral division of the optic tract, did so also after regeneration; and in the tectum the fibres remained in the parallel layer until they reached the correct site of termination, when they formed a plexiform layer.

These very elegant observations confirm the general finding that fibres

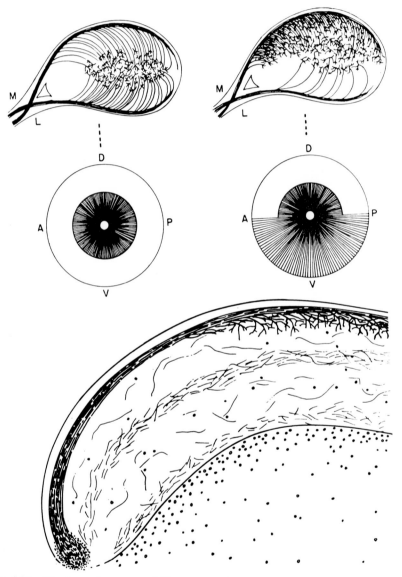

Fig. 4.22.   The type of regenerated fibre pattern obtained with removal of the peripheral retina. Below, enlarged detail of the result as viewed in a transverse section of the tectum. From Attardi and Sperry, 1963.

may get back to their proper places, and suggest that a rather high degree of chemotactic specificity may operate to allow the fibres to choose their correct paths as well as the appropriate destinations. However it is well to be cautious in evaluating these results from this form of histological staining. Tne colour differences between newly-regenerated fibres and normal ones do undoubtedly exist and may even be demonstrated (sometimes) by the less tricky Holmes' silver method (Gaze, unpublished observations); but the decision whether a particular fibre is old or new rests on a rather subjective interpretation of the histological picture. Furthermore any silver method can only show up fibres, or groups of fibres that are large enough to be identified with the light microscope. In this context two points are relevant: firstly, the work of Grainger et al. (1968) indicates that, in a tissue-culture situation, what appears by light microscopy to be a single fibre may, when examined with the electron microscope, turn out to be a bundle of fibres, some so small as to be beyond the limits of light microscopic resolution. It would seem reasonable that this may be the case also in vivo; secondly, during regeneration of the optic nerve in the goldfish, the regenerating fibres are all initially unmyelinated (T. J. Horder, personal communication). And we will expect that some or all of the regenerating fibres will be initially considerably smaller in diameter than the normal nerve fibres. Thus again, there may well be difficulty in seeing such regenerating fibres with the light microscope. Even in the normal goldfish optic tectum, all the fibres in the most superficial layer are unmyelinated and very fine (Fig. 4.23). With these facts in mind, we should perhaps conclude that the histological observations of Attardi and Sperry (1963) can show only a part of the picture; the positive findings are highly relevant and support previous ideas; but the absence of fibres demonstrable by this technique in certain places may not be taken as good evidence that some fibres do not exist there. Again we must say that only selective staining methods for degenerating fibres or electron microscopy can answer this question clearly. This point is emphasized by Fig. 4.24 which shows (in a frog) that, after regeneration of the optic nerve, the appearance of the affected tectum may be very different from normal, with *apparent* absence of the optic fibres; in this animal, however, there was a full restoration of the visual map across the deafferented tectum, including a full pattern 4 projection (see later: Analytical experiments on the mode of reconnection of optic nerve fibres).

The precision with which the retinotectal projection is restored

Any statement one may make about the accuracy of restoration of the visual projection will depend on the mode of assessment used. Thus if we use tests of visual function, and assume that normality of function is linearly related to normality of fibre projection (an assumption that is certainly not justified), we find that visual acuity may be restored to 78%

of normal fish: (Weiler, 1966). And in experiments involving colour discrimination in fish, when the optic nerve had been cut in untrained animals, the learning curves obtained after regeneration of the optic nerve did not differ significantly from those obtained in normal, unoperated fish. Furthermore, when fish that had been trained in colour discrimination before section of the optic nerve were tested again after regeneration, under conditions that excluded relearning, they gave 18 or more correct responses in their first 20 trials, a level of performance equal to that in normal animals (Arora and Sperry, 1963).

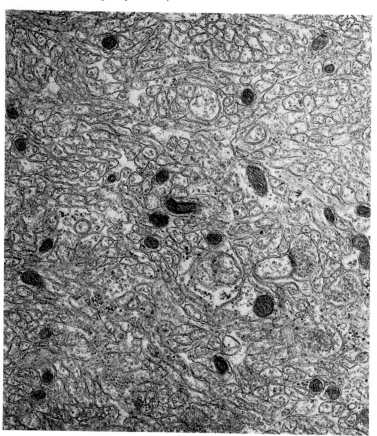

FIG. 4.23.   Electron micrograph of the most superficial layer of the goldfish optic tectum. × 15,000. (From photograph by Margaret Wilson.)

We may say, therefore, that in its tested spatial and chromatic aspects, visual function after regeneration of the optic nerve may achieve between 80–100% of normal performance. This does not permit us to say that the retinotectal fibre connections have been restored to the same degree of precision. In the first place, we have no information about the functional fibre redundancy in the visual system. It is conceivable that visual function, normal to all our rather crude methods of testing, could be achieved with only a small proportion of the optic nerve fibres connected. Observations pointing in this direction are the intriguing experiments of Galambos *et al.* (1967) where a considerable degree of pattern recognition was achieved by cats after section of 98% of the fibres in the optic tract. Proper restoration of visual function strongly suggests that the proper *pattern* of retinotectal connections has been re-established but it can tell us little about the density of the reinnervation, since we do not know the

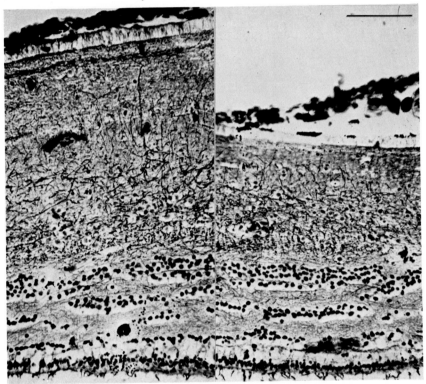

FIG. 4.24. Photomicrographs of similar regions in the normal tectum (left) and the affected tectum (right) after section and regeneration of one optic nerve. The superficial layers of the affected tectum are greatly reduced in thickness in comparison with the normal side, and the affected tectum shows no signs of the optic fibre layers which are conspicuous on the normal side, near the surface. Despite the obvious abnormality of the affected tectum, a full pattern 4 projection was recorded from it. It may be noted that the thickness of the cellular layers is almost identical on both sides. Calibration 100 μ.

minimal density required to provide normal function as assessed by our tests.

Similar difficulties attend any attempt to assess quantitatively the completeness of restoration of the retinotectal projection, using electrophysiological data. The restoration of a normal projection pattern, where the map of the visual field covers the tectum as completely as in a normal animal, can give us no useful information about the proportion of fibres that have got back to their proper places. Optic nerve fibre counts in animals with regenerated nerves will not help, since we have no assurance that all the fibres which have regenerated to fill the nerve at the site of counting, have made tectal connections. Seemingly the only way to obtain this quantitative information would be to perform synaptic counts of optic fibres terminations, and this has not been done and may not even be feasible.

In a normal adult frog there are nearly half a million fibres in each optic nerve (Maturana, 1959) and approximately the same number of neurons in each tectum (Lázár and Székely, 1967), all of which may probably be influenced by the optic input. Those optic fibres which terminate superficially in the tectal neuropil have arborizations about ten microns in diameter, whereas the optic fibres that end deeper in the superficial neuropil each may arborize over 50–70 microns (Lázár and Székely, 1967). The corresponding receptive field diameters for these fibres are approximately 3° for the most superficial fibres and 15° for the deepest ones (Maturana et al., 1960). In the electrophysiological mapping of a frog's retinotectal projection it is customary to place the electrode serially at positions some 200 microns apart on the tectal surface. The dorsal surface of the tectum, which is the only part that is directly accessible for mapping, is some three millimetres in diameter; thus, under optimal conditions, a tectal map may comprise some 50 recording positions; occasionally more, but always less than 100. If we assume that the optic nerve fibre terminations are uniformly spread over the surface of the tectum, then we may have approximately 700 overlapping terminations strung out in a line across one axis of the tectum ($\sqrt{490,000}$). Of these, some 350 would cover the part of the tectum accessible for recording. And these 350 terminals would be sampled by approximately 5–10 electrode positions. The calculations cannot be carried to any meaningful conclusion since there are too many assumptions involved and we do not know what proportion of terminals are superimposed to give the normal depth-distribution of the various classes of visual unit. The point emerges, however, that the recording procedure, although the most accurate available, provides but a poor sample of the tectal innervation. And, most relevant, an unknown proportion of optic fibres could be unconnected and we would be unable to detect it by any method yet devised; provided always, of course, that the missing fibres were evenly spread across the projection map. The technique of electrophysiological recording merely tells us that those fibres we actually record got back to those particular places from which we recorded them. Moreover, in view of the work of Wickelgren and Sterling (1969), we must recognize that the absence of an electrical response at a certain position need not imply that no fibres go there; the possibility of inhibitory gating exists.

From the results of mapping experiments, therefore, we may not make statements about the proportion of fibres that succeed in reinnervating the tectum. We may, however, make meaningful statements about the *pattern* of the restored projection. It has been shown, for example, that the probability of obtaining a normal retinotectal map, on the basis of a random walk from position to position in the visual field, is less than 0·000001 (Gaze and Jacobson, 1963c).

ANALYTICAL EXPERIMENTS ON THE MODE OF RECONNECTION OF OPTIC NERVE FIBRES

The development of the regenerated projection

The evidence discussed so far shows that regenerating optic nerve fibres can re-establish their proper terminal distribution in the optic tectum. Various experiments have been performed with a view to finding out how this could occur. One approach used has been to take a series of "time-sections" through the process of regeneration, with the intention of observing different phases of the restoration of connections (Gaze and Jacobson, 1963c). A large series of frogs with sectioned optic nerves was examined electrophysiologically, each animal at a different post-operative interval. The retinotectal projections recorded from these animals were found to be classifiable into four different varieties of pattern, three of which were abnormal.

The animals giving tectal responses to visual stimulation soonest after operation (23–33 days) all yielded an abnormal retinotectal projection. Instead of the visual field being represented in a regularly extended fashion over the tectum (see normal, Fig. 4.13), responses were elicitable only from one or two localized regions of the visual field (Fig. 4.25). These regions tended to lie towards the nasal and temporal poles of the field. Within each effective field region the various points were confused; but each field region projected to about half the tectum. For instance, in Fig. 4.25, the electrode at any of the numbered positions on the lateral half of the tectum was able to record activity from stimulation anywhere within the nasal group of field positions, but from nowhere else in the field. Conversely, the medial tectal positions were related in a similar way to the temporal field positions. In several animals there was a central region of tectum from which responses could be obtained following stimulation of either field district.

Some of the frogs giving this type of retinotectal projection (called pattern 1 by Gaze and Jacobson) showed the two retinal regions as indicated in Fig. 4.25; others showed only one or the other.

All such pattern 1 projections were thus grossly abnormal and the only order apparent in the projections was that the nasal field positions projected rostrolaterally on the tectum while the temporal field positions projected medially. The nature of the individual responses from these animals was also abnormal. Jacobson has since reported that if, in such an animal showing pattern 1 regeneration, the medial brachium of the optic tract is cut, the responses from the medial half of the tectum (temporal group of field positions) disappear (Jacobson, 1966). This would suggest

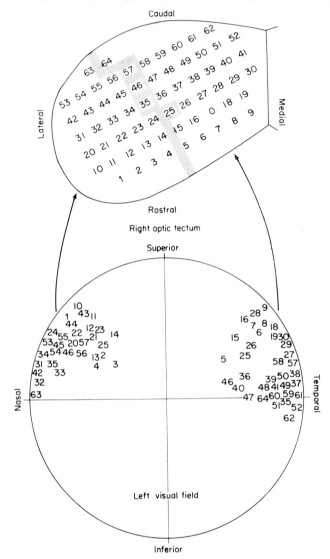

Fig. 4.25. A 'pattern 1' projection recorded from a frog 68 days after section of the left optic nerve. As indicated by the arrows, stimulation within each of the effective regions of the field gave rise to activity in the corresponding half of the tectum. Electrode positions on the stippled strip of tectum gave responses to stimulation at either of the field groups. From Gaze and Jacobson, 1963c.

that each group of field (retinal) positions connects to the tectum via its appropriate branch of the tract. Fourteen out of 67 animals showed pattern 1 (Gaze and Jacobson, 1963c).

Another group of animals showed a pattern that was abnormal in that there was some evidence of proper organization of the projection across the latero-medial tectal axis but none across the rostrocaudal axis (Fig. 4.26). This partial ordering of the projection (pattern 2) was found only at the rostral region of the tectum and was seen in 4 out of 67 animals. A third pattern of projection seen in 12 out of 67 animals, was an approximate restoration of the normal map.

The fourth and final class of projection pattern described by Gaze and Jacobson (1963c) involved a partial or complete restitution of the normal contralateral projection, together with an anomalous but retinotopically organized projection from the nasal part of the field to the rostrolateral tectum (Fig. 4.27). The anomalous nasal field positions in these animals represent part of the "ipsilateral" visual projection (Gaze, 1958b; Gaze and Jacobson, 1962; Gaze and Jacobson, 1963a) which has here appeared on the wrong tectum.

Although all the direct retinotectal fibres in a normal frog are crossed, there is nevertheless an ipsilateral visual projection (Gaze, 1958b; Gaze and Jacobson, 1962). The path taken by the impulses from the eye to the ipsilateral optic tectum involves initial passage to the contralateral tectum, followed by an intertectal link. This is indicated by the fact that localized destruction of the appropriate point on the contralateral tectum (A) selectively abolishes the ipsilateral response at the other tectum (B) to stimulation from the same point in visual space, without interfering with either the contralateral input to tectum B from the same place in the visual field, or the ipsilateral projection from other points in the field at other points on the tectum (Gaze and Jacobson, 1963a; Keating and Gaze, 1970). Furthermore, the ipsilateral visual response is always of longer latency than the contralateral response to the same stimulus. The inter-tectal linkage involved in this ipsilateral projection involves fibres which pass rostrally and cross in the postoptic commissures (Keating and Gaze, 1970).

The pattern 4 projections found in some animals after regeneration of the optic nerve had all the characteristics of an "ipsilateral" projection: the latency of the responses from the anomalous field positions was longer than that from the normal field positions; the retinotopic arrangement of the anomalous positions was a mirror-image of the normal ipsilateral projection; and destruction of the corresponding (same field position) point on the *ipsilateral* tectum resulted in disappearance of the anomalous responses at the appropriate positions on the contralateral tectum (Gaze and Jacobson, 1963c).

In view of the fact that the normal ipsilateral projection involves passage of the pathway through the contralateral tectum, what are we to make of these pattern 4 projections, where the "ipsilateral" projection has ended up on the contralateral side? Gaze and Jacobson (1963c) showed that, in one animal with a pattern 4 projection (F172), as well as the anomalous "ipsilateral" which went to the contralateral tectum, there was an

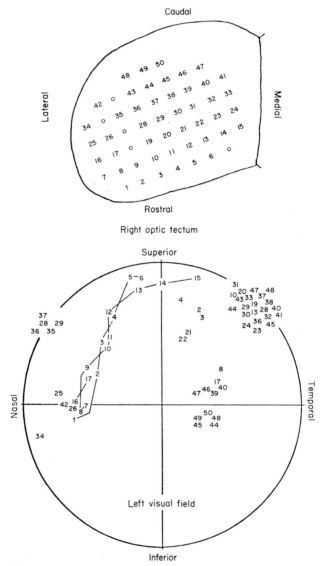

FIG. 4.26. A "pattern 2" projection recorded from a frog 246 days after section of the optic nerve. This projection is muddled with the exception of the rostral two rows of tectal positions, where the corresponding field positions show ordering in one axis but not the other. From Gaze and Jacobson, 1963c.

anomalous "contralateral" projection which went to the ipsilateral tectum
(Fig. 4.28). Further investigation of the pattern 4 type of projection (Gaze
and Keating, 1970a) has shown that (1) pattern 4 only occurs when the
optic nerve has been cut; never when the nerve has been crushed and the

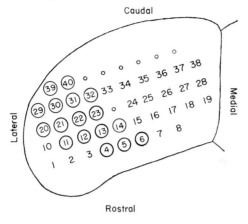

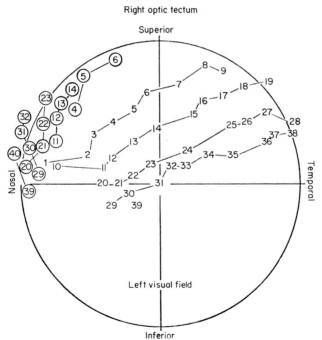

FIG. 4.27. A "pattern 4" projection, recorded from a frog 243 days after section of the
optic nerve. Here the contralateral projection (unringed numbers) is properly restored
but there is, in addition, a retinotopically-organized projection (ringed numbers) from
the far nasal field to the rostrolateral tectum. As described in the text, this anomalous
contralateral projection, indicated by the ringed numbers, represents a projection which
should normally appear on the ipsilateral tectum. From Gaze and Jacobson, 1963c.

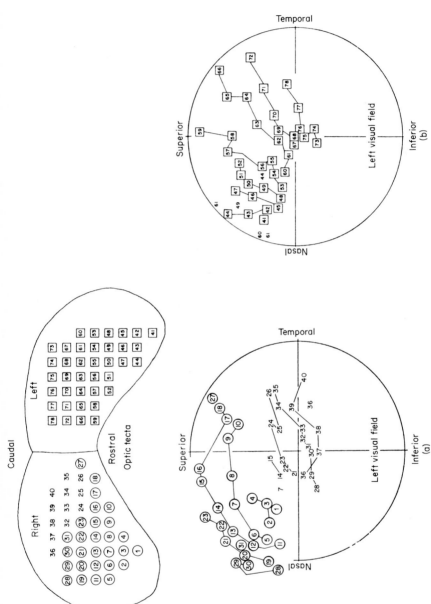

FIG. 4.28 A full, or double pattern 4 projection, recorded from a frog 172 days after section of the optic nerve. Both perimeter charts refer to the left visual field. It may be seen that there are three projections from the left eye: (1) a restored projection to the contralateral (right) tectum, shown by the unringed numbers in the field; (2) a "contralateral" projection to the ipsilateral tectum, shown by the numbers in squares; and (3) an "ipsilateral" projection to the contralateral tectum,

sheath left intact. This suggests that a factor in the production of pattern 4 is the escape of some of the regenerating fibres from the confines of the nerve, close to the chiasma, and their entry into the diencephalon on the same side as the eye. Fibres entering the brain ipsilaterally have been reported both by Gaze and Jacobson (1963c) and Gaze and Keating (1970a). These fibres we assume to continue up the ipsilateral optic tract and form a "contralateral" projection across the ipsilateral tectum. (2) In all cases of pattern 4 which have been investigated in sufficient detail, the anomalous "ipsilateral" projection is accompanied by an anomalous "contralateral" projection (Gaze and Keating, 1970a); as, indeed, would have to be the case if our present views on the nature of the ipsilateral projection are correct (Fig. 4.29).

The question of the significance to be attributed to these various patterns of regeneration is difficult to answer in relation to patterns 1 and 2 and fairly straightforward in the case of patterns 3 and 4. Gaze and Jacobson (1963c) found that there was some evidence of a temporal progression through the patterns, in numerical order, during regeneration. Thus all the earliest responses after nerve section showed varieties of pattern 1, while pattern 4 occurred more frequently the longer the interval between nerve section and recording. Patterns 2 and 3 appeared to be intermediate in time. The time-differences between the patterns suggested that perhaps patterns 1 and 2 were stages in the normal process of restoration of an organized projection. The only way in which this suggestion could be properly tested would be to record several times in the same animal and to observe one type of projection actually change into another with the passage of time; this has not been done so far, since it is very difficult to keep the animals alive after decerebration, curarization and a prolonged recording session. In four cases double recording was successfully performed but these animals did not provide an answer; in three of them the first recording was negative in that it was attempted before the optic nerve had regenerated to the tectum; and in the fourth animal the only progression found between the recordings (which were separated by 85 days) was that pattern 1 had apparently later developed a pattern 4, while preserving some of the features of pattern 1 (Gaze and Jacobson, 1963c).

The responses recorded in cases of pattern 1 were mostly abnormal; they were of considerably lower amplitude than normal, were difficult to localize, and could not usually be separated into identifiable unit-types. For these reasons we must be somewhat cautious in assigning these responses to any particular structures in the tectum. It would seem reasonable, however, to assume that the abnormal pattern 1 responses came also from optic nerve fibres, which in this case had not (yet?) formed their normal types of termination but which were rather widely arborized over the tectum. A wider than normal terminal arborization, while the fibres are perhaps searching for an adequate site at which to terminate,

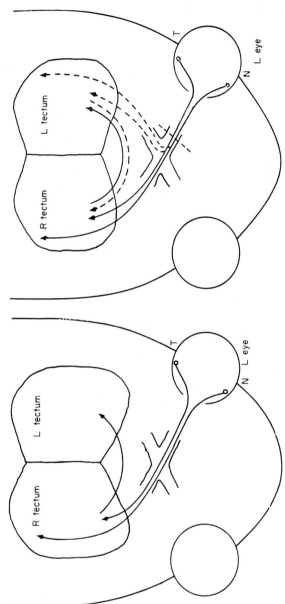

Fig. 4.29. Left: Summary of the normal contralateral and ipsilateral projections in a frog; Right: Summary of the full "pattern 4" projection, after nerve regeneration. Some of the nerve fibres have regenerated properly back to the contralateral tectum and thus restore the contralateral (and hence, the ipsilateral) projection. Some fibres, however, enter the brain ipsilaterally at the site of section and thus give rise to a "contralateral" projection on the ipsilateral side, and thus also an "ipsilateral" projection on the contralateral side.

could account both for the lessened amplitude and lack of localization shown by these responses.

The grouping of pattern 1 stimulus positions in the visual field (retina) would indicate that, initially, not all regions of the retina connect with the tectum simultaneously. There appear to be regions of retina, one nasal and one temporal, from which the first tectal connections are made. Apart from the fact that nasal field (temporal retina) tends to project in pattern 1 to lateral tectum and temporal field (nasal retina) to medial tectum, this type of projection shows no order. The first sign of organization in the projection may occur in pattern 2, where those field positions projecting to the rostral part of the tectum are ordered in their distribution across the mediolateral axis of the tectum but not across the rostrocaudal axis. It is not at all obvious why there should be such an axial difference in these pattern 2 animals; conceivably it represents the effects of mechanical and temporal factors acting on the regenerating fibres as they approach the tectum from in front; alternatively the axial differences may manifest something of the nature of the inherent "specification" of the tectum, which, during neurogenetic differentiation, probably becomes specified separately across the three axes of space.

Patterns 3 and 4 are much more straightforward. In these cases the nature of the recorded responses may be normal and our original arguments concerning the origin of the potentials will apply: these patterns indicate fibre distributions. Two points stand out from a consideration of patterns 3 and 4. The first is that pattern 3, the restoration of a "normal" retino-tectal projection occurs in comparatively few cases—12 out of 49 animals (Gaze and Jacobson, 1963c). This does *not* indicate, however, that three out of every four animals with regenerated optic nerves show failure of an organized projection to return. The series of intervals studied by Gaze and Jacobson (1963c) was chosen to catch the process of regeneration in various stages of completeness. And the results would strongly suggest that, in *all* cases where sufficient time is allowed, organized regeneration will occur. However, the pattern that tends to be restored eventually following *section* of the nerve is not a normal projection nor yet a deficient one; it is supernormal. In these animals (pattern 4) the eye connects directly not only with its contralateral tectum but also with its ipsilateral tectum; and a secondary result of this is that, from the operated eye, there is an "ipsilateral" projection to both sides of the brain.

The occurrence of pattern 4, given that fibres may enter the dien-cephalon ipsilaterally, merely tells us that the two sides of the brain (tectum) are equivalent as far as concerns pattern formation by the fibres from an eye. The tecta are mirror-symmetrical in whatever controls the terminal distribution of optic nerve fibres. This, of course, had previously been shown, by inference, by the results of Sperry's (1944) experiments in which he uncrossed the optic chiasma. Each eye was in that case able to

6*

form "appropriate" connections with its ipsilateral tectum and the functional result was that the animal misdirected its visual responses symmetrically about the midsagittal plane. The work of Gaze and Jacobson (1963c) and Gaze and Keating (1970a) shows that it is not necessary to uncross the chiasma to achieve this spectacular abnormality of connection; it is sufficient merely to cut the optic nerve near the chiasma and the animal will do the rest.

The equivalence of the two tecta for the restoration of the projection pattern does, however, bring into sharp relief another problem of very considerable interest: what causes the optic nerve to connect with its *contralateral* tectum in any case? This question is, of course, part of the wider one of the mechanism of crossing of nerve pathways in general. The problem of neural decussations was extensively discussed by Cajal (1899; 1952), from a largely teleological point of view, but the most interesting attempt to account for nerve crossings in terms of mechanism was in the more recent work of Szentágothai and Székely (1956). From their observations of the directions taken by optic nerve fibres growing back from various types of Cyclopean eyes and eyes in other abnormal relations to the brain these authors felt compelled to postulate specific properties belonging to the various ganglion cells which, in combination with guiding structures in the optic stalk or brain itself, induce the fibres to cross in certain cases.

That any factors inducing fibres to cross cannot be very powerful is suggested by the ease with which eyes can be made to connect with the ipsilateral tectum. It seems likely that here the developing system takes into account a variety of factors, including original direction of growth, timing, fibre specificity and so forth. Upset or alteration in any one of these factors could then lead the fibres to behave abnormally only if the extent of the alteration outweighed the conservative effects of the other factors.

The possible existence of inherent cellular factors inducing certain fibres to cross the midline is made more likely by the recent evidence that not all frog optic nerve fibres are crossed (Knapp *et al.*, 1965; Scalia *et al.*, 1968). All fibres from the eye going to the tectum do appear to cross in the chiasma, but there is a considerable projection of fibres from the eye to the ipsilateral diencephalon. Nothing is as yet known about the time of ingrowth of these ipsilateral fibres during development, so the possibility remains that simple mechanical factors, associated perhaps with different timing, could account for the differential distribution of the optic nerve fibres to the two sides of the brain. It is equally possible, and perhaps more likely, that individual fibres somehow know whether they are to cross or not.

A final question concerning the pattern 4 projections relates to the distribution of "contralateral" fibres at their site of entry into the diencephalon. Some optic nerve fibres go up the normal contralateral optic tract, having crossed the chiasma in the normal fashion; others enter the diencephalon on the same side and pass up the ipsilateral optic tract. It would be interesting to know whether the fibres running up ipsilaterally are separate axons or branches of those passing contralaterally. It is quite possible that, at the site of section, some fibres branch and provide the double contralateral projection in this fashion; the evidence is so far insufficient to enable us to determine this point.

The results of Gaze and Jacobson (1963c) showed that regenerating optic nerve fibres could, if given sufficient time, re-establish equivalent patterns on both sides of the brain; and moreover they suggested that, in the early phases of regeneration the ingrowing fibres initially came from localized regions of the retina and arborized widely at the level of the tectum. This latter point received no support from the work of Attardi and Sperry (1963), which showed only a restoration of the original distribution, with no evidence of wider arborization of the regenerating fibres. However, as was mentioned previously, the technique used by Attardi and Sperry would be inadequate to demonstrate aberrant fibres, particularly if these were of small diameter, as would be expected of exploratory arborizations. In this situation the positive evidence obtained by electrophysiological methods may be accorded more weight than the negative histological results. Attardi and Sperry (1963) were, of course, using goldfish; it is quite possible that species differences may occur here. An attempt to resolve this difference between the histological results of Attardi and Sperry and the recording results of Gaze and Jacobson was made by Westerman (1965). In goldfish Westerman removed three of the four retinal quadrants, then cut the optic nerve and allowed it to regenerate. Later he investigated the retinotectal projection from the remaining retinal quadrant by electrical stimulation of the retina and recording from the tectum. He found that the quadrantic projection was restored after regeneration in his animals, with no extraquadrantic overlap. Thus Westerman found no evidence of widespread arborization of regenerated fibres in the tectum. While the possible existence of species differences in this context cannot be ignored, it is possible that an extensive time-series of fish experiments, comparable to those of Gaze and Jacobson on the frog, might reveal an analogous phenomenon in the fish (see next section).

Retinotectal size-disparity in adult goldfish

Apart from such a time-series of experiments as that discussed in the previous section, observations on the restoration of the visual projection from a normal eye to a normal tectum are likely to be somewhat unrewarding in that they can tell us little about the nature of the mechanisms that may be involved. There are many different ways in which optic nerve fibres *could* get back to their proper places in the tectum and we are unlikely to be able to decide what mechanisms are at work merely by studying the end result. If we could introduce a controlled abnormality into the relationship between retina and tectum we might have a better chance of distinguishing between the various possibilities. This was the basis of the experiments of Attardi and Sperry (1963). Electrophysiological experiments, using a comparable approach, have led in some cases to somewhat different results.

The retinotectal projection may be looked upon as the anatomical manifestation of a topological relationship between two surfaces, that of the retina and that of the tectum. If, during regeneration, the retinotectal projection could be artificially constrained so as to "compress" it at the tectal end, or alternatively could be manipulated so as to make the tectal end relatively larger than the retina, then one might investigate the "rigidity" of the mechanism that links retina to tectum. If this mechanism is modifiable to any extent, one might look for a compressed map of the visual field on the tectum in the one case and in the other case an expanded map. I have previously pointed out the difficulties of interpretation that may result when ordinary histological methods are used to tackle such problems.

Jacobson and Gaze (1965) used three different experimental approaches to this problem in adult goldfish. Firstly the retinotectal projection was mapped electrophysiologically before and immediately after lateral hemisection of the optic nerve close to its origin from the retina. At this position in the nerve the fibres are still arranged in an orderly retinotopic fashion, and the field projection to the appropriate half of the tectum was found to be absent after lateral hemisection of the nerve. In another group of fish the nerve was hemisected as before and crushed proximal to the site of section. The animals were then mapped at various intervals after operation. The object of this procedure was to find a stage when regeneration had occurred only of those fibres from the half of the optic nerve that had been crushed but not of those fibres that had been cut as well as crushed. This was an attempt, therefore, to allow half the optic nerve to reinnervate the tectum. The result, while difficult to assess because of the unknown regeneration rates in the various circumstances, suggested that in some cases there was a partial restitution of the field projection to the appropriate part of the tectum. In a third group of animals either the lateral or the medial half of the optic tectum was removed and the corresponding optic nerve crushed. Later electrophysiological mapping indicated that the projection had become appropriately restored to the residual medial or lateral half of the tectum (Fig. 4.30).

Thus these results did not show any kind of plasticity in the regenerating fish retinotectal projection; the findings agreed with the histological work of Attardi and Sperry (1963) and suggested that a rigid place-specificity controlled the regeneration of the optic fibres back to the tectum. There was no evidence of compression of the visual field map when a whole

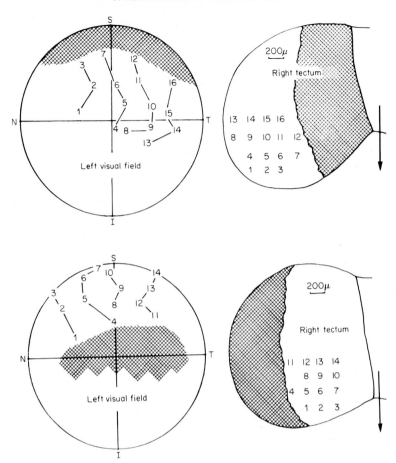

FIG. 4.30. (upper) The projection from the left visual field to the residual lateral part of the tectum in an adult goldfish, mapped 118 days after removal of the medial half of the tectum and crush of the optic nerve. Cross-hatching indicates the extent of the tectal lesion and the corresponding field deficit; (lower) The converse result, 127 days after removal of the lateral half of the tectum in another fish. From Jacobson and Gaze, 1965.

retina regenerated fibres towards the medial or lateral half of the tectum (the other half having been removed at the time the nerve was crushed), nor was there any suggestion of expansion of the map when half the retina was allowed to reinnervate the whole tectum. In each situation only the appropriate part of the visual field map was restored when the fibres regenerated.

Very different results were obtained when a whole optic nerve was allowed to innervate the *rostral* half-tectum in adult goldfish (Gaze and Sharma, 1968; 1970). The considerations leading to this variation on the theme of size-disparity were several. Firstly, the fact that the retina becomes polarized separately along the nasotemporal and dorsoventral axes suggests that the corresponding axes (rostrocaudal and mediolateral) in the tectum may also polarize separately during its development and if so, possibly such axial differences may be manifest during nerve regeneration. It has, in fact, been shown that the rostrocaudal axis of the neural plate becomes polarized before the mediolateral axis (Roach, 1945). Secondly, the occurrence of pattern 2 (Fig. 4.26) during regeneration of the optic nerve in the frog (Gaze and Jacobson, 1963c) suggests axial differences in the control of regenerating fibres. Furthermore, removal of the lateral or medial half of the tectum involves massive injury to the lateral or medial branches of the optic tract and this may affect the nature of the result.

After removal of the caudal half of the optic tectum in adult goldfish (Gaze and Sharma, 1970) without other injury to the optic nerve fibres, the retinotectal projection, mapped over 100 days later, consistently showed reduplication of field positions as they projected to the tectum (Fig. 4.31). The projection from the nasal field to the residual rostral

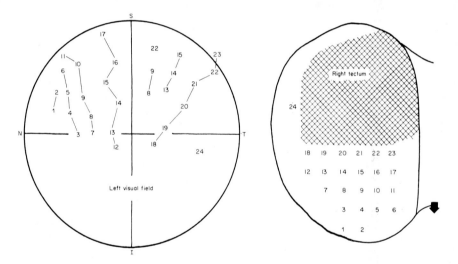

FIG. 4.31. The retinotectal projection 137 days after removal of the caudal half of the right tectum in an adult goldfish. The optic nerve in this experiment was not cut or crushed. Field positions 1–6 are approximately correct. Some of the field positions in rows 7–11 and 12–17 are reduplicated by positions in the temporal field. Positions 18–23 in the field are abnormal in that these positions should project to caudal tectum. The hatched area indicates the tectal lesion. From Gaze and Sharma, 1970.

half-tectum was preserved (points 1–6) but there was also a partial restoration of the "missing" field projection, which went, however, to the residual rostral half-tectum. These positions in the temporal field were found to project in correct sequence across the mediolateral axis of the tectum but were misplaced rostrally along the rostrocaudal axis. When there was more than one row of these temporal field positions, the rows projected to the residual rostral tectum in correct mutual order (Fig. 4.31). Thus several points on the residual rostral half-tectum each received input from two positions in the field; the "correct" field position and a field position which should have projected to the absent caudal half-tectum. In some cases, tectal positions at the caudal end of the residual rostral half-tectum gave responses only from the abnormal temporal field positions.

In these cases the optic nerve was not crushed; the projection to the rostral part of the tectum was therefore not deliberately upset. The only fibres that were cut were those passing to the extirpated caudal region of the tectum. Yet some of these fibres eventually redistributed themselves across the rostral, foreign, tectum, in correct sequence. The nasal part of this projection is presumably made up of the original (uncut) fibres; the central positions in the field are reduplicated, while the far temporal positions project to central tectal positions which do not show responses from their proper places in the field. Thus the projection to the caudal part of the residual rostral half-tectum is inappropriate and these abnormal connections appear to have *displaced* the appropriate ones. When the removal of the caudal half of the tectum was combined with crush of the optic nerve, commonly the result was that the entire visual field projection was compressed onto the residual rostral half-tectum (Fig. 4.32).

The results of these experiments thus suggest that the regenerating fish optic nerve behaves differently according to whether a tectal deficit involves mediolateral halves or rostrocaudal halves. The observations (Gaze and Sharma, 1970) in cases of caudal tectal removal exclude, unequivocally, a rigid place-specification along the rostrocaudal axis of the goldfish tectum. Displaced optic nerve fibres may find their way to a foreign part of the tectum and may there distribute themselves in appropriate retinotopic order. This could not happen if the regenerating fibres were solely specified for certain places on the (missing) caudal half of the tectum. Moreover, we might perhaps have expected the fibres displaced from the caudal tectum to innervate that part of the residual rostral tectum nearest to their home territory. Thus temporal field positions 8 and 9 (Fig. 4.31) would, after displacement from the caudal half-tectum, go to positions 20 and 21 on the residual rostral tectum. This type of distribution of the displaced fibres was never seen; in all cases (although to a greater or lesser extent) the fibres which previously projected to the caudal tectum became redistributed across the residual rostral tectum in "correct" sequence, i.e. nasal to temporal field lying from rostral to caudal on the tectum.

These results could suggest that what happens during nerve regeneration in this situation is not so much that a cell-to-cell interlinkage between retina and tectum is restored, rather the restoration is one of projection-pattern. This is what might be expected to occur if the mode of connection-control were some mechanism working in a graded fashion across the

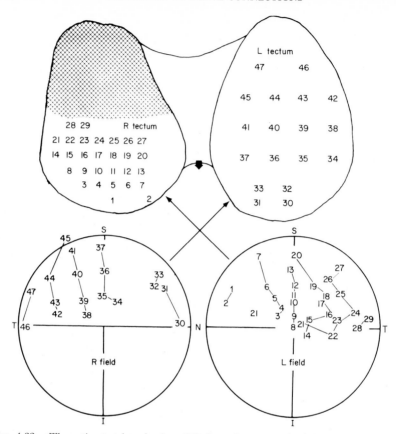

Fig. 4.32. The retinotectal projections 173 days after removal of the caudal half of the right tectum and crush of the left optic nerve in an adult goldfish. The projection from the right eye to the left (normal) tectum shows that the entire dorsal visual field is extended over the entire dorsal surface of the tectum. The projection from the left eye to the operated right tectum is seen to cover approximately the same extent of field although the tectum is reduced by half. It may be seen that, although the spacing of the tectal positions on the left tectum is twice that on the right half-tectum, the spacing of the field rows is comparable in the two cases. From Gaze and Sharma, 1970.

relevant axis of retina and tectum. Thus we could consider that most nasal field (most temporal retina) should connect with most rostral available tectum; and most temporal field (most nasal retina) with most caudal available tectum. In this case, after crushing the optic nerve, we would expect the entire visual field to project (in a compressed fashion rostro-caudally on the tectum) to the residual rostral half-tectum, since most temporal field should project to most caudal tectum, which is now the caudal edge of the residual rostral half-tectum. Either a strict location-specificity or a graded and more plastic control mechanism would give a normal projection, of course, if both eye and tectum were normal; but the projections found in animals with caudal half-tectal removals fit the plastic mechanism better. Our present knowledge of how the retinotectal projection becomes restored during optic nerve regeneration is obviously unsatisfactory; there are too many contradictions about. Yet this state is much to be preferred to an unjustified sense of complacency.

TRANSPLANTATION OF EYES, RETINAL TISSUE AND OPTIC TRACTS

Embryonic eyes have been transplanted to many different sites on the body and for a variety of reasons. Thus Stone (1960) transplanted an eye to the side of the body in *Amblystoma* at stage 36 (Harrison) and later regrafted the eye back into an orbit so as to study the ability of the organ to continue its differentiation in an abnormal site. This experiment could have been made much more interesting if the eye had been explanted before the time of axial polarization and replanted some considerable time afterwards. Detwiler (1928) and Detwiler and Van Dyke (1934) transplanted eyes to a position just caudal to the forelimb, in order to investigate the effect of these grafts on the outgrowth of the limb nerves. Eyes have also been transplanted onto the tails of premetamorphic amphibians and have survived the resorption of tail tissue (Schwind, 1933). In none of the cases just mentioned was any attempt made to study the functional properties of eyes in these abnormal positions; and it would not be expected that optic nerve fibres, even if they succeeded in reaching the central nervous system, would be capable in these situations of finding their suitable intracentral connections. In cases where an eye is transplanted to an abnormal site on the head, however, the possibility exists that the ingrowing optic nerve fibres could make effective connections and permit visual function; it would be worthwhile in such cases to study the central pathways followed by the fibres.

The ingrowth of optic nerve fibres leads to a cellular hyperplasia in the region of brain so innervated. This phenomenon will be discussed in relation to the normal development of the optic tectum (p.183 *et seq.*); here we need only note that it has been shown (May and Detwiler, 1925) that an eye grafted in place of an ear leads also to central enlargement, this time in the medulla. Harrison (1929) has demonstrated that a large eye grafted in place of a normal small one leads to overdevelopment of the optic tectum and a comparable effect has been found when a supernumary eye is added (Pasquini, 1927).

It would be expected that if a grafted supernumary eye were able to establish fibre connections with the brain of the host, it should show visual function. There appears to be only one report, up to the present time, showing that this may happen. Hibbard (1959) transplanted an extra eye on the top of the head in embryos of *Rana pipiens* at stage 17 (Shumway). The operation was such that a piece of donor brain was transplanted with the eye. One of the experimental animals was later shown to have positive optokinetic circling reactions to stimulation of the extra eye, after both normal optic nerves had been cut. This case is not completely satisfactory, however, in that for some reason the animal could only swim in counter clockwise circles. Thus the fact that during stimulation with a striped drum the animal turned more than twice as frequently as when the drum was stationary may merely indicate some form of effective visual input and not necessarily an ordered one. A more or less randomly patterned increase in activity in the brain could perhaps have given the same result.

When an extra eye is transplanted in a *Xenopus* embryo at stage 32 to a site between the two normal eyes, the transplant may in some cases be shown subsequently to connect with the brain. If the optic nerve fibres from the transplant come near the normal course of the optic pathway, they may be seen to join with the normal fibres and apparently head for the tectum (D. Johnston, personal communication). The fibres behave here as though, when they come sufficiently close to part of the normal pathway, they recognize and follow it. When deliberately misled, at a local level, by cross-transplantation of the medial and lateral branches of the optic tract in goldfish, optic fibres tend to cross back into their own pathway (Arora and Sperry, 1962); if the fibres are prevented from uncrossing again by being deeply inserted into the wrong tract, they have been observed to continue in this tract and cross the foreign tectum until they reach their appropriate zones of termination (Arora, 1963).

These findings, taken along with the demonstrated ability for optic fibres to get back to their "proper" places in the tectum, suggest that the fibres may be under the influence of positional information all the way along the central part of the optic tract. Given a chance, optic fibres will follow the correct path to their destinations; prevented from so doing, they may still be able to terminate appropriately, provided that they come close enough to their target. How close this has to be for the fibres to be able to pick up the directional information again is a matter for further experiment. Most interesting in this respect is the work of De Long and Coulombre (1967), who grafted small pieces of embryonic chick retina on to the surface of the optic tectum in somewhat older chick embryos and later observed the direction of outgrowth of fibres from the retinal explants. They found that fibres from a particular quadrant of the retina (explanted) grew preferentially towards specific areas of the tectum (Fig. 4.33) and that the target areas accorded with the known normal distribution of retinal fibres. Regardless of the site of the graft on the tectum the direction taken by outgrowing fibres correlated with the retinal site of origin of the graft. The normal eye had been removed before its fibres grew into the tectum. For both these reasons, the fibres from the graft could not have been simply following the channels that would be taken by normal fibres over the tectum. De Long and Coulombre discounted the possibility that randomly searching pioneering fibres might find matching terminal fields by trial and error, with secondary enlargement of the successful tract by "selective fasciculation" and atrophy of the unsuccessful fibres. They found no evidence of randomly straying fibres; and although the histological method they used (Protargol impregnation) may have been

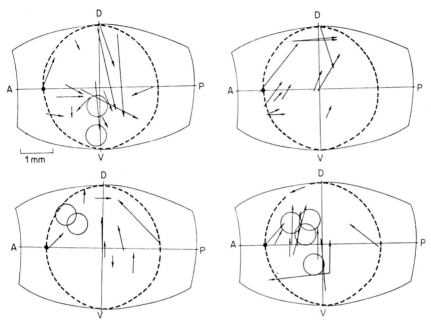

FIG. 4.33. Diagram showing the origin, direction and length of fibre fascicles arising from retinal grafts on the surface of the chick embryonic tectum. The small circles represent grafts whose fibres penetrated directly into the tectum beneath the graft. The results obtained with retinal grafts from each quadrant of the eye are presented separately: Top left, Seventeen grafts of dorsal retina; Bottom left, Eleven grafts of ventral retina; Top right, Ten grafts of nasal retina; Bottom right, Fifteen grafts of temporal retina. The fibres appear to head for the appropriate region of tectum. From De Long and Coulombre, 1967.

inadequate to allow fine fibres to be followed, yet the fascicles seen ran in straight lines towards the target regions. This suggests that the fibres were guided throughout their course; moreover, it suggests very strongly that the guidance mechanism functions on axial gradient, or coordinate-system principles, and not on the basis of individually specified cells.

REGENERATION IN THE URODELE VISUAL SYSTEM

Whereas in anurans the retina remains virtually intact after section of the optic nerve, in urodeles this is not so. In these animals, after optic nerve section and after eye transplantation, the entire retina degenerates and is eventually replaced by regeneration from the cells of the ciliary margin of the retina (Gaze and Watson, 1968). Burgen and Grafstein (1962; Grafstein and Burgen, 1964) have used this phenomenon in an investigation of the effects of various operations on the eye in *Triturus viridescens.* They removed the front portion of the eye, removed the retina from the back of the eye, then replaced the front part either with or without various degrees of rotation with respect to the back of the eye. In some

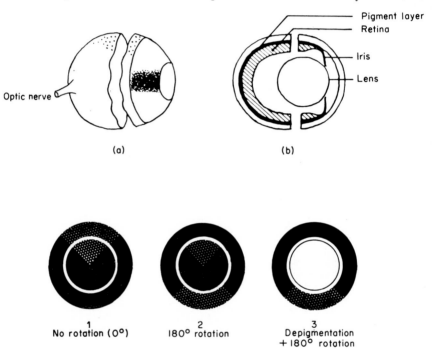

FIG. 4.34.   Types of operation on the newt eye in the experiments of Burgen and Grafstein; (a) Diagram of right eye transected a short distance behind the cornea-scleral junction, seen from its posterolateral aspect: (b) Diagram of longitudinal section through eye after transection, indicating the structures on the inside of the eye attached to each portion of the eyeball: 1, 2, 3: Diagrammatic representation of pigment layer following various experimental procedures, with dotted region indicating position of original superior quadrant. (1) Corneal part of eye replaced in its original orientation, central part of pigment layer left intact. (2) Corneal part of eye rotated through 180°, central part of pigment layer left intact. (3) Corneal part of eye rotated through 180°, central part of pigment layer removed. From Grafstein and Burgen, 1964.

cases they removed the pigment epithelium from the back of the eye as well (Fig. 4.34). The animals were kept for 4–7 months and then were used to map the electrophysiological projection from regenerated retina to the tectum.

In four animals in which the pigment epithelium had not been removed from the back of the eye, and the corneal part of the eye had been replaced in normal orientation, the regenerated retinotectal projection was normal.

After rotation of the front part of the eye a variety of abnormal projections were, however, found (Fig. 4.35). In nine out of 12 animals in which the front of the eye had been rotated, the tectal representation of the central region of the retina was displaced but in all cases the orientation of central and peripheral projections was similar; i.e. if the central projection was rotated, so was the peripheral projection and if the one was normal, so was the other. Among 11 animals in which the pigment layer had been removed from the back of the eye, three had also had the front of the eye rotated; and two of these showed a normally oriented visual projection.

These results are extremely interesting; but it is difficult to make a coherent story out of them—and this is made more difficult by the way in which the authors present their data. Grafstein and Burgen (1964) assume that the regenerating retina comes from the underlying pigment epithelium. The autoradiographic studies of Gaze and Watson (1968) however, show that this is probably not so. The new retina that regenerates after degeneration of the old one originates mainly in the cells of the ciliary margin which is also the region from which the continued growth of the adult new retina occurs (Fig. 4.36). This could account for the observation that the central part of each projection showed in each case the same orientation as the peripheral part.

The results of Burgen and Grafstein, and those of Gaze and Watson, serve to focus our attention on the question of the origin of retinal place specificity. If we accept the need for some form of retinal specification in order to account for non-random regeneration, how might this specificity spread over the array of retinal ganglion cells? In the developing retina, as will be discussed shortly, the number of these cells present at the time axial polarization occurs is very small compared to the number present in the adult. Most of the retinal ganglion cells develop *after* retinal polarization has occurred. These cells would then have to acquire their specificities in some way different to the original mode of axial specification. Conceivably these ganglion cells become specified via their close relationships to other cells in the eye, for instance the pigment epithelium; or perhaps they acquire their characteristics during the orderly process of cell division in the germinal zone at the retinal margin.

If specificity is to be assigned to the retinal ganglion cells in Sperry's sense, the events taking place during retinal regeneration and restoration of the retinotectal projection in adult newts become even more intriguing. Most of the new retina comes from the cells at the ciliary margin; the first cells to appear move in across the back of the eye and take up positions near the centre of the eye; later cells add on nearer the retinal periphery. Thus those cells near the fundus are in this sense "older" than the cells at the edge of the retina.

One would like to know what happens to the specificity characteristics of these new retinal cells as they progressively alter their retinal position.

A suggestion as to what may be happening comes from the work of Cronly-Dillon (1968), who investigated the retinotectal projection at various intervals after removal of the newt retina. The normal newt retinotectal projection has already been illustrated (Fig. 4.16). Cronly-Dillon found that,

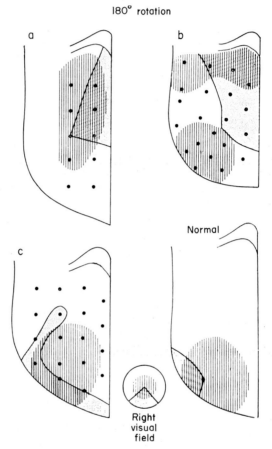

FIG. 4.35.   Types of visual projection formed after retinal regeneration in the newt. A, B, C: Diagrams of some patterns of retinal projection, observed in different animals after retinal regeneration following 180° rotation of corneal portion of pigment layer with central portion of pigment layer left intact. The vertically hatched region indicates the representation of the central visual field, extending to 50° from the centre. The dotted region indicates the representation of the inferior quadrant of the visual field. The large dots indicate the recording points on each tectum. The parallel rows of recording points are 200 microns apart; (a) Case no. 5. Representation of central field abnormally located; orientation of representation rotated (only part of tectum explored); (b) Case no. 44. Dual representation of central field; orientation of part of representation rotated; (c) Case no. 88. Representation of central field normally located; orientation of representation unrotated. Normal: Diagram of normal tectum, with only one recording point, representing the centre of the visual field indicated. Inset diagram represents right visual field, showing portions of field whose tectal representations are indicated. From Burgen and Grafstein, 1962.

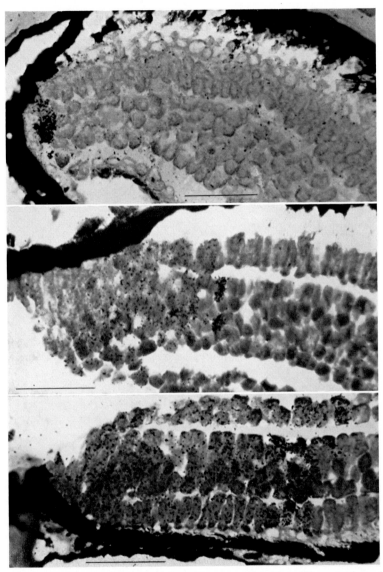

FIG. 4.36.   The continued growth of the adult newt retina. Top: The animal was killed 24 hours after administration of ^{3}H-thymidine. A couple of cells are labelled at the retinal margin, but there is no label anywhere else in the retina; Middle: Autoradiograph from an animal 91 days after it had received ^{3}H-thymidine. All cells near the retinal margin are labelled. Bottom; 168 days after administration of ^{3}H-thymidine. The label has spread further along the retina and is heaviest where the labelled region joins the un-labelled retina. Calibrations 50 μ. After Gaze and Watson, 1968.

some five months after operation, the multi-unit receptive fields recorded from the tectal regions receiving input from the peripheral parts of the retina were larger than normal; whereas receptive fields from the tectal region to which the central retina projected were more or less normal in size (Fig. 4.16). The receptive field characteristics of single optic fibres at this time were normal. By nine months and one year after operation the multi-unit receptive fields were generally smaller and more uniform in size over the entire retinotectal projection, which was nearly normal topographically by this time.

These observations are consonant with the findings (Gaze and Watson, 1968) that central retina is older than peripheral retina in the regenerated newt visual system. The central ganglion cells have been in existence longest, and have had the longest time to establish tectal connections. The peripheral ganglion cells, on the other hand, are more recent and have had less time for retinotectal connections to form. It may be that the accuracy of tectal localization shown by regenerating optic nerve fibres in this situation varies inversely with the "maturity" of the ganglion cells.

THE DEVELOPMENT OF THE RETINOTECTAL PROJECTION AND THE FOOTBALL FIELD PROBLEM

Regeneration of the optic nerve may lead to the recovery of visual function. Before there is any point in asking how such functional recovery is achieved, it will be as well for us to consider further *what* is restored during optic nerve regeneration. Many aspects of visual performance are certainly recovered, both on behavioural and electrophysiological criteria. But the question of most concern is what is happening to the regrowing fibres themselves. The evidence so far discussed indicates that these get back to their proper places in the tectum. So we can now usefully ask, what is meant by the term "proper places"? The reason for asking this question can be illustrated by what I call (with apologies to Lewis Wolpert) the Football Field Problem. This problem can be expressed in the following fashion: in Association Football a team consists of a certain number of men who each have their proper playing positions on the field. When they run out at the beginning of a game, the members of the team each take up their appropriate standing positions. How do they know where to go?

There are four main categories of method, whereby the footballers could determine their positions of the field: (1) Each man could go and stand on his own square of turf, appropriately and recognizably labelled for him; (2) Each player could decide his proper place with reference to the totality of the group as a whole and not with reference to numbered positions on the ground. In this case the team would need to have some reference points on the field itself to permit them to orient the group with relation to the field. But apart from these field reference points, the group would be a self-organizing system with relation to their individual positions. There are, of course, many ways in which such self-organization could be achieved within the group of players; the "numbering off" procedure by which a military unit attains a ceremonial drill formation is one. (3) The team members could be positioned on the field by some form of "ballistic" control; an individual player could be told to run so many steps straight out on to the field, then turn 90° left (or right), run a further series of numbered steps, then stop. (4) Each player could have a particular starting place in the pavilion, and a certain orientation; on the word "go", he would run out blindly, bouncing from side to side of the alley leading to the field, and end up running in a direction determined by the sum total of his ricochets. He would either stop when he ran out of wind or else *be* stopped by being tripped over a raised piece of turf, cunningly arranged beforehand by providence in the form of the team-manager.

In our neurological context we can at once forget mechanism (3), the ballistic programme; the evidence from optic nerves grown back to the tectum via abnormal paths (Gaze, 1959; Hibberd, 1967), from rotated embryonic eyes, and the selection of appropriate terminal depths in the tectum by regenerating fibres despite the fact that the tectum is thinner than normal (Gaze and Keating, 1969) exclude this form of control. It is highly likely that we can also ignore mechanism (4), which biologically corresponds to the "accident of development" approach. The same experiments that excluded mechanism (3), together with the observations on the direction of growth of fibres from retinal grafts on the tectum (De Long and Coulombre, 1967) appear to rule out mechanism (4). This leaves us with mechanisms (1) and (2).

The relevance of these two approaches to team arrangement on the football field is that they both deal with pattern formation and they each give a different answer in different situations. On the "numbered place" mechanism, the team will be in trouble if some adjacent landowner decides to chop a bit off the field on one side. In this case, some of the team's numbered positions will be gone and there is no provision for reallocating the displaced men. Likewise, on this mechanism the team would be unable to cope with its situation if the game were to be played "seven-a-side". On the other hand, if the team used one of the self-organization methods for allocating field positions, there would be no difficulty in closing up the pattern to cope with a decreased size of field, or opening up the pattern to provide for an increase in playing space. This consideration of the Football Field Problem suggests some questions that we might usefully ask of the system of regenerating (or developing) optic nerve fibres; and these matters are discussed in the following sections. Before we can consider further the question of regeneration, however, it will be helpful if we look at the normal development of the visual system.

The development of the eye, optic nerve and retinotectal projection

The eyes develop as outgrowths from the developing forebrain and the early stages of this process do not concern us at the present time; they are dealt with in detail by Lopashov and Stroeva (1963). We are interested particularly in the mode of development of the connections between eye and brain with special reference to the setting up during neurogenesis of the topographical retinotectal map.

The early work of Sperry (1943b; 1944; 1945b) and the later electro-physiological experiments discussed previously show that in adult amphibians (and fishes) the normal point to point projection from the retina to the tectum may be restored during regeneration of the optic nerve. This topographical relationship between eye and tectum however, only becomes determined, in the embryological sense, at a certain stage of embryonic development. Stone (1960) rotated the eye and cut the optic nerve in *Amblystoma* at various stages of development. He found that if the operation was performed after stage 36 (Harrison) the animals later had reversed vision; whereas animals in which the operation was performed earlier (up to late tail-bud stages) developed with normal vision. Thus prior to stage 36 the system is capable of "regulation"; but at or about this stage something happens in the developing retina which is later manifest as a specification of the retina in terms of the tectal connections it forms. After stage 36 in these animals the retina is polarized such that from then on nasal retina will only connect with caudal tectum and temporal retina with rostral tectum.

The polarization of the retina occurs separately along the three axes of space. As was suggested by Sperry (1945b) and shown by Székely (1954b), the retina of *Triturus* acquires its definitive nasotemporal axis before it is specified along the dorsoventral axis. This has since been elegantly confirmed by Jacobson (1967a; 1968a) for *Xenopus* by electrophysiological recording. This author rotated eyes at various stages from 28 to 35 (Nieuwkoop and Faber, 1956) and later mapped the retinotectal projections after metamorphosis. Animals in which the eye had been rotated 180° before stage 30 showed normal projections; those in which the rotation had been performed at stage 30 gave a map in which the projection was inverted in the nasotemporal axis but normal in the dorsoventral axis (Fig. 4.37). When the eye was rotated after stage 30 the result was complete inversion of the tectal projection across both axes. Thus in *Xenopus* nasotemporal polarization occurs at around stage 30 and dorsoventral polarization very shortly afterwards, within a period of a few hours. Polarization of the retina across the third dimension (inner-outer) has been shown to occur (in *Hyla*) later still (Eakin, 1942).

At stage 30–31 therefore, some events of differentiation occur which specify the retina in terms of surface position; and Jacobson has further correlated these events with the cessation of DNA synthesis in the ganglion cells (Jacobson, 1968b). Using autoradiography of embryos labelled at various stages with tritiated thymidine, Jacobson showed that DNA synthesis ceased in the ganglion cell layer at stage 29. Thus all the cells that will form ganglion cells and hence become specified by stage 30–31 have ceased DNA replication some hours previously; and Jacobson suggests that neuronal specification of this sort may thus involve the synthesis of specific macromolecules.

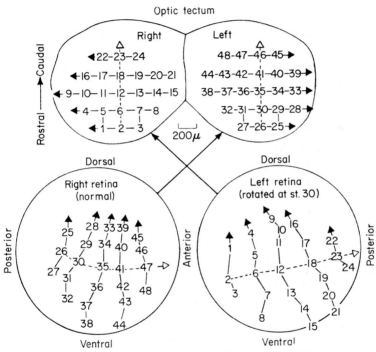

FIG. 4.37. The retinotectal projection in adult *Xenopus* to the left tectum from the normal right retina, and to the right tectum from the left retina which had been rotated 180° at larval stage 30. The projection from the left retina is normal in the dorsoventral axis but is inverted in the anteroposterior axis. From Jacobson, 1968a.

At the time at which retinal polarization occurs there are some 500 or so ganglion cells in the developing retina, none of which has yet put out an axon. In adult *Xenopus*, on the other hand, there are some 50,000 fibres in an optic nerve and, presumably, a similar number of ganglion cells in the eye. Thus the number of ganglion cells increases 100-fold between the time of polarization and adult life in *Xenopus*; and in *Rana* the factor is probably nearer 1000, since each optic nerve in the adult contains nearly half a million fibres. Those ganglion cells that originally populated the retina at stage 30, if they still exist in later life, must make but a small contribution to the adult retina. Where then do all the remaining ganglion cells come from, and how do they become specified appropriately?

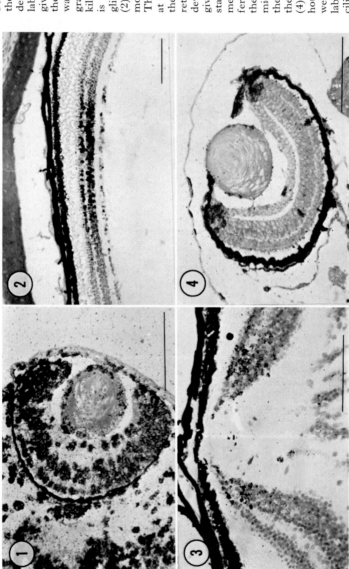

FIG. 4.38. The development of the retina in *Xenopus laevis*. The developing retina was pulse-labelled with ³H-thymidine, given as a single injection into the embryo or larva; the animal was later killed for autoradiography. (1) Injected stage 30, killed stage 40. Most of the eye is labelled. Some central ganglion cells are not. Bar, 100 μ. (2) Injected stage 30, killed 3 months after metamorphosis. This shows the site of the label at the very back of the fundus; the whole of the rest of the retina was unlabelled, i.e. had developed *after* the label was given. Bar, 100 μ. (3) Injected stage 30, killed 3 months after metamorphosis. This is a different (adjacent) section from the same animal as the previous micrograph. This section shows the localization of the label at the optic nerve head. Bar, 100 μ. (4) Injected stage 45, killed 3 hours later. The retina is by now well formed and the site of the label shows that the cells at the ciliary margin are incorporating thymidine. Bar, 100 μ.

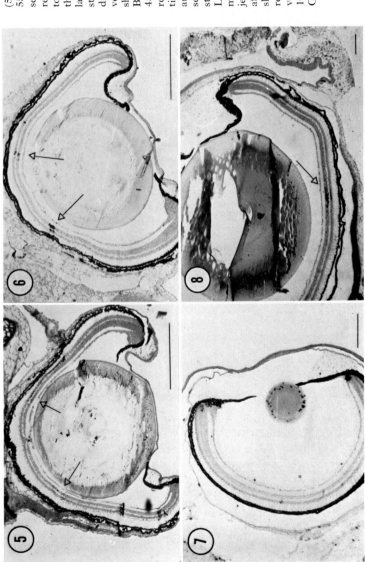

(5) Injected stage 45, killed stage 55. The label is confined, in the section, to two small regions of retina, closer to the fundus than to the ciliary margin. Thus the fundal retina between the labelled areas developed before stage 45, whereas the retina distal to the labelled areas developed after stage 45. Arrows show the two labelled regions. Bar, 300 μ. (6) Injected stage 45, killed stage 61. Again, two regions of label (arrows). This time the distal regions of retina are larger than in the previous section. Bar, 300 μ. (7) Injected stage 58, killed 12 hours later. Labelled cells only at the retinal margins. Bar, 200 μ. (8) Injected stage 58, killed 3 months after metamorphosis. The arrow shows a region of retinal label; retina distal to this has developed later than stage 58. Bar, 100 μ. From Straznicky and Gaze, 1970.

The answer to the first of these questions is that virtually the whole of the adult amphibian retina is formed by mitosis of cells at the ciliary margin; this mitosis taking place after the stage at which the retinal anlage becomes polarized. The existence of this germinal zone at the ciliary margin was emphasized by Glucksmann (1940) and Stone (1959); and autoradiography with tritiated thymidine (Straznicky and Gaze, 1970) shows that the increase in the size of the retina of *Xenopus* tadpoles is due to the addition of new cells from the retinal ciliary margin (Fig. 4.38). When the label is given as a single dose later than stage 50 the eventual localization of the marked cells in the postmetamorphic retina is some distance in from the ciliary margin, indicating that all the lightly-labelled and unlabelled cells nearer the margin were formed after the administration of the thymidine. When the label is given early in larval life, shortly after the time of retinal polarization, little label is to be found in the retina later than stage 50 and what there is to be found is all at the back of the fundus. The role played by cell death in the development of the retina is not clearly understood. Glucksmann (1940; 1965) has drawn attention to waves of cell degeneration that occur in the developing frog retina at stages up to the time of overt histological differentiation. An interesting and presently unsolved question is why these retinal cells should degenerate and one is tempted to compare the retinal situation with that of the dorsal root ganglion or the ventral horn, discussed in a previous chapter.

The fact that the amphibian retina is continually adding cells to increase its size throughout larval, and into adult life, raises interesting problems about cell specification and retinotectal connections. It is usually assumed that, in these animals, during the initial ingrowth of optic fibres to the tectum, the adult projection pattern, or something close to it, is straightway set up. While this may be so, we must emphasize that there is as yet no evidence whatever for this assumption. Argument from the nature of visual function to the type of fibre connection cannot be used in this situation and the earliest electrophysiological recordings deal with the projection in late larval and early postmetamorphic life.

The only relevant evidence available on the early development of the retinotectal projection in amphibians comes from the eventual results of eye rotation in embryonic life. The fact that rotation of the eye by 180° after retinal polarization, and rotation between the times of nasotemporal and dorsoventral polarization, in both cases before optic fibres grow out to the tectum, results in complete inversion of the field projection, or inversion across a single axis respectively, shows clearly that the tectal distribution of the optic nerve fibres is not a mere reflection of mechanical guidance factors or timing differences in the ingrowth of the fibres. Thus even in the original development of the retinotectal projection there is strong evidence in favour of a specific topological relationship between retinal surface and tectal surface which cannot be accounted for in any simple fashion. And during larval life, after the time of retinal polarization, new ganglion cells are continuously being added to the retinal margin as the eye grows larger. Retinotectal connections probably first appear in *Xenopus* at about stages 35–38; and the evidence from optic nerve fibre counts (Gaze and Wilson, unpublished) and autoradiography of the retina (Straznicky and Gaze, 1970) shows that extensive increase in the number of ganglion cells occurs after this time. We may assume, although this has never been demonstrated, that the newly developing ganglion cells send their fibres to the growing periphery of the tectum. This would be expected, since the new ganglion cells appear at the ciliary margins of the retina and these project, in the adult, round the topological "neck" of the tectum; that is, along the dorsomedial edge and its continuation ventromedially. Since the newly added ganglion cells thereafter behave, when regenerating, as if they are specified in terms of retinal position, we have to assume that whatever form of cell specification may occur here is either transmitted to daughter cells during mitosis in some fashion or else is impressed on the new cells by close contact with, for instance, the pigment epithelium. Since this latter is also increasing in extent during development of the eye we are driven back to the idea that cell specificity is transmitted by some form of asymmetric cell division at the retinal margin.

Development and differentiation in the tectum

Sperry's hypothesis of neuronal specificity involves an intercellular recognition phenomenon. Specified retinal ganglion cells produce specified axons, which eventually connect up with specified tectal cells. Such a hypothesis requires that the tectum as well as the retina be specified, and in a complementary or matching fashion. As a result of operations on the eye anlage performed at various stages of development (Székely, 1954b; Jacobson, 1967a; 1968a) we now know the stages at which retinal polarization occurs—and with considerable precision in the case of *Xenopus*. When does the tectum become polarized, and is tectal polarization related to the ingrowth of optic nerve fibres?

Obviously the simplest and most direct way of answering these questions would be to do for the tectum what has so successfully been done for the eye: rotate it at various stages and observe the effects on the retinotectal projection. Unfortunately this has not so far proved feasible. Crelin (1952) rotated one optic tectum in *Amblystoma* at stages from 23 to 35 (Harrison) and later investigated the vision of the operated animals. He found that tectal rotation up to stage 35, although giving increasingly deficient function the later the operation was performed, did not qualitatively alter visual response. Operation at later stages was unsuccessful on account of technical difficulties. Thus Crelin's experiments suggest that tectal polarization had not taken place by stage 35, although the existence of considerable tectal regeneration after operation makes the result unreliable.

Tectal rotations have been attempted also in larvae of *Xenopus* at various stages (G. Székely, R. M. Gaze, L. Beazley and M. J. Keating, unpublished) with no success; histological examination of operated embryos shortly after tectal rotation mostly failed to show evidence of successful grafting; and electrophysiological recording from some operated animals gave no indication of the existence of a graft, rotated or otherwise. Unfortunately negative evidence here is without value and we must conclude that tectal rotation experiments have so far not been successful in throwing any light on the question of the time of tectal polarization.

There is considerable evidence that optic nerve fibres arriving at the tectum play an important role in its further differentiation, whether or not they are concerned in tectal place specification. Harrison (1929) transplanted eyes between embryos of *A. punctatum* and *T. tigrinum* and found that the larger eye of *tigrinum* in a *punctatum* host led to increase in size and cellular hyperplasia of the corresponding contralateral tectum; and conversely when a small eye was transplanted into a large host. The existence of some form of reciprocal effect on the eye was suggested by Harrison's observation that, in those eyes that failed to connect with the brain, the ganglion cell counts were considerably lower than in the normal eye.

The cellular differentiation of the optic tectum is intimately related to the ingrowth of optic nerve fibres. In *Rana pipiens* the early optic tectum is composed of cells alone, but as optic fibres arrive at embryonic stage 23 (Shumway), cells start detaching from the embryonic central gray to become the first cells to populate what later will be the superficial layers of the tectum (Kollros, 1953); the rim of optic nerve fibres slowly advances over the surface of the tectum, but not until larval stage IV (Taylor and Kollros) does a thin layer of fibres cover the caudal pole of the lobe. Enucleation of an eye before it connects with the tectum leads to hypoplasia of the corresponding tectum. Histochemical study of the developing tectum of *Rana pipiens* shows that, at stage 25, when the optic fibres have begun to cover the rostral pole, there is already considerable cholinesterase present in the rostral half of the tectum; whereas the enzyme can only be found in the caudal tectum by stage VI. Enucleation of an eye at stage 23 resulted in marked hypoplasia of the contralateral tectum by stage XII and along with this there occurred also a substantial reduction in the specific cholinesterase activity of the affected lobe; thus part of the cholinesterase development in the optic tectum is in some way dependent on the presence of optic nerve fibres (Boell *et al.*, 1955).

Removal of an eye at a time when nervous connections with the brain have already been established is also followed by deficient development of the contralateral tectum in amphibians, as shown by the observation that dendrites on the affected side are shorter and branch less profusely than those on the normal side (Larsell, 1931). The effect of temporary interruption of the optic nerve during larval life on the development of the tectum was studied by McMurray (1954) in *Xenopus*. She found that the pattern of innervation in the normal animal was similar to that described for *Rana pipiens* by Kollros (1953). Enucleation of an eye before the optic fibres reached the tectum resulted in hypoplasia of the affected tectum to the extent that, at metamorphosis, there were only 54% of the normal complement of tectal cells present. McMurray showed that the movement of tectal cells out into the superficial layers was in all probability a direct effect of the ingrowth of optic nerve fibres, since temporary interruption of the optic nerve, by crushing, gave a rapid suppression of migration of cells from the deep layers of the tectum. Information is thus transferred to the tectum by the presence of optic nerve fibres; and it is tempting to speculate on the possible relationship between this information and the passage of substances along the optic nerve, which has been demonstrated autoradiographically (Grafstein, 1967). The fact that section of the optic nerve in the adult fish or amphibian, when tectal development may be expected to be complete, leads to a diminution in tectal thickness, suggests that some differentiated cells may degenerate under these conditions; this effect has been demonstrated in the young mouse by autoradiography with tritiated thymidine (De Long and Sidman, 1962); most neurons had undergone final mitotic division by embryonic day 13 and after enucleation at birth some 40% of these neurones disappeared on the affected side. Most neuroglial cells, in the other hand, arose after birth; and about 45% of those due to appear on post-natal day three failed to form on the deafferented side. Thus here many deafferented neurones degenerated and many cells due to form later failed to do so, as a result of enucleation.

The most successful attempt so far to demonstrate independent tectal specification during development has been the work of De Long and Coulombre (1965) on the chick embryo. Using a modified Bodian Protargol staining method these authors first determined the timing of the innervation of the optic tectum in normal embryos. They found that the first optic fibres reached the rostroventral region of the tectum by 6 days of incubation and that there was thereafter a steady progression of fibres across the tectum until by 12 days the entire tectal surface was covered by optic fibres. Next, De Long and Coulombre demonstrated that localized retinal lesions made at day 3 of incubation could be repaired; and the resulting tectal projection was normal when examined at 12 days; the eye at day 3 is still capable of regulation. In contrast to the findings with operation at day 3, localized (quadrantic) retinal lesions made at day 4–5 yielded permanently scarred retinae and abnormal tectal projections (Fig. 4.39). There was in each case a deficit in tectal innervation which corresponded with the quadrant of retina which had been removed. Since the retinal lesions were made at day 4–5, that is, *before* the first fibres had connected with the tectum, the systematic abnormalities found in the tectal coverage suggest that the

7

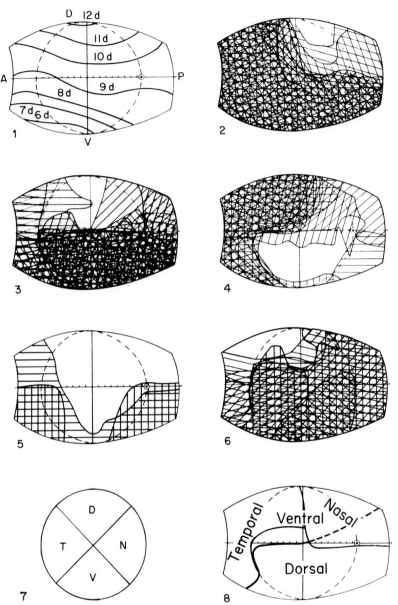

FIG. 4.39.　The development of the retinotectal projection in the chick. (1) The mode and timing of innervation of the tectum by optic nerve fibres. This, and the other diagrams, represent equal area representations of the tectal surface. The lateral aspect of the surface is shown between the dashed lines; the hidden medial surface has been folded out to obtain a two-dimensional representation. The left tectum is shown in this figure with the directional orientation (anterior, posterior, dorsal and ventral) as shown. The advancing border of optic nerve fibres growing onto the tectal surface in normal development, as determined from silver-stained specimens, is indicated by the lines labelled with the days of incubation. The tectum is completely covered by 12 days.

[Caption continued at foot of page 187]

tectum had already become specified before the optic fibres reached it; or anyway that tectal specification was independent of the influence of the ingrowing optic nerve fibres.

The Football Field Problem and the Retinotectal Projection: The effects of introducing a retinotectal size-disparity in the embryo

The essence of the problem under discussion is, in biological terms, whether during regeneration of the optic nerve the various fibres get back to their proper places on a "place to place" basis, with each fibre seeking its uniquely labelled termination site in the tectum; or whether what is restored is the *pattern* of the projection, with the various fibres sorting out at tectal level with respect to the positions of all the others, and with orientation of the pattern with relation to the tectum. I must state at the outset that the evidence bearing on this matter is conflicting and further-more, if we are to present the facts adequately we must consider the results of some embryological experiments on the visual system.

In neuroembryological work on visual localization, Székely (1954a) demonstrated that animals which had been given surgically-constructed "double-nasal" (NN) or "double-temporal" (TT) eyes at the appropriate stage of development, later behaved, in their visual pursuit reactions, as if the entire visual field were temporal, or nasal. After destruction of the rostral half of the tectum (to which the temporal retina (nasal field) normally projects), the animals with TT retinae (NN visual field) behaved as if they were totally blind; whereas animals with NN retinae (TT visual field) became blind when the caudal half of the tectum was destroyed.

These results could thus be taken as suggesting that the fibres from each (similar) half-eye grow only to the appropriate part of the tectum; nasal retina to caudal tectum; temporal retina to rostral tectum, leaving the other half of the tectum in each case without optic afferents. Later electro-physiological analysis of the retinotectal projection from compound eyes in *Xenopus*, however, as discussed below, showed that this is not the case. The observations on compound eyes show clearly the inadequacy of such behavioural experiments for the determination of the nature of fibre projections.

(2–6). Distribution of optic fibres on the left tectum following ablations of segments of the contralateral retina at 4–5 days. The area covered by fibres in an individual specimen is indicated by parallel ruled lines; several specimens are superimposed on diagrams 2, 3, 4 and 6; two specimens are superimposed on diagram 5. (2) Ablation of nasal quadrant of retina; the posterodorsal quadrant of tectum is bare of fibres; (3) Ablation of ventral quadrant of retina; the dorsal tectum is bare; (4) Ablation of dorsal quadrant of retina; the ventral tectum is bare; (5) Ablation of both dorsal and ventral quadrants of retina; both dorsal and ventral tectum are bare; (6) Ablation of temporal quadrant of retina; the anterodorsal tectum is bare; (7) Diagram of the right eye showing the designation of retinal quadrants used in this work. D, dorsal; N, nasal; V, ventral; T, temporal; (8) Composite map of the optic fibre projection on the optic tectum in the 12 day embryo. The labels refer to the retinal quadrants. From De Long and Coulombre, 1965.

The projections from NN and TT compound eyes

In a series of experiments on *Xenopus* the retinotectal projections from compound eyes were investigated electrophysiologically (Gaze *et al.*, 1963; 1965). Operations were performed on embryos at stages 30–32 (Nieuwkoop and Faber, 1956), when the nasotemporal axial polarization of the retina had already occurred, but before any nerve connections had yet formed between the developing eye and the brain. The operation involved cutting one eye cup vertically into a nasal and a temporal half; the temporal half was removed and replaced by a nasal half taken from another animal, to form a NN compound eye; and conversely to form a TT eye. The operated animals were then reared beyond metamorphosis and later used to map the electrophysiological projection from the operated eye to the optic tectum.

The retinotectal projection in a normal *Xenopus* has been illustrated in Fig. 4.14. The entire dorsal surface of the tectum is taken up by the retinal projection, with nasal field (temporal retina) projecting rostrally and temporal field (nasal retina) projecting caudally. The contralateral projection from a NN compound eye (TT field), however, turns out to be very different (Fig. 4.40). The original nasal half retina (original temporal field) projects, in appropriate order, across the *whole* dorsal surface of the tectum, which in a normal animal receives input from the entire retina. Thus the projection of the original half-retina is normally organized across the lateromedial axis of the tectum (dorsoventral axis of the visual field) but is spread-out or extended over a greater-than-usual extent of tectum in the rostrocaudal axis. Similarly, the transplanted half-retina connects, also in appropriate order, with the whole of the tectum; but the order of projection is now appropriate to the *original* nasal position of this half-eye, and *not* to its actual temporal position in the orbit. Thus (Fig. 4.40) each tectal position receives input from two positions in the visual field (retina) and these tend to be disposed symmetrically about the vertical meridian of the field.

The contralateral projection from a TT compound eye (NN field) shows the same type of systematic abnormality; but in this case it is the original temporal half-retina (nasal field) which projects in appropriate order across the whole of the tectum, with a mirrored projection from the transplanted temporal half-retina (Fig. 4.41). The ipsilateral visual projections in animals with compound eyes may also show systematic abnormalities (Gaze *et al.*, 1965; Gaze *et al.*, 1970), and these are discussed in the next chapter.

The nature of the retinotectal maps from compound eyes (Figs 4.40 and 4.41) suggest that the tectal arrangement of fibres from ganglion cells distributed along the intact axis of the eye (dorsoventral) is normal, whereas ganglion cells distributed along the cut axis (nasotemporal) spread out their tectal terminations to cover the full extent of the rostrocaudal tectal

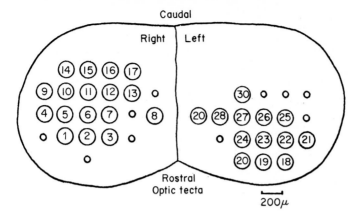

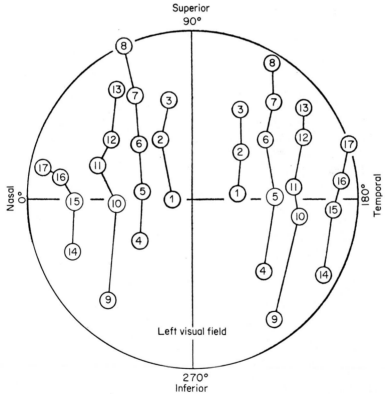

FIG. 4.40.   The contralateral retinotectal projection from a compound NN eye in *Xenopus*. The left eye, which is NN, projects contralaterally to the right tectum. The numbers on the left tectum refer to a different field chart not shown in this illustration. Small open circles on the tecta are positions from which no responses could be obtained. It may be seen that each half of the compound eye effectively connects with the whole of the contra-lateral (right) tectum and that the order of the projection is correct for the temporal half-field (nasal half-retina) and reversed for the other half-field. From Gaze, Jacobson and Székely, 1963.

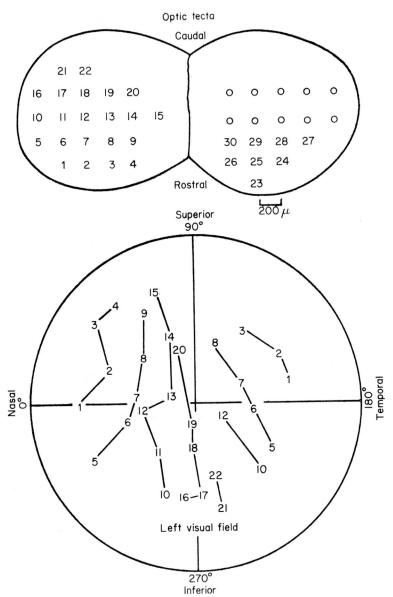

FIG. 4.41.   The contralateral retinotectal projection from a compound TT eye in *Xenopus*. The left eye, which is TT, projects contralaterally to the right tectum. The numbers on the left tectum refer to a different field chart not shown here. It may be seen that each half of the compound eye effectively connects with the whole of the contralateral (right) tectum and that the order of the projection is in this case correct for the nasal half-field (temporal half-retina) and reversed for the other half-field. From Gaze, Jacobson and Székely, 1963.

axis. Thus ganglion cells in each half of a compound eye appear to be able to "slide" their connections across the tectum. In terms of the Football Field Problem, the compound eye is analogous to a football team that has been cut in half along a line running between the two goals, and the team reconstituted by putting two similar halves together. Thus there would be two "left forwards", two "left backs", etc. The field (that is, the tectum) is considered to be normal size. Any team constituted in this fashion, provided that it was made up of reasonably intelligent players, would at once reorganize itself so that the "grafted" half-team took over the functions of the missing half-team. Thus the extra left half-team would "respecify" themselves and take on the character of a right half-team. Such a team, in other words, would be expected to be able to alter its polarity.

This is not what happens in the retinotectal situation. Here, the analogy would be with a football team that had to retain its left-right polarity. Thus if the first man orients in relation to the edge of the field, each other player numbers off from his proper team-mate on the left, and the resulting team pattern has to adjust to the size of the field, then, with a compound LL team, made up of unintelligent players, we would expect to find the characteristic pattern of the left half of a team reproduced, and spread across the field, but with two players at each position. Density of players at a particular point, it seems, is irrelevant.

To return to the biological situation: both normal development and neural regeneration lead to the setting-up of a consistent normal pattern of retinotectal connections. Sperry's hypothesis states that these orderly connections reflect the existence of matching neuronal specificities in retina and tectum. The specificity hypothesis may be formulated in various ways. For instance, we may postulate that the distinctive differences between parts of the retina are specificities of a discontinuous nature (rather like the locking mechanisms of a sophisticated jig-saw puzzle) as could be the case if an immunological type of specification were involved. Such a system appears to me to be inherently unlikely in this situation; and moreover the compound eye projections indicate that such a hypothesis is incorrect, at least in the assumption of a parallel and independent development of tectal specificities. In normal *Xenopus* fibres from the temporal half of the retina go to the rostral part of the tectum and fibres from nasal retina go to the caudal part of the tectum. Yet in an animal with an NN retina fibres from this nasal retina go to virtually the entire contralateral tectum (Fig. 4.40) and the same is true for fibres from the TT retina (Fig. 4.41). Thus one and the same part of the tectum appears to be capable of forming appropriately organized connections with either temporal or nasal retina (Fig. 4.42). Yet the form or pattern of the projection, either NN or TT is correct within itself. In each case the projection formed from the original half-eye is correct, but has spread rostrocaudally over the whole tectum.

An alternative approach to the specificity hypothesis is to assume that

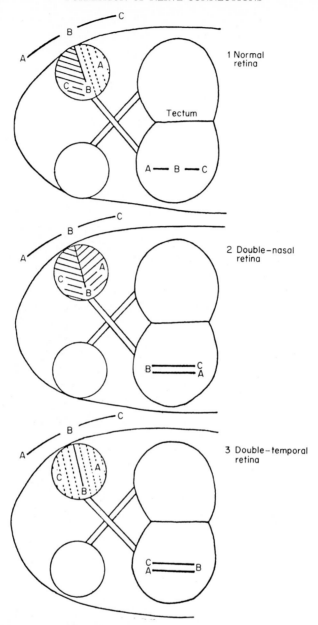

Tectum

1 Normal
retina

2 Double–nasal
retina

3 Double–temporal
retina

FIG. 4.42. The relationship between field, retina and tectum in normal, double-nasal and double-temporal eyes. Nasal retina is indicated by hatching with solid lines, temporal retina by hatching with dotted lines.

(1) With normal eye the points A, B, C, in the visual field are represented in that order rostrocaudally on the contralateral tectum.

(2) With the double-nasal retina (double-temporal visual field), the points B, C, in the temporal field are represented in their correct order on the contralateral tectum, but the representation is spread out rostrocaudally to cover the entire tectum. The projection of the nasal field mirrors the temporal field about the midline (B).

[*Caption continued at foot of page* 193]

the cellular differentiation in the retina should be orderly and continuous (Sperry, 1943b), such that neurons further apart in the retina should differ more than those closer together. On this assumption any retinal point could be completely identified by reference to only two differential "gradients", one in each major axis of the retina. Thus each ganglion cell could be adequately specified by two parameters; for instance, one representing the "gradient" value along a nasotemporal axis, the other representing its value along a dorsoventral axis (Gaze et al., 1963) (Fig. 4.43). I must confess to a certain diffidence in using the term "gradient" here, since this is a word that has long been overused and underdefined in embryological literature. I would emphasize, therefore, that the word "gradient" is here used in a mathematical rather than a biological, chemical, physical or any other sense; we have no idea with what sort of physical reality these "gradients" correspond. However, the word is very useful for two reasons: firstly, it suggests experimental approaches to the subject (Wolpert, 1969) and secondly, it can describe quantitatively what happens in the experiments on compound eyes (and in various other developmental situations—Lawrence, 1966; 1970). In the gradient system envisaged here it is the relative position of a cell on the gradient that matters; whether point A is uphill or downhill from point B. If such a gradient is halved, the gradient will still be complete in that it runs from maximum to minimum, but it will be compressed in space. If we assume a system of such gradients to be operative in specifying the retina and a similar system to specify the tectum, then if half the retina is removed we should expect the remaining half to spread its connections out so as to cover the entire tectum (Fig. 4.43). This is what seems to happen in the compound eye experiments.

Interpretations of NN and TT projections: Spreading versus tectal overgrowth

There is, however, an interesting embryological objection which could be raised to this interpretation (Sperry, 1965). It could be argued that since, effectively, only half a retina is sending fibres into the developing tectum, and since we know that the arrival of optic afferents is related to the cellular differentiation of the tectum, as described in a previous section, then perhaps only the appropriate half of the tectum continues to develop. In this case, for NN eyes, only the caudal half of the tectum would develop properly, while for TT eyes it would be the rostral half of the tectum. And since the developing half of the tectum would receive a double complement of fibres (being supplied by two similar half-retinae) it would grow larger than normal and thus come to resemble a normal

(3) With the double-temporal retina (double-nasal field), the points A, B, in the nasal field project in the correct order to the tectum, but the representation is spread out to cover the entire tectum rostrocaudally. The projection of the temporal field mirrors the nasal field about the midline (B).

In each double eye the order of tectal projection is correct for the original half-retina and reversed for the foreign half-retina. From Gaze, Jacobson and Székely, 1963.

7*

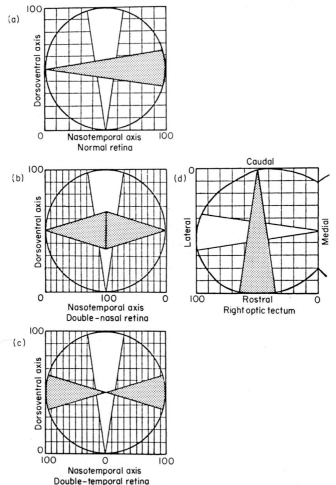

Fig. 4.43.   Diagram of the gradient system postulated by Gaze, Jacobson and Székely as specifying the retina and tectum. (a) Normal retina superimposed on a grid giving the values of the gradient in nasotemporal and dorsoventral axes. These values are to be thought of as extending from minimum to maximum; they have been expressed as 0–100 %; (b) Double-nasal retina. The dorsoventral (DV) gradient is unchanged but the eye has been halved so that the entire extent (0–100%) of the nasotemporal (NT) gradient now occupies the nasal half of the NT axis. Since the other half of the eye is also a nasal half, the same applies here, and the two gradient maxima meet in the midline. The retinal distance represented by each "step" on the DV gradient is normal, while the retinal distance represented by each step on the NT gradient is halved; thus there are twice the normal number of steps across the NT axis of the retina. (c) Double-temporal retina. The DV gradient is unchanged but the eye has been halved so that the entire extent (0–100%) of the NT gradient now occupies the temporal half of the NT axis. Since the other half of the eye is also a temporal half, the same applies here, and the two gradients start outwards from the midline. Again, the number of steps along the NT axis of retina is twice the normal number; (d) Diagram of the contralateral tectum showing the order in which the retinal gradients are represented along tectal axes. Since in operated animals the tectum was not halved, the gradients here still extend over the entire surface; thus 0–100% in each retinal diagram corresponds to 0–100% on the tectum. From Gaze, Jacobson and Székely, 1963.

tectum; the two half-retinae would thus connect, not with a whole tectum, but with an overgrown half-tectum. The distinction between these possible modes of development of the compound eye projection is very relevant to an understanding of the mechanism of formation of neuronal connections between eye and tectum. If the former alternative is true, and the fibres from each half-retina spread out rostrocaudally on an otherwise normal tectum, this would support the gradient hypothesis mentioned above; if the latter alternative is true, and the fibres from each half-retina are restricted to the appropriate half of the tectum, which then becomes hypertrophied, this would suggest that a more rigid type of place-specificity was controlling the selective termination of fibres from the various parts of the retina.

The first attempt to settle the spreading/not spreading controversy was the work of Gaze *et al.*, (1965), who compared the retinotectal magnification factors (MFs) from normal eyes and from compound eyes. The MF is the number of microns of tectum, measured linearly, representing one degree of retina, measured meridionally. The MF is thus a measure of the relative amounts of tectal representation of different parts of the retina. In a normal *Xenopus* the MF measured along the horizontal meridian of the field is approximately equal to that along the vertical meridian, whereas from a compound eye (NN or TT) the ratio MFH/MFV is nearly 2. This suggests that the retinotectal projection from each half-eye is spreading out across the rostrocaudal extent of the tectum. Such measurements are inconclusive, however; it is possible that such a ratio might also occur on the basis of an overgrown half-tectum.

The effects of uncrossing the chiasma in animals with one NN or TT eye

The question of whether the fibres from each (specified) hemiretina in a compound eye spread over an essentially normal tectum, or whether the retinal fibres go selectively to their appropriate half of the tectum, which then overgrows, can be investigated by uncrossing the optic chiasma. On Sperry's (1965) suggestion (overgrowth of a specified half-tectum), each half of the compound eye should then connect with only the appropriate half of the normal tectum, leaving the other half vacant; and conversely, only half of the normal eye should connect with the whole of the "compound eye tectum", since in terms of fibre specificities it is only half a tectum.

This experiment has been performed (Gaze *et al.*, 1970a) with very intriguing results. A series of *Xenopus*, each with a compound eye (NN or TT) was prepared and, just after metamorphosis, the chiasma was uncrossed by the simple expedient of cutting it along the midline and inserting a barrier of Millipore filter to prevent the optic nerve fibres from crossing as they regenerated (Fig. 4.44). This procedure has the effect of making each eye connect with the tectum on its own side, with the result that the compound eye connects with the normal tectum while the normal eye connects with the "compound eye tectum". The result was that the compound eye, consisting essentially of half an eye (but with perhaps twice as many fibres as half an eye) spread the connections from each hemiretina over the entire *normal* tectum (Fig. 4.45). This was the case whether the compound retina was NN or TT. Moreover the normal eye, which in its connection to its own normal tectum would give a full normal projection, also did so when forced to connect with the "compound eye tectum".

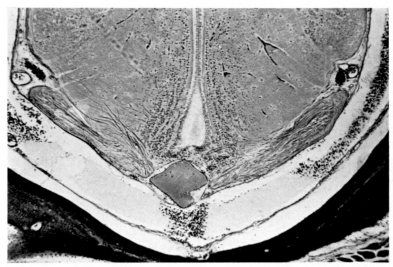

FIG. 4.44.   Photomicrograph of *Xenopus* brain with uncrossed optic chiasma, showing the small piece of Millipore filter in position at the chiasma, with the optic nerves approaching from each side. Coronal section, 15 microns, Holmes' silver stain. From Straznicky, Gaze and Keating, in preparation.

This result can be interpreted in various ways, which I shall enumerate here and leave any attempt at assessing the merits of the various possibilities until I have discussed some other, relevant, experiments. Thus we may say:

(1) If, at the time of formation of the compound eye, it was rigidly determined in respect to its nasotemporal polarization; and if it remained so at operation, then the results of uncrossing the chiasma show that the connections from a specified half-eye can spread over a whole normal tectum. In this case the retinotectal relationship is plastic in that the tectal connections of optic nerve fibres, originally destined for certain regions of the tectum, can move to other positions in an ordered fashion. If we allow that such "sliding connections" may exist, then we could also expect perhaps that the connections from a whole normal eye could move in a comparable fashion, but in the opposite sense, so as to take up orderly

positions on an overgrown half-tectum. Acceptance of the idea that the connections from each half-eye can spread over a whole normal tectum, and thus that tectal connections can shift, immediately prevents us from determining whether the tectum connected to a compound eye is normal or an overgrown half-tectum. Either could be the case and this experiment would be inadequate to decide the issue.

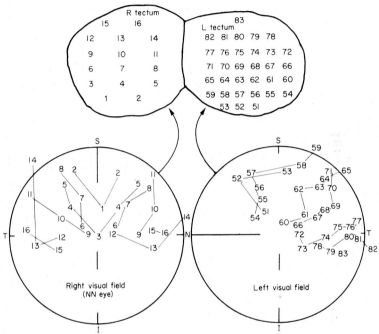

FIG. 4.45. Retinotectal projections after uncrossing the optic chiasma in a *Xenopus* with a right NN compound eye. The compound eye was formed at stage 32 and the chiasma uncrossed shortly after metamorphosis. Each eye now projects directly to its ipsilateral tectum. It may be seen that the NN right eye gives a typical NN map across the whole extent of the (normal) right tectum. Each half of the compound eye projects over the entire rostrocaudal extent of this tectum. Furthermore, the normal left eye forms an approximately normal map across the entire extent of the "NN" left tectum. From Straznicky, Gaze and Keating, in preparation.

(2) During development the normal eye connects up in such a fashion that the nasal extremity of the retina goes to the caudal extremity of the tectum, while the temporal extremity of the retina goes to the rostral extremity of the tectum. If we now half the embryonic eye down the vertical midline (as in a stage 32 *Xenopus*, when making compound eyes) and remove the temporal half, we are left with a half-eye that extends from the nasal extremity to the (old) midline; but the midline is now the temporal extremity of this half-eye and, in the compound eye situation, this part of the eye in fact behaves as if it were the normal temporal extremity; that is, it connects with most rostral tectum; and correspondingly for the transplanted half of the compound eye.

We could thus assume that the specificity-characteristics (in Sperry's sense) of the ganglion cells near the (divided) medial edge of each half-eye had undergone a form of "pattern regulation" and taken on the specificity-characteristics of the normal missing end of the eye. Thus instead of ganglion cells which are specified for rostral end of tectum lying at the temporal extremity of the normal eye, they will now lie at the temporal extremity of the half-eye, i.e. at the mid-line; and likewise for the transplanted half-eye. Such a compound eye would thus comprise, in terms of neuronal specificities, two "normal eyes" stuck together in this somewhat unusual geometrical arrangement.

If such were the case, then after uncrossing the chiasma we should expect that each half of the compound eye, since each is a whole eye in terms of specificities, would connect across the entire extent of the ipsilateral (normal) tectum; thus there should occur a reduplicated field projection of the sort one normally sees with compound eyes that innervate their own tecta. And conversely, we should expect the normal eye to make a normal map across its own ipsilateral tectum, which was formerly connected to the compound eye. It will be seen that the results of uncrossing the chiasma in animals with one compound eye fit exactly the predictions made on the basis that the compound eye consists of two mini-eyes put together with opposite nasotemporal polarity.

If we follow this line of argument we may say that the observation that a normal eye, connected with a "compound eye tectum", gives a normal projection map and not merely half a map, suggests strongly that the tectum is normal insofar as it relates to optic nerve fibres. Thus if we consider the eye as possessing a Sperry-type specificity structure, then the tectum under discussion displays a normal specificity structure. This in turn suggests that each half of the compound eye, which formerly covered the same tectum, has also a complete specificity structure. In other words, each half-eye has undergone "pattern-regulation" following the operation, although not size- or shape-regulation. And this again fits the second observation, that each half of the compound eye, when connected to a normal tectum, gives a full and orderly coverage.

Before we conclude that such a pattern regulation is what occurs in these compound eyes, however, we have to consider the results of certain other varieties of operation.

"Regulation"? The projections from half-eyes

We may now consider what happens when a half-eye, during development, connects with the tectum. This experiment was originally performed by Székely (1957), who removed the nasal half of the eye anlage in a tail-bud embryo of *T. vulgaris*, then rounded-up the remaining temporal half of the eye to form a complete sphere. This, after healing, was transplanted to the contralateral orbit of another embryo in reversed orientation, so that the original temporal pole became topographically nasal and the topographically temporal pole was the one formed by the fusion of the (unspecified) dorsal and ventral poles (Fig. 4.46). Eyes of normal shape but

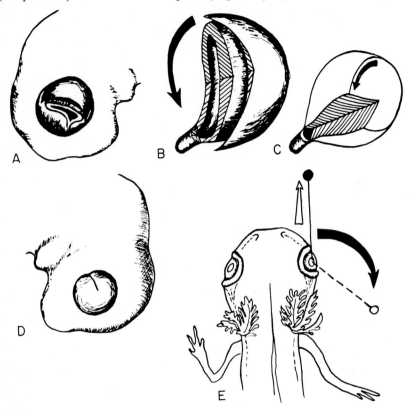

FIG. 4.46.   Diagram representing the operative procedure and the visual reflexes from the eye made of a half-eye primordium. A: Removal of the nasal half of the eye primordium. B and C: The edges of the remaining temporal half are pressed together to form a spherical body. D: Transplantation of the half eye primordium in the place of the contralateral eye of another embryo with reversed anteroposterior axis. The scar of the united edges is in temporal position; the original temporal pole is in nasal position. E: Visual reflexes of the operated right eye. A lure presented in the anterior visual field (filled circle) evokes a turn to the side, and the animal tries to catch the lure presented in the posterior visual field (empty circle) with a forward jump. From Székely, 1957.

half the normal size developed under these circumstances; and later behavioural tests of vision indicated that the unspecified new pole had come to manifest the characteristics of a "nasal" pole, despite its temporal position. If, despite our scepticism concerning the validity of such behavioural tests, we accept these results for the sake of our further discussion, then this experiment indicated that the eye is still capable of a certain "regulation" under these circumstances; and that the existence of a

specified pole (nasal or temporal; both varieties were used) at one side of
the eye can give rise to the development opposite it of the complementary
pole, the other end of the nasotemporal axis. This effect is of considerable
theoretical interest, since normally the nasotemporal axis of the eye is
presumably polarized by the inductive effect of the tissues surrounding
the orbit; yet here the unspecified eye tissue in temporal position became
specified as *nasal* pole (in terms of the functional connections it eventually
formed), even though in the normal course of events, if the specifying
influence of the surrounding tissues were still active, one would have
expected a temporal pole to develop here. In other words, the specifying
influence of the already-determined pole may be more effective than the
influence of the environment.

   Similar operations to those described above have been performed on
Xenopus embryos at stage 32, after biaxial polarization of the eye had
occurred (Straznicky *et al.*, 1970a). A nasal half-eye was rounded-up to
form a complete but smaller eye and this was left *in situ* in the orbit. When
the retinotectal projection was later mapped, after metamorphosis, the
results, from some of the animals, confirmed the previous observations of
Székely (1957) in that an apparently complete eye of normal polarity
projected in the appropriate fashion to the tectum (Fig. 4.47). Thus the
original dorsal and ventral poles became respecified as nasal, while new
dorsal and ventral poles appeared. The projection covered the whole of
the tectum, which was apparently of normal size. In this case, since the
operated eye is effectively a complete eye in miniature, the projection would
be expected to extend its tectal connections in both axes to match the
retinal and tectal pattern maps of specificity and the result should be
comparable to that previously demonstrated by Harrison when he grafted
a small eye into a large host (Harrison, 1929). The fact that the tectum
appeared to be of normal size is irrelevant. If the half-eye contained a
smaller number of ganglion cells than a normal eye, then the tectum
presumably would contain a decreased population of cells; but this would
not necessarily be obvious to the naked eye.

   While this form of regulation has been the result in some such experiments, in others the half-eye does not regulate. The projection pattern
that then results is just what would be expected on the basis of a simple
geometrical deformation of the specified half-eye (Fig. 4.48). Thus the
retinal pole opposite the line of section projects in a fairly normal fashion
to the tectum while the field projections corresponding to the "wrapped-
round" part of the retina give an appropriately deformed projection. The
difference between this unregulated retinal projection and that shown in
the previous figure gives support for the existence of regulation in this
latter; the visual field projection is behaving differently in the two cases
and the difference is directly related to the nature of the retinal operation.
If we now consider that such an unregulated half-eye comprises half the

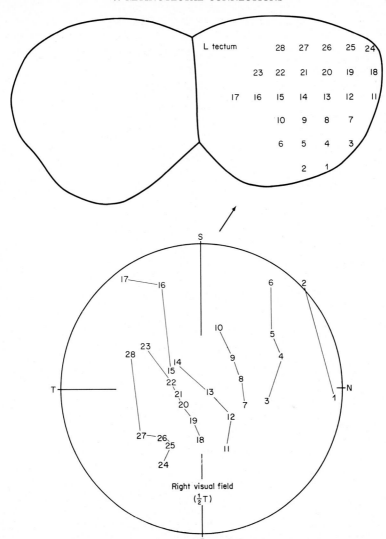

FIG. 4.47. The retinotectal projection from a temporal half-eye in *Xenopus*. The nasal half of the eye was removed at stage 32 and the remaining nasal half was rounded-up to form a sphere. The projection was mapped some months after metamorphosis. The affected tectum appears normal in size and the projection appears to be a normal projection. "Regulation" of the operated eye thus seems to have occurred. From Straznicky, Gaze and Keating, in preparation.

normal range of neural specificities, in Sperry's sense, then it is conceivable that the tectum, which shows complete coverage by such a projection, is in fact a half-tectum in terms of specificities, although it may appear normal in size. Alternatively we would have to postulate that the tectum is normal in range of specificities, in which case "sliding" retinotectal connections are

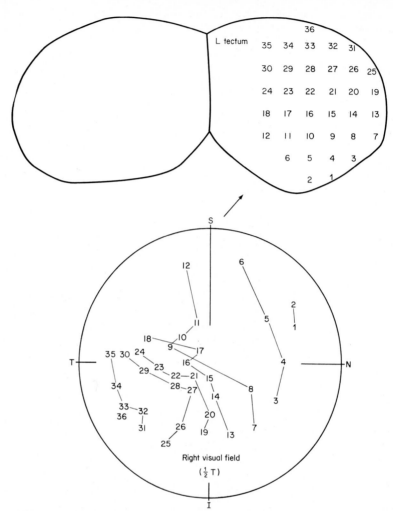

FIG. 4.48.   The retinotectal projection from a temporal half-eye in *Xenopus*. The half-eye was formed at stage 32 and the projection mapped after metamorphosis. In this case the "hooking" of the rows of field positions (19–24; 25–30) indicates a lack of regulation in the operated eye. From Straznicky, Gaze and Keating, in preparation.

occurring, in that part of the eye which normally connects with mid-tectum now connects with one or other extremity of the rostrocaudal tectal axis. This form of dichotomy (which will probably turn out to be mis-leading) could perhaps be investigated by uncrossing the chiasma in animals with one half-eye; since if the term "unregulated" means anything in this context, such a pattern, on a *normal* tectum, should only connect with half the tectal area. Unless, of course, sliding connections were to occur at the tectum. Thus, in this hypothetical situation, complete tectal coverage would not enable us to distinguish between the proposed mechanisms; whereas restricted tectal coverage would.

These experiments on half-eyes may tell us something relevant to the mechanism of axial specification. We say that the eye becomes specified at about stage 30–31 in *Xenopus*. Experiment shows that this process of specification takes place separately in time along the nasotemporal and dorsoventral axes of the eye. Specification in this sense appears particularly to be a process of polarization of the eye, the appearance of polarity in respect to the connections that will later form. Thus if we consider the eye, and in particular its nasotemporal axis, this represents an axis of polarity. To specify this nasotemporal axis, we must either have nasal and temporal ends or one of the ends and a direction. If we represent such a polarized axial array as a series of unitary objects ordered in a row, the two modes of ordering may perhaps be visualized as if, in the one case, the objects are strung out on a piece of string under tension. In this case we need the two ends to preserve the ordering; if we cut the string in the middle, the ordering is at once lost. If, on the other hand, we consider the objects arranged along a rigid wire supported at each end and then consider what happens if we cut the wire in the middle, we obtain quite a different result. In this case *one* end of the axis, together with the direction given by the rigidity of the wire, is sufficient to preserve the axial ordering of the objects in the remaining half.

The half-eye experiments suggest that the nasotemporal axis can be adequately preserved by one end only, together with, presumably, a vector. In the rounded-up half-eye we have removed one end of the existing polarized axis; the system regulates by the production of the missing end, from unspecified (or even from DV specified) tissue. And moreover, the tissue used to form the new pole had, originally, some of the quality (polarity, position on gradient) of the *other* pole. For instance, if the half-eye is a residual temporal half, then all its tissue sits in the temporal half of the polarity axis or gradient; yet, when the upper and lower margins are fused to form a new pole, this acquires the character of the nasal pole (despite temporal position). Furthermore, we can say that it does not matter which end of the axis we retain; with either, the resulting new pole is the opposite one.

There is yet a further variant on the half-eye theme; one that I mention with diffidence because I cannot yet be completely certain that it is not due to an experimental artifact. In some few animals the projection from the "half-eye" turned out to be reduplicated in the fashion of that from a compound eye. It is conceivable, though unlikely, that animals with compound eyes escaped and became mixed with half-eye animals. The following points are relevant but inconclusive: (1) the half-eyes were nasal halves and each of the reduplicated "compound" projections was double-nasal; (2) proper compound eyes are usually normal in size, whereas the "half-eye" ones were all small, as are proper half-eyes; (3) no mixing of animals in the opposite direction has been found; (4) a major catastrophe of animal-mixing would be unlikely to pass undetected in view of the precautions taken. Thus, while no weight can be put on this phenomenon until the experiments are repeated, it is at least possible that here we have a form of reduplication akin to that which has previously been reported for limb buds, ears and certain other structures (Harrison, 1921, 1936, 1945; Swett, 1937; Waddington, 1940; Waddington, 1956, pp. 424–428).

The projections to half-tecta formed in larval life

The converse of the half-eye projection is that from a whole eye to a half-tectum; this approach has been used both in larval and adult life, with very different results in different types of animal. Here, we consider the results when the operation is performed in larval *Xenopus*. If, at stage 53 (Nieuwkoop and Faber, 1956) the rostral or the caudal half of one tectum is removed and the animal then allowed to survive until a few months after metamorphosis, the eventual retinotectal projection shows that only the appropriate part of the retina (visual field) projects to the residual piece of tectum (Fig. 4.49). Which half of the tectum is removed in later larval life does not matter; in each case only the proper region of tectum connects (Straznicky *et al.*, 1970b). Thus in this situation the projection does not show evidence of plasticity and the results appear to support the idea of a rigid, unmodifiable specificity mechanism active in the formation of retinotectal connections. This matter will be considered further on p. 207 *et seq*.

The projections from double-ventral compound eyes

Up to the present we have considered operations separating the retina into two halves across the nasotemporal axis; and the corresponding (rostrocaudal) tectal axis. It is, of course, possible to divide the retina across the dorsoventral axis instead, and thus to produce double ventral (VV) or double-dorsal (DD) eyes. Both varieties have been formed (Gaze *et al.*, 1970b) and their behaviour investigated. Since the ventral fissure is apparently necessary for the formation of an optic nerve, and since DD eyes contain no ventral fissure, it is to be expected that such eyes will not have an optic nerve; and this is the case.

When the compound eye is formed of two ventral halves, however, it does form a connection with the brain; and the retinotectal projection from such VV eyes is different in kind to that from NN or TT eyes (Gaze *et al.*, 1970b). In a normal *Xenopus*, ventral retina (dorsal field) projects across the dorsal surface of the tectum while dorsal retina (ventral field) projects round the lateral edge of the tectum. In the projection from a VV eye, however, many positions on the dorsal surface of the tectum each receive input from two positions in the field, one dorsal and one ventral;

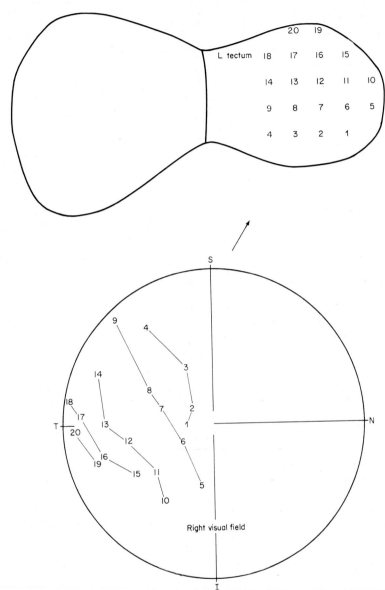

FIG. 4.49. The projection from a whole (i.e. unoperated) eye to the residual caudal half of the tectum in *Xenopus*. In this animal the rostral part of the left tectum was removed at larval stage 53, just before metamorphosis. It may be seen that only the appropriate part of the visual field (retina) projects to the residual caudal half of the tectum. From Straznicky, Gaze and Keating, in preparation.

and such reduplicated field positions tend to be symmetrically arranged about the horizontal meridian of the field (Fig. 4.50). Thus far the phenomena are comparable in kind, if not in axial direction, with those found in NN and TT projections.

Electrophysiological mapping of the visual projection is normally carried out only across the exposed dorsal surface of the tectum. And whereas this

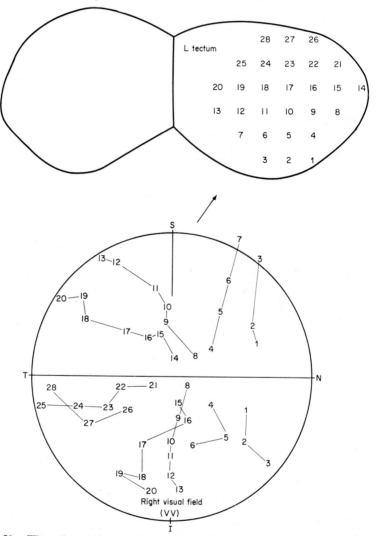

FIG. 4.50. The retinotectal projection from a double-ventral compound eye in *Xenopus*. The compound eye was formed at stage 32 and the projection was mapped after metamorphosis. Positions in the dorsal field are reduplicated by those in the ventral field. The ordering of the projection is correct in the nasal half of the field but in the temporal half the rows of field positions, both dorsal and ventral, show a strong tendency to curve towards the temporal pole. From Straznicky, Gaze and Keating, in preparation.

includes the entire extent of the nasotemporal field projection, it does not include the entire extent of the dorsoventral field projection. The most ventral positions of the field project round the lateral edge of the tectum. In the projection from a NN or TT eye, the fibres from each hemiretina appear to extend their connections in a uniform fashion across the entire rostrocaudal extent of the tectum. If a comparable phenomenon were to occur with VV eyes, we would expect that each hemiretina would extend its connections uniformly across the entire mediolateroventral extent of the tectum. And if this were the case, then since recording is normally only made from the *dorsal* surface, there should be a strip of field projection, above and below the horizontal meridian, which is missing from the projection maps; this is because that particular part of the field from a VV eye would be expected to project to the most lateral part of the tectum, out of reach of the recording electrode. No such gap in the field projection from the VV eye has, however, been seen. In each case the field positions continue to appear on the map, right up to the horizontal meridian. Thus whatever may be happening to account for this distribution of connections from a VV eye, the end result is different from that with NN or TT eyes.

Furthermore, in a normal *Xenopus*, with tectal recording positions running lateromedially across the dorsal tectum, the corresponding field positions run ventrodorsally. It may be seen from Fig. 4.50 that such a simple state of affairs does not obtain in the VV projection. Mostly, the nasal extremity of the field is fairly normally organized in this fashion, but as we progress across the field, so the rows of field positions tend to curl around in a temporal direction. The most obvious immediate cause of this is that there is, in these animals, an extended tectal representation of the *centre* of the visual field. But why this should be so, and what happens to the lateral part of the tectum, are points that as yet are far from clear.

It will now be helpful if we consider again, in the light (or perhaps I should say under the shadow) of these results, the possible courses of events during the development of the retinotectal projection. I should emphasize that the developmental programmes outlined are largely hypothetical since we yet lack adequate information on these matters.

Further considerations on the development of retina and tectum

Normal eye to normal tectum. The apparent course of events is illustrated in Fig. 4.51. We consider the situation at certain selected stages of development. At stage 32 the eye has become polarized in its major axes but has not yet connected to the tectum *anlage*. The horizontal, or nasotemporal axis of the eye that is shown in the diagram, would at this stage contain some 20–50 ganglion cells. By stage 39 the eye would have enlarged somewhat (1000 fibres in the optic nerve, Gaze and Wilson, unpublished) and the initial retinotectal connection will have formed. The assumption in the diagram, that nasal retina connects to caudal tectum and temporal retina to rostral tectum, while valid for the adult, is not proven for the larva. At stage 54 the enlargement of the retina and tectum has increased further; there are now perhaps 14,000 fibres in the optic nerve and the new cells added to the retina are produced at the ciliary margins, so the eye increases in size by continually adding to its edges. As the diagram indicates, we assume that the newly formed tectal connections become arrayed in concentric circles as the tectum develops, around the originally innervated position. Finally the situation in the young adult is shown,

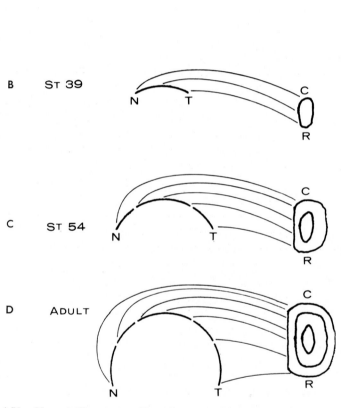

Fɪɢ. 4.51.   Normal *Xenopus* eye: Hypothetical scheme for the mode of development of retinotectal connections. (A) At stage 32 the eye has become polarized along the NT and DV axes, but has not yet sent any axons to the tectum. The diagram represents the NT axis of the eye; (B) At stage 39 the eye has grown somewhat in size and the first tectal connections have formed. These are represented as they are found in the adult, with temporal retina connecting with rostral tectum and nasal retina with caudal tectum; (C) By stage 54 the eye has increased considerably in size, with the newly-formed retina adding on at the retinal margin. The diagram shows the tectal connections that may be formed by the newly-developed marginal retina; (D) Shows the tectal projection of the NT axis of the retina, as revealed in the adult.

with the normal retinotectal projection. The diagrams oversimplify the developmental sequence by showing a four-dimensional system in two dimensions only; we assume the newly developing retinal fibres from the eye margin to connect with the topological "neck" of the tectum, where the tectum contacts the rest of the brain, since this is the actual site of the marginal projection in the adult. We thus assume the tectum to be produced rather as is a handknitted sock; continually new surface is being added at the neck and the original piece of tectal surface becomes progressively more displaced as the new surface increases all round it. These diagrams make no statement about mechanisms; they merely indicate what may spatially be the case at various stages of development; and their interest lies in their contrast to the other eye-tectum relationships, where the situation appears to be very different.

Compound (TT) eye to its contralateral tectum. At stage 32 the eye has been made compound but otherwise appears normal (Fig. 4.52). As soon as the eye connects with the tectum, however, we start running into trouble. The figure shows the central retina connecting to caudal tectum and the two temporal edges to rostral tectum. This is the case in the adult and we merely assume it to be so at this stage of development. The difficulty starts as soon as we consider the mode of growth of the eye and how this might relate to the tectum. The normal eye grows by adding to its ciliary margins; we assume (and at present this is only an assumption) that the compound eye also grows at the edges. The *central* part of the eye apparently does not take part in this growth. Yet since the eye undoubtedly gets bigger, with more fibres running to the tectum, which itself also increases in size, a retinotectal distribution fitting with what we know to be the case in the adult could occur as shown in the diagrams for stage 54. If we assume that the tectum increases in size symmetrically around the original innervation area, then to account for the continued presence of the central retinal representation at the caudal tectal margin, we have to assume "sliding" connections in the tectum; the connections of the central regions of the retina will have to move caudally as the tectum grows. Alternatively, as shown in the right-hand diagram, we may assume that the connections of the central region of the retina stay put; in which case the tectum will have to grow asymmetrically to accommodate towards its rostral part the incoming fibres from the two *temporal* retinal margins. This, obviously, is a variety of the "overgrown half-tectum" hypothesis. The final stages, according to these two mechanisms, are shown in the bottom diagrams.

We may now consider further the interpretation of the uncrossed-chiasma results:

(1) If we assume that each half of a compound eye (NN or TT) has become specified in a rigid fashion, prior to operation, such that each ganglion cell can thereafter only connect with its corresponding tectal

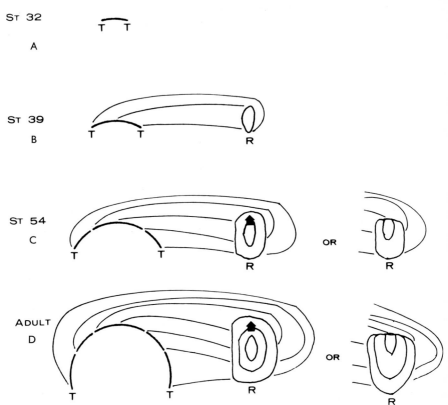

FIG. 4.52.   Compound (TT) *Xenopus* eye: Hypothetical scheme for the mode of development of retinotectal connections. (A) At stage 32 the eye has become polarized along NT
and DV axes and the operation to form a TT eye has been performed. No retinotectal
connections have yet formed; (B) At stage 39 the first tectal connections have formed.
On the assumption that these connections show the same ordering that is found in an
adult TT eye, each temporal pole of the eye is shown connecting with the rostral tectum,
while the midline of the retina connects with caudal tectum; (C) At stage 54 the eye has
enlarged considerably, by the addition of new cells at the retinal margins. This is so in the
normal eye and the assumption is made here that the mode of growth of a compound eye
is similar; If the order of connections at this stage is similar to that in the adult, the vertical
midline of the retina will connect with the caudal pole of the tectum. To achieve this, if
we assume the tectum to grow symmetrically, by adding tissue all round the previously
developed piece (see B), then with the assumed mode of retinal growth (i.e. at the margins),
the tectal connections of those midline retinal cells that have previously reached the tectum
(see B) will have to "slide" further caudal. Alternatively we may postulate that the asymmetrical ingrowth of two sets of temporal fibres may lead to asymmetrical growth of the
tectum, as on the right hand side of the figure; (D) Similarly in the young adult: to account
for the continued presence of the projection from the retinal midline at the caudal
extremity of the tectum, we must either postulate "sliding" tectal connections or asymmetrical growth of the tectum.

region, then we have to postulate asymmetrical growth of the tectum to account for the nature of the compound eye projection. But in this case the results of uncrossing the optic chiasma indicates that the specificity-relationship between retina and tectum can alter. Tectal cells that originally connected with central retinal cells now do so with ganglion cells at the margin of the retina. Further, if this form of plasticity can occur, it is difficult to see the need for the postulated rigidity in the first place. If connections from a normal eye can "slide" across a "compound eye tectum", one might assume that connections from half an eye (i.e. one half of the compound eye) could similarly "slide" across a normally-developing tectum. Moreover, under this hypothesis of rigid retinotectal specification we have to accept that these plastic changes in the retinotectal connection pattern can occur after metamorphosis.

(2) If we assume that each half of a compound eye (NN or TT) undergoes a form of pattern regulation such that it becomes, in terms of retinotectal specificities, a miniature normal eye, then we have further difficulties. In the first place, that part of the normal retina which goes to the caudal extremity of the tectum is the nasal pole. On a regulation hypothesis we would have to consider that the "nasal pole" of a TT eye was the vertical midline of the retina; and likewise this is the "temporal pole" of a NN eye. And whereas topologically we may accept that a "pole" may be an extended line, *biologically* it is difficult to see how this peculiar geometrical arrangement could work.

Secondly, the regulation hypothesis does not get us out of the difficulty of having to postulate either "sliding specificities" or "sliding connections". To show that this is so, we merely have to consider the known mode of development of the retina. The retina grows at its edges, not in the centre. In *Xenopus* cells are continually being added at the retinal margin, until some unknown time after metamorphosis. And since we know that the central part of a TT eye projects to the caudal end of the tectum, whereas the "nasal" and temporal extremities of the retina project to the rostral part of the tectum, we find ourselves faced again with the possibilities, in Fig. 4.52: either sliding connections occur or otherwise half the tectum overgrows. But *in either case* the "centre" of the half-eye, in which regulation is assumed to occur, shifts in relation to the centre of the whole compound eye, as retinal growth takes place. When the nasotemporal axis of the half-eye is only 30 cells in length, its centre is 15 cells from the geographical centre of the whole eye; when the half-axis is 100 cells long, its centre is 50 cells away, and so on. Since the half-eye is growing only at one end of the nasotemporal axis, the centre of this axis has to move continually down the line. Whereas in the development of the normal eye (Fig. 4.51) the "centre" of the eye remains more-or-less constant in position in the eye and cells are added on all round it.

On the regulation hypothesis we postulate that each half of the compound eye (NN or TT) has a full range of specificities, from most nasal to most temporal; this we would conclude from the fashion in which both the compound eye and a normal eye can each connect with one and the same tectum. During the development of a normal retinotectal projection the projection of the centre of the retina probably remains constant and later

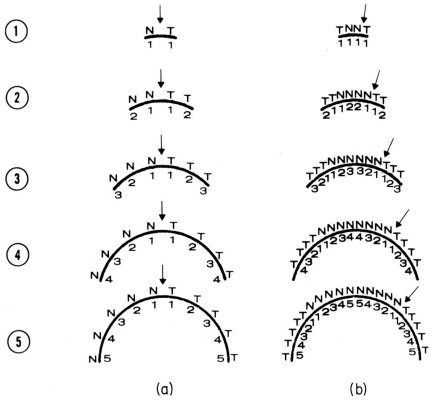

FIG. 4.53. The distribution of cell specificities in a normal eye and in a "regulated" compound eye. Arrows indicate the centre of the normal retina and the centre of the half-eye. Ringed numbers (1)–(5) indicate stages in the growth of the eye. (a) The normal retina grows at the edges. Its midline remains in the same place; (b) The centre of each half of the compound eye moves away from the geographical centre of the whole eye, as the latter grows. Thus if each half of the compound eye is considered to comprise a complete range of "specificities", then one and the same cell, at the geographical centre of the whole eye, must change its label (from N_1 to, eventually, N_5) as the eye grows.

developing rings of retina project to later developing rings of tectum. In the projection from a "regulated" compound eye, on the other hand, the tectal region receiving input from the centre of the post-larval half-eye only develops fairly late and the specificity-characteristics of the half-eye should change as the eye grows.

As shown in Fig. 4.53 the normal eye increases in size by adding cells at the retinal margin. Eventually, in the adult, the most recently-added nasal cells project to the caudal extremity of the tectum, while the most recently-added temporal cells project to the rostral pole of the tectum. If we depict the normal full range of nasotemporal specificities in the young adult eye as $N_5N_4N_3N_2N_1T_1T_2T_3T_4T_5$, then ganglion cells with specificity N_1 or T_1 were among the first to develop and N_5 and T_5 the last to develop. If we now consider the case of a regulated half-eye (making up half of a compound eye), then we may postulate that each half-eye comprises a full range of specificities. Initially, shortly after the time of operation, the constitution of the compound eye may be represented as $T_1N_1N_1T_1$. At the next stage another cell is added to the margin on each side (in reality, all round the eye) and the constitution of the eye would then have to be represented as $T_2T_1N_1N_2N_2N_1T_1T_2$. Addition of a further cell at each side would then result in the arrangement $T_3T_2T_1N_1N_2N_3N_3N_2N_1T_1T_2T_3$ and so forth. The eventual arrangement would be as shown in Fig. 4.53, where it can be seen that the cells at the centre of the compound eye systematically change their *name* (specificity) as the eye grows. In the developing *normal* eye this does not have to happen, since as the retina adds cells at its edges, these new cells may be considered to acquire the new specificities appropriate to their situations. But in the compound eye (as in the normal eye) the cells at the centre of the retina are probably the original ganglion cells dating from the beginning of the eye development. Thus, since the cells do not disappear and become replaced by new ones bearing the needed new specificities, we have to consider that the same cell changes its specificities as the eye increases in size.

In view of my previous comments on behavioural techniques, I should perhaps mention, in fairness to those experimenters who prefer to use behavioural methods for the investigation of neural organization, that the question of whether or not a compound eye consists of two "regulated" normal eyes put together, could perhaps be usefully investigated in this way. Thus, if in a TT eye the midline is to be considered as the joined nasal poles, stimulation with a lure in the centre of the visual field should result in the animal striking to the temporal extremity of the visual field (since nasal retina corresponds to temporal field), while stimulation at either the temporal or the topographically-nasal edge of the retina should give responses directed to the nasal extremity of the field. If the middle region of a compound TT retina did in fact show the behavioural quality of a nasal pole in this fashion it would tend to support the "regulation" hypothesis. At present this form of evidence is not available.

(3) There is probably, however, a fallacy in all this, which I am tempted to describe as the fallacy of the undistributed middle. My arguments have all been based on the assumption that the setting-up and regeneration of orderly retinotectal connections is based on the mechanisms of neuronal specificity, which would require that each ganglion cell, during development, acquires a unique chemical label. And whereas this may be so, it

remains but one out of several possibilities. In particular it would perhaps be worth-while to investigate the applicability of self-ordering mechanisms in neural development and regeneration. Since we are concerned with the projection from retina to tectum, however, both retina and tectum are involved and any self-ordering mechanism for growing optic nerve fibres would, by itself, be inadequate. There must also exist a means of relating the fibre pattern to the tectum; that is, there has to be a "tectal anchor" for the projection. A map is only useful if it can be oriented with relation to the terrain. There are several ways of doing this in the visual system; one such could involve the place-specification of each ganglion cell in terms of its *relative* position in a system of crossed gradients.

CONCLUSIONS

My main conclusion when I consider the experimental evidence that has been discussed in this chapter, is that this is the wrong time to attempt to write in a synoptic fashion about the formation of retinotectal connections. Only a few years ago the situation looked neat and tidy; fibres got back to their proper places on the basis of a cell-to-cell recognition phenomenon which was to be explained by a refined differential chemospecificity of the elements involved. At the present time (1969) the answers are by no means so obvious and we can safely say that the phenomena of the genesis and regeneration of neural connections between retina and tectum now seem much less straightforward than was formerly thought to be the case.

It is valid to say that the *pattern* of the retinotectal projection may be restored in all cases where the eye and the tectum are otherwise normal. It is also true that the *pattern* is restored in the case where a half-eye or a compound eye grow into an unoperated tectum. By "pattern" in this context I mean the appropriate distribution of fibres from the entire nasotemporal extent of the eye or part-eye, across the entire rostrocaudal extent of the tectum. In all cases, it appears that the topological order of the projection is maintained. Thus in this situation fibres from the eye or part-eye distribute themselves in an orderly fashion so as to fill the available tectal area, which in turn probably develops with a specific dependence, spatially, on the retinal connections. And when half the tectum is removed in *Xenopus* at stage 53, the projection, when mapped after metamorphosis, shows that only the appropriate half of the retina has connected with the half-tectum. In adult goldfish we may have a different result; here there is evidence of compression of connection from the whole retina on to a residual rostral half-tectum. These various results appear inconsistent with one another. Yet, within one class of experiment, on one type of animal, at one developmental stage, the results are highly consistent. We are not dealing here with mere random processes giving fortuitously one type of result or another. It is now possible to predict accurately what will be the result if another experiment of the type mentioned above is performed. Thus the visual system in each case is following some rules relating to how it should connect; unfortunately for us, however, the rules seem disconcertingly different in the various situations considered.

I believe sufficiently in the effectiveness of causal analysis in neurogenesis to think that the various conflicting pieces of evidence will eventually fall into place. But this will await better experiment and more rigorous thought. As in human converse, so in experiment: a stupid question often leads to a stupid answer. In the experimental situation a stupid question is one that is not properly aimed; and it leads, as often as not, to an answer which is largely useless in that it does not advance our analysis at all, or merely tells us, in different form, what we already know. Unfortunately, many of our experiments fall into this class. Rarely, we ask the right question by accident; even more rarely, by intention. An example of the former case would be the initial question about the nature of the retinotectal projection from a compound eye; an example of the latter case would be the question as to the effect of uncrossing the optic chiasma in an animal with a compound eye.

5. INTRACENTRAL CONNECTIONS

Thus far I have discussed those neuronal connections that can be called primary inputs and outputs of the nervous system. I have dealt, in some detail, with the arguments that specifically localized connections, a mapping of the sensory or motor surface on to the nervous centre, is necessary to permit adequate function in these parts of the nervous system. When dealing with primary inputs and outputs we are able to consider the entire extent of the nervous system involved; our experiments may deal with only a narrowly selected aspect of input or output, but we have no difficulty, in principle, in extending our observations to include the sum total of the peripheral connections of the nervous system. The complexity of the situation is in each case limited by the number of dorsal root fibres, of ventral root fibres, or, for instance, the number of fibres in the optic nerve. Moreover the numbers of fibres involved are not vastly different for frog or man and we may have little conceptual difficulty in generalizing our ideas on mechanisms, obtained from work on amphibia, to the higher vertebrates.

The situation is very different when we consider *intracentral* connections. In man the number of primary inputs and outputs are somewhat comparable to those in the lower vertebrates; but with the extensive encephalization that accompanies ascent of the phylogenetic scale the numbers of neurones involved in intracentral connections has increased by many orders of magnitude. In terms of mechanisms of connection-formation, this enormous increase in numbers of elements appears to pose major problems; such a quantitative change may well involve extensive qualitative differences in the way cells connect with one another. And whereas it is no problem to show that the arrangement of primary inputs and outputs is normally highly organized in a topographical fashion, we have as yet little idea of the precise connections within the deeper parts of the central nervous system; once we get beyond the visual input to the occipital cortex, for instance, the interconnections have so far proved too complex to unravel. The connections within the central nervous system of a higher vertebrate, when considered at the level of detail, seem chaotic. What we would like to know is whether they are in fact chaotic or whether they merely appear so.

The classical hypothesis of neuronal specificity was developed in relation to studies on the primary inputs and outputs of the amphibian nervous system (Sperry, 1951a). As I have described in the previous chapter, there are difficulties inherent in this hypothesis even when it is applied to the systems from which it was derived. We may well ask whether, if we provisionally accept the hypothesis of neuronal specificity, it can be usefully applied to the patterning of synaptic relations in the more central parts of the nervous system—which become relatively larger and more important as we go up the animal scale. Sperry (1951b; 1958a,b; 1963; 1965) maintains that this is so. The local-sign specificity that is impressed on afferent fibres by the process of differentiation is presumed by him (e.g. 1958a) to determine the type of second-order neurones which the growing fibre-tips will find acceptable for synapsis; and this inference implies the existence of a similar refined qualitative specificity among the central neurones.

Some of the difficulties inherent in any attempt to extend the hypothesis of neuronal specificity to cover *all* intracentral connections have been considered by Sperry in his early papers and are further discussed by Székely (1966). Thus any such scheme of selective central connections must allow for considerable plasticity in function and even for complete reversal of response; furthermore, the establishment of both excitatory and inhibitory linkages on the basis of interneuronal affinity brings complications for the hypothesis (Sperry and Miner, 1949). In this context Sperry (1958a) considered that neurons appear, as a rule, to have affinities for a variety of other neurone types; and furthermore he suggested that the synaptic predispositions of a given fibre may be conditioned by its surroundings and may thus differ as the growing fibre enters different regions of the central nervous system.

The conception of a nervous system that is engendered by the hypothesis of neuronal specificity is one in which the system is extensively prewired. It is a nervous system of Sherringtonian character, where the precision of determined interneuronal connections is extended beyond the spinal cord to include the whole of the central integrative system. A nervous system built in this fashion would have many switchboard-like characteristics; and such a system is anathema to many neurophysiologists. With rigidly determined interconnections, how could one account for the very extensive functional plasticity of the normal higher animal? Our difficulty in envisaging how such a system could work stems less from any fundamental inadequacy of the Sherringtonian approach than from our inability (or unwillingness; it amounts to the same thing) to bring our ideas on switchboards up to date. Arguments about the deficiencies of switchboard neural systems frequently tend to assume that the switchboard in question

8

is analogous to a turn-of-the-century telephone exchange; but a more valid analogy would be a modern computer, which is also a form of switchboard. A computer is a machine for handling information; and the "memory" capacity of a machine, more than anything else, determines the complexity of its possible behaviour (Turing, 1948).

Sperry (1958b) had reached somewhat similar conclusions when he pointed out that, with facilitatory sets operating in a switchboard or fibre circuit system, the functional patterns, though still dependent on specific connections, become much less a direct reflection of the underlying structural design. With a morphologically rigid circuit system *of sufficient complexity*, it is possible to obtain an almost unlimited variety of different responses from the same stimulus, merely by shifting the distribution of central facilitation and inhibition; i.e. by opening or closing certain central pathways at one time and others at another time. Sperry's point of view has been expressed in this fashion:

"It now appears that the complicated nerve fiber circuits of the brain grow, assemble, and organise themselves through the use of intricate chemical codes under genetic control. Early in development the nerve cells, numbering in the billions, acquire and retain thereafter individual identification tags, chemical in nature, by which they can be recognised and distinguished one from another.

As the maturing neurons and their long pulse-carrying fibers begin to form functional interconnections to weave the complex communication networks of behavior, the growing fibers become extremely selective about the chemical identity of other cells and fibers with which they will associate. Lasting functional hookups are established only with cells to which the growing fibers find themselves selectively matched by inherent chemical affinities.

The outgrowing fibers are guided by a kind of probing chemical touch system that leads them along exact pathways in an enormously intricate guidance program that involves millions and perhaps billions of different chemically distinct brain cells. By selective chemical preferences the respective nerve fibers are guided correctly to their separate channels at each of the numerous forks or decision points which they encounter as they travel through what is essentially a multiple Y-maze of possible channels.

Each fiber in the brain pathways has its own preference for particular prescribed trails by which it locates and connects with certain other neurons that have the appropriate cell flavor. The potential pathway and terminal connection zones have their own individual chemical flavors by which each is recognised and distinguished from all others in the same half of the brain and cord. Indications are that right and left halves are chemical mirror maps of one another. . . . Cytochemical differentiation in terms of gradients and fields is basic all through the central nervous system. Cells close together within a given nucleus or cortical area are similar and those farther apart are increasingly different as the separation increases. The tendency for fiber projections from one central field to another to interconnect opposite poles of the two gradients appears so frequently in central nervous organisation as to suggest that this affinity between opposites may be a rather direct reflection of the nature of the underlying chemical affinities, a complementarity principle perhaps (Jehle, 1963). The dorsal retina, for example, connects to ventral tectum, the lateral somatic thalamus connects to medial cortex, the medial nucleus gracilis projects to lateral thalamus, and so on." (Sperry, 1965).

Most of the examples discussed so far have been from the primary inputs and outputs of the nervous system. Within the visual system, these include, for lower vertebrates, the retinotectal pathways; while for mammals they include the entire path through the lateral geniculate and up to the visual cortex. I have described, in the previous chapter, the nature of the retinotectal projection in lower vertebrates, and the evidence that this is established without relevance to visual function. The same probably applies to the mammalian primary sensory inputs, since it has been shown that, in neonatal kittens, geniculate cells, optic-tract fibres and cells in the visual cortex may show approximately normal receptive-field organization and functional architecture (Wiesel and Hubel, 1963a; Hubel and Wiesel, 1963). Since binocularity was one of the cellular characteristics investigated, it seems very likely, although this has not directly been shown, that the topography of the retinocortical projection, that is, the cortical map of the visual field, was also established previsually. And I would surmise that the same will be found to apply to the other primary sensory inputs in the mammalian brain.

Thus far we are on familiar territory; it has merely been established that, in all vertebrates so far examined, the primary sensory inputs and the primary motor outputs are organized according to a pattern which is determined prefunctionally. However, increasingly as we ascend the phylogenetic scale, we find that more and more of the brain lies, as it were, between the primary inputs and outputs. And in these parts of the brain, sometimes called the "association areas", we have no adequate information on the nature or precision of the neural interconnections.

There are certain regions in the brain where a wealth of information exists about connectivity; this is particularly true for the cerebellum (Eccles et al., 1967; Szentágothai, 1967) and the archicortex (Andersen, 1966). In these situations there is evidence for a high degree of selectivity in the connections that are formed; this is perhaps most dramatically illustrated in the hippocampus, where, in region CA1, the most peripheral parts of the hippocampal apical dendrites are activated from the entorhinal area; the next sections receive the Schaffer collaterals; below this come the commissural inputs; while the somata are exclusively affected by the basket cell terminals. However, these regions of the brain have been chosen for this sort of study for this very reason, that they show a marked lamination and obvious structural order.

We have no such detailed information yet for the neocortex. Sholl (1956) has calculated that the cortical arborization of a single geniculate visual fibre may encompass some 5,000 neurones, and he maintains that, although it is unlikely that all the neurones within the spread of the branches of the fibre would be affected, yet the effect of the impulses incoming along one such fibre must be diffuse and not punctate. Unfortunately, for those who study neural connectivity, both "diffuse" and "punctate" have become emotive terms. We may agree with Scholl that the incoming activity may be widely distributed; but this need not imply lack of order in the distribution. An advertisement for a scientific book, arriving on my table in the morning, has probably also arrived also at the houses of some 50 other biologists at about the same time. This does not mean that the company sending out the advertisement has just scattered them around Edinburgh; grocers and housepainters will not receive them. Widespread is not the same as random.

Sholl's book on the organization of the cerebral cortex represents perhaps the first modern attempt to reach some form of understanding of the relationship between structure and function in the brain. As such it is immensely valuable as well as very readable. Unfortunately it is also somewhat misleading in certain respects. Sholl holds, for instance, that histological studies show that no theory of brain function relying on specific circuits can be maintained and that the alternative approach must depend on statistical considerations in which the connections of individual neurones are of less concern and the connectivity pattern of the neuronal aggregate is studied. Two points can be made here: the first is that the histological studies considered by Sholl (or even those more recently) certainly do not show that specific circuits are unnecessary for proper function; indeed it is doubtful to me whether it would even be possible, in principle, for histological studies to lead to this conclusion. The second point is that, while many neurophysiologists use statistical methods for the most adequate description of some electrophysiological results (Burns, 1968), this does not necessarily imply that the neural connections underlying the electrical activity are themselves random; the connections could be well-ordered but of such complexity that only a statistical treatment of the functional results is feasible.

The randomness or otherwise of neural connections is being widely discussed at the present time and I have the distinct impression that some of the discussion misses the mark, mistakes shadow for reality. This point has been well made by Siebert (1962):

"A random process is a *mathematical model*, not a physical reality. To say that some set of data can be usefully considered for some purposes *as if* it came from a certain random process is not by any means the same as saying that the physical process involved *is* that random process. Indeed the physical process need not actually be 'random' at all in any ordinary sense. The problem may merely be so complex in formulation or analysis (for example, the flip of a coin, behavior of gas molecules, height of ocean waves, and so on) as to render the calculation of presumably deterministic effects unfeasible.

The theory of random processes bears the same relationship to the 'real world' as does any other mathematical theory, such as geometry. Whether an observed shape can be usefully considered as a triangle and, if so, what values to assign to the angles are problems in surveying, not geometry."

There is also a very real sense in which to describe the structure of any nervous system as "random" is an improper usage. The term "random" could probably only be usefully applied to certain neural connections *before they are formed*; once the connections exist they are no longer random. Some of the difficulties inherent in the concepts of randomness and order are discussed, with relation to biology, in a most interesting paper by Bohm (1969). When a biologist talks of "random" connections in part of the nervous system, he probably means not that the connections are unordered, but that it does not matter, from the point of view of function, what the order is. The issue of specific versus random connections is unresolved and is perhaps most pertinently stated by Kennedy *et al.* (1969), who make the good point that, since we cannot distinguish formally between the alleged randomness of connections and our own ignorance about them, the matter will have to await further experiments.

Sholl (1956) achieved a considerable simplification in his treatment of neuron types to be found in the cortex; and his study of cortical connectivity led him to conclude that the statistical distribution of fibres was of paramount importance in determining their detailed connections. To an arguable extent he oversimplified the structure of the cortex in his attempt to see underlying principles of organization. A reassessment of the work of Cajal (1952) in the light of recent anatomical techniques (Colonnier, 1966) suggests that, in particular, the stellate cells show very considerable specialization (Fig. 5.1). The connectivity of these cells indicates that not only do axons go selectively to certain areas of cortex but they may also be specific for certain cells or parts of cells. Synapses could then still be considered random only insofar as they are established on all cell bodies or all dendrites or all pyramidal or all stellate cells that they meet in a specific layer or at a specific distance from the cell of origin. Axons do not contact randomly in the sense that they synapse indiscriminately with any neuronal surface along their course (Colonnier, 1966).

The aim of the present volume is to discuss the formation of nerve connections; however, as I argued in the introductory chapter, we can only investigate meaningfully the formation of nerve connections if we know what connections are formed. And as far as concerns the greater part of the cerebral cortex, this we do not know. Our ignorance in this matter has one great advantage—it helps us to keep an open mind on the question of the structural requirements for intelligent behaviour.

Over recent years, since the early work of McCulloch and Pitts (1947) and Turing (1948) there has been a great upsurge of interest in the design of models that have various of the attributes of brains. Prominent among the factors leading to this situation has been the work of Lashley (1929) with its general implication that learning was dependent on the *amount* of functional cortical tissue and not on its anatomical specialization. So confusing did Lashley find his own results that, after some 30 years of

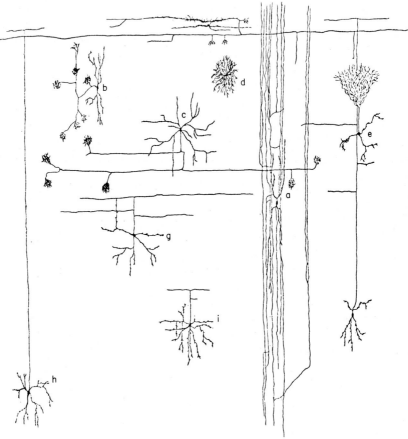

FIG. 5.1.   Composite drawing showing the configuration of various stellate cells in the cortex, after Cajal. From Colonnier, 1966.

investigation into learning and memory, he felt tempted to come to the conclusion that the phenomena he had been studying were just not possible! (Lashley, 1950).

The apparent equipotentiality of cortical tissue revealed by Lashley's work, together with anatomical evidence which suggests that there is a continued and extensive loss of neurones from the cortex during adult life (reviewed by Burns, 1958) has led biomathematicians to the conclusion that the vertebrate central nervous system as a whole shows, in its performance, a *system* error-rate which is much lower than the error-rate of its components (Cowan, 1962). Furthermore the mammalian cerebral

cortex appears to be a highly redundant system in terms of its functional
connections: *redundancy*

> "Consider the eye. Each of its hundred million rods and cones may at one
> moment fail to fire with much light, and at the next, fire with almost none
> (Hecht, 1955). If this be by chance it may be ignored in large groups of
> contemporaneous impulses. We detect the agreement of these signals by their
> coincidence on the ganglion cells and relay only that information to the brain.
> Thus we pay for certainty by foregoing information that fails to agree with
> other information. No machine man ever made uses so many parallel channels
> or demands so much coincidence as his own brain, and none is so likely to go
> right." (McCulloch, 1950).

The field of machine intelligence and the functions of artificial "neural"
nets is, of course, a rapidly-expanding area of study and its very extensive
literature can not be dealt with here. My object in discussing, however
briefly, these cybernetic considerations, is to show that the work of the
model-builders is indeed highly relevant to our own study of neural
connectivity. Thus a recent review of the field (Arbib, 1965) surveys the
attempts that have been made to design reliable networks from unreliable
components, up to the work of Cowan and Winograd (1963). Arbib (1965,
p. 48) notes that "if a modular net, designed for a specific function, is
transformed to minimize its susceptibility to errors due to the malfunction
or death or neurons, the resultant network has a detailed randomness
which is closely akin to that found in the detailed anatomy of the brain".
This statement to some extent begs the question, since as I have already
argued, we do not know to what extent the detailed structure of the brain
is ordered or random. In view of these results, however, we may now
reverse the argument: redundancy and especially randomization of connections were built into these automata partly because it was thought that
connections in real neural systems were redundant and somewhat random.
Automata so built can be shown to work; therefore we would do well to
consider whether, in certain of its parts, the nervous system might not
show some "randomness" of connection also. And so—back to biology and
the investigation of whether localization of function always goes along
with specificity of connection.

As I have mentioned previously, experiments by Hubel and Wiesel
(Hubel and Wiesel, 1963; Wiesel and Hubel, 1963b) would indicate that
the topographical nature of the mammalian visual projection to the cortex
is established without the aid of visual function; and it is very likely that
the other primary inputs and outputs of the mammalian nervous system
are also established prefunctionally. The organization of these pathways
could well depend on a chemospecificity mechanism as suggested by Sperry.
If so, then we would expect these pathway connections to manifest
properties of rigidity and unmodifiability comparable tc those shown by

experiments on the amphibian visual system. Furthermore if we contem-
plate a nervous system *completely* specified in Sperry's sense, then the whole
system will be expected to be morphologically rigid (Sperry, 1958b). And
whereas such a system could, as my previous arguments have attempted to
show, display a very large repertoire of reactions and much functional
plasticity, yet we have to consider also the possibility that certain forms of
behavioural plasticity, notably those related to learning and memory, may
involve synaptic changes between neurones (Ungar, 1968; Gaze and Keating,
1970b).

Even in man, by far the greater proportion of intracerebral connections
are formed after birth. This follows from observations on the development
of the morphology of cerebral cortical neurones. During the first two years
of life the weight of the human brain increases by about 350% (Coppoletta
and Welbach, 1933). We do not know to what extent the number of
neurones increases during the same period in man although it is of interest
that in some other mammals, Altman (1967) has shown that the "microneurones" are mainly of postnatal origin, in parts of the brain other than
the neocortex. Information on the time of development of cerebral cortical
microneurones is not yet available and it will be interesting to see whether
these also are developed after birth; particularly so since these neurones
include the stellate cells, which appear to play a major role in the functional
relationship between specific afferent fibres and cortical pyramidal cells
(Colonnier, 1966; Szentágothai, 1967). Part, at least, of the postnatal
increase in brain size in man is due to the morphological development of
the already-existing neurones (Fig. 5.2). Thus in the neonate there are few
if any dendrites present (De Crinis, 1934) and the time of their appearance
varies in different parts of the cortex. According to De Crinis dendro-
genetic maturity first occurs in the primary sensory and motor projection
areas, and only later occurs in other parts of the cortex. This observation
agrees well with my earlier suggestion that the primary inputs and outputs
are organized prefunctionally. Since most cortical dendrites only develop
after birth it follows that their connections can only appear after this time.
It is a major unsolved problem whether these late-appearing dendritic
connections are formed under the control of innate specificity mechanisms
or some other, perhaps functional, influence.

The observation that brief exposure to light in otherwise dark-reared
rats may lead to significant alterations in the synaptic morphology of the
visual cortex (Cragg, 1967) suggests that some aspect of function exerts an
effect on the development of dendritic connections. Similarly, the
commonly-instanced ability of neonatal animals to survive brain damage
with minimal after-effects on function (Lenneberg, 1967) indicates the
effectiveness of postnatal cerebral organization; and this presumably
includes the patterns of connectivity which, to an unknown extent, must
underly specific function. In this context we can agree with Arbib (1965)

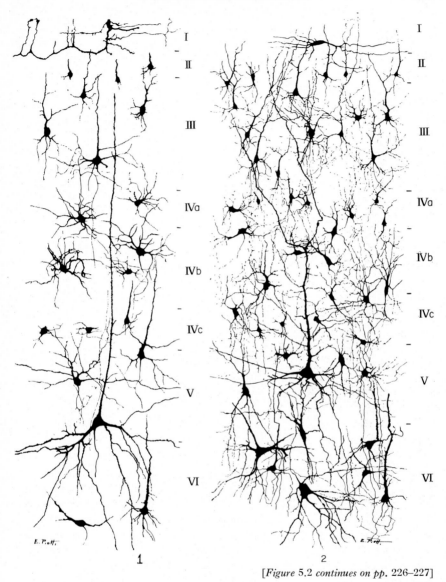

[*Figure 5.2 continues on pp.* 226–227]

FIG. 5.2. The development of dendritic arborizations in the human visual cortex. (1) Neonatal; (2) 1 month; (3) 3 months; (4) 6 months; (5) 15 months; (6) 24 months. Reprinted by permission of the publishers from Jesse L. Conel "The Postnatal Development of the Human Cerebral Cortex", Cambridge, Mass: Harvard University Press, copyright 1939, 1941, 1947, 1951, 1955, 1959 by the President and Fellows of Harvard College.

on brain-simulation experiments, that *complete* randomness of connections is not a helpful concept:

8*

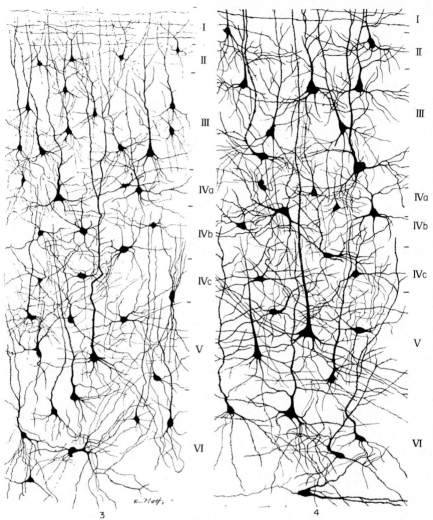

3   4

"There are intellectual acts open to a human child which are forever denied to a gorilla—and these must be due, it would seem, to genetically determined differences in structure. Darwinian evolution took aeons to build the capability for pattern recognition into our brains—it would be surprising if a random network should evolve such a capability in a few hours of learning" (Arbib, 1965, p. 48).

In the remainder of this chapter I intend to discuss two situations where a functional control appears to be exerted over the behaviour of neural connections. In the first of these situations, the mammalian visual cortex, the genesis of properly organized connections between the incoming fibres of the optic radiation and the cells of the visual cortex seems to be independent of visual function but the maintenance of some of these connections in a functional state is dependent on visual interaction between the

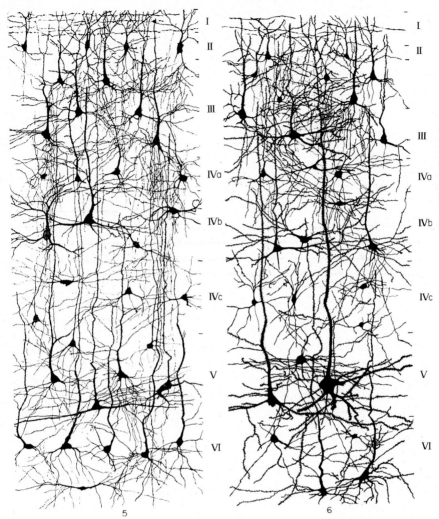

two eyes. In the second situation, the development of the intertectal connections that form part of the anuran ipsilateral visual projection, the evidence at present available suggests that a functional interaction between the two visual inputs is the mechanism that *determines* the topographical order of the intertectal projection.

EFFECTS OF FUNCTION ON THE DEVELOPMENT AND MAINTENANCE OF MAMMALIAN VISUAL CONNECTIONS

The work of Cragg previously cited indicates a role for function in the development of synaptic morphology. Mice reared in darkness show changes in nuclear size in the upper part of the visual cortex (Gyllensten, 1959; Gyllensten *et al.*, 1965), whereas animals brought up in a visually

enriched environment show increased dendritic branching in the visual
cortex (Holloway, 1966; Diamond *et al.*, 1964). Thus *some* aspect of visual
function appears to be playing a part in postnatal structural changes in the
visual cortex. But from these experiments we cannot gain any precise idea
of what aspect is involved. More helpful in this respect is the work of
Hubel and Wiesel, on young kittens.

Studies on the receptive-field characteristics of cells in the cat's visual
cortex suggest that the connections between the lateral geniculate nucleus
and the striate cortex, and those between individual visual cortical cells
are highly specific (Hubel and Wiesel, 1962); moreover, as I have previously stated, the cortical responses of visually inexperienced kittens
closely resembled those of mature cats in the receptive-field characteristics
of individual cortical cells (Hubel and Wiesel, 1963). A major difference
between the cortical activity of these visually inexperienced kittens and
that of adult cats was that the young kittens showed a much lower level of
maintained activity under conditions of steady, diffuse, background
illumination; and responsive cells fatigued quickly and responded sluggish-
ly to the most effective stimuli. It would be interesting to know to what
extent these differences were correlated with lack of dendritic maturity in
the newborn kittens. Except for this sluggishness of response, cortical cells
of visually inexperienced kittens resembled those of mature cats in their
responses to patterned stimuli; similarities included field orientations,
columnar arrangements of cells with like receptive-field orientations, and
binocular interaction; as in an adult cat (Hubel and Wiesel, 1962), the great
majority of cells recorded in immature kittens could be influenced from
each eye separately from, apparently, the same point in visual space. The
subdivision of responsive cells in terms of ocular dominance was also
similar to that in the adult animal (Fig. 5.3).

These observations would suggest that the visual input to the cortex is
already partly connected up in visually inexperienced kittens; and yet
kittens appear to be quite unable to use their eyes at the time of normal
eye-opening, which usually occurs between the sixth and the tenth day.
Visually guided avoidance of objects appears about the 14th day, while
pursuit, following movements and visual placing reactions only appear by
20–25 days. Thus, since the input distribution to the cortex appears to be
present from the time of eye-opening, the inability of young kittens to use
their vision appears to be related more to a lack of effective visuomotor
connections than to an inadequate visual cortical input (Hubel and Wiesel,
1963).

Normally organized visual input to cortical cells thus exists at the onset
of visual experience. It will be obvious, however, that this statement
concerning the results of Hubel and Wiesel applies to *functional* connections. I shall assume, for the purpose of my further discussion, that these
functional connections represent anatomical connections. We do not know

whether this is so since in the mammalian visual system there have as yet
been no analyses of the visual projection adequate to allow us to equate
morphological and electrophysiological results in young animals. The
advisability of caution in the attempt to deduce fibre connections in the
cortex from such electrophysiological work is suggested by the observations

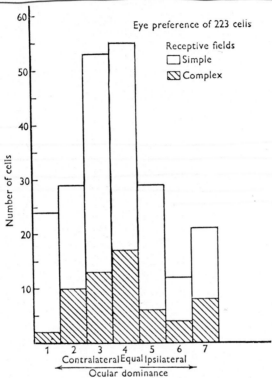

FIG. 5.3. Distribution of 223 cells recorded from the cat visual cortex, according to
ocular dominance. Histogram includes cells with simple fields and cells with complex
fields. The shaded region shows the distribution of cells with complex receptive fields.
Cells of group 1 were driven only by the contralateral eye; for cells of group 2 there was
marked dominance of the contralateral eye, for group 3, slight dominance. For cells in
group 4 there was no obvious difference between the two eyes. In group 5 the ipsilateral
eye dominated slightly, in group 6, markedly; and in group 7 the cells were driven only
by the ipsilateral eye. From Hubel and Wiesel, 1962.

of Horn and Hill (1969); these authors tilted cats while recording cortical
responses to visual stimulation and they found, in one animal, that a new
"receptive-field" appeared, in a different part of the visual field. And while
the orientation of the axis of the original receptive-field was tilted when the
animal was tilted (but not to the same extent as the tilt of the animal),
the orientation of the axis of the secondary receptive-field was similar to
the original, untilted, orientation of the first receptive field.

   Although the pattern of visual cortical responses is largely normal in
visually inexperienced kittens, if one eye is deprived of pattern vision from

the time of eye-opening the result is a grossly abnormal visual cortex (Wiesel and Hubel, 1963b) in that virtually all the cortical cells recorded are then completely uninfluenced by the deprived eye (Fig. 5.4); whereas in a normal mature cat, or a visually inexperienced neonatal kitten, about four fifths of the cells in the striate cortex are binocularly influenced.

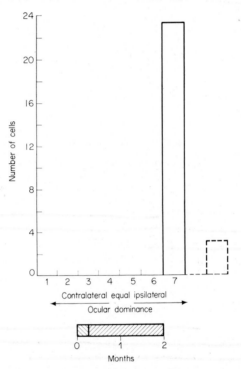

Fig. 5.4.   Ocular-dominance distribution of 26 cells recorded in the visual cortex contralateral to the deprived eye. This 2-month-old kitten had had its right eye covered from the time of normal eye-opening by a translucent contact lens; the left eye was normally exposed. Twenty-three cells were driven by the normally exposed (left, or ipsilateral) eye, and were therefore assigned to ocular-dominance group 7. Three cells could not be activated by either eye (interrupted lines). From Wiesel and Hubel, 1963.

Monocular deprivation thus provides physiological defects in a system that was once capable of functioning. It appears that the deprivation must continue for a period of ten days or more for these cortical abnormalities to occur; for in one animal which has been monocularly deprived from the time of normal eye-opening up to 19 days after birth, the ocular dominance pattern of cortical cells was still normal (Hubel and Wiesel, 1963). The animals which did show cortical abnormalities had been monocularly deprived for periods of 2 months from the time of eye-opening. If one or two months of normal visual experience preceded one to four months of monocular deprivation, the cortical cells still behaved abnormally, although less so than in animals that had been deprived from the time of eye-opening. Three months of monocular deprivation in an adult cat, however, led to no detectable changes in the pattern of ocular dominance in cortical cells (Wiesel and Hubel, 1963b). In these experiments on kittens, the cortical impairment was just as marked after deprivation with a translucent occluder, which prevented pattern stimulation but reduced diffuse illumination by only 1–2 log units, as it was with lid-closure, which prevented form vision and also reduced diffuse illumination by 4–5 log units. The significant deprivation thus seems to be pattern vision.

The abnormal ocular dominance pattern revealed by these experiments on monocular deprivation, is due to interference with normal binocular *interaction*. This is shown by a further series of experiments where kittens were deprived binocularly by lid suture at 6–18 days after birth, for periods of $2\frac{1}{2}$–$4\frac{1}{2}$ months. The previous results on monocular eye closure could have led one to expect that binocular closure would give areas of cortex containing no responsive cells at all; yet in these animals after binocular deprivation, although the cortex was by no means normal, most cells not only responded to visual stimuli but over half of those that did respond did so normally. Thus interference with one visual input gives gross cortical abnormality while interference with both leaves the cortical cells more normal in this respect.

Further evidence that the cortical abnormality after monocular deprivation is not merely due to a decrease in excitation arriving at the cortex via the occluded eye was provided by experiments in which both eyes were left open but a squint was produced by section of the medial rectus at 8–10 days after birth. The visual cortices of these animals, recorded some three months later, showed a very abnormal picture of ocular dominance with much less binocular interaction than normal (Hubel and Wiesel, 1965). Most cells were driven by one eye only, some by the ipsilateral eye, some by the contralateral; furthermore there were regions of complete contralateral or ipsilateral dominance in which one eye drove cell after cell as well as the unresolved background activity, with no trace of a response to stimulation of the other eye. Advance of the electrode would lead to the region dominated by one eye giving way to a region dominated by the other (Fig. 5.5). In these experiments therefore, the abnormal ocular dominance patterns shown by the cortical cells were brought about by the existence of a squint which kept the two eyes from working together, without cutting down the input to either eye. Comparable abnormalities of cortical function was seen when alternate eyes were occluded daily in otherwise normal kittens (Hubel and Wiesel, 1965).

In a normal cat the two receptive fields of a single cortical cell are similar in arrangement and occupy corresponding positions in the two eyes. Small disparities in the receptive field positions have been analysed by Barlow *et al.*, 1967; Nikara *et al.*, 1968; Pettigrew *et al.*, 1968a,b and

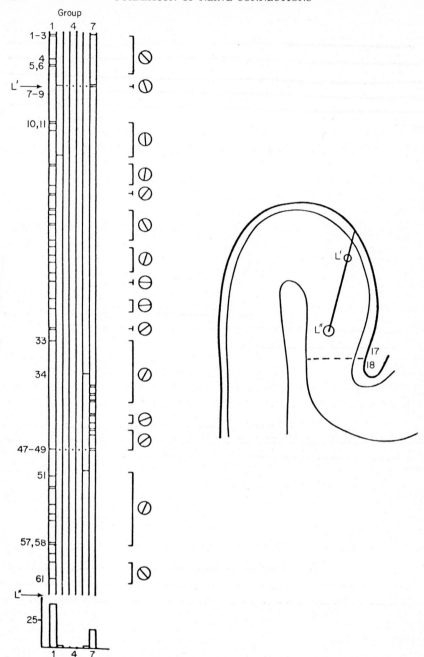

Fig. 5.5. Reconstruction of a penetration through right hemisphere of a 12-month-old cat with divergent strabismus from birth (cat 2). To the right is shown a coronal section through the right postlateral gyrus. The electrode track is shown passing through two

[Caption continued at foot of page 233]

appear to form part of a mechanism for binocular depth discrimination. With corresponding fields, an object in visual space will tend to affect a cortical cell in the same qualitative way via either eye and with a nearly synchronous input to the cell. Absence of this close synchrony, together with activation of at least one of the convergent afferent pathways seems to be the prerequisite for the breakdown of the normal ocular dominance pattern. On the basis of these experiments Hubel and Wiesel (1965) suggested that, in some systems at least, the maintenance of a synapse depends not only on the amount of incoming impulse activity but also on a normal interrelationship between activity in the different afferents.

N.B.

The first few months of postnatal life in the kitten appear to be a critical period for the establishment of a normally maintained binocular input to visual cortical cells. Animals with one eye closed for three months from birth showed no evidence of recovery of a normal pattern of binocularity when studied after a further period of several months with the previously closed eye open and the other eye shut (Wiesel and Hubel, 1965b). The three months period of closure of the previously open eye had little or no effect on that eye's ability to drive cortical cells; whereas simple closure of one eye after several months of normal vision produced a marked cortical defect (Wiesel and Hubel, 1963b).

Summarizing these experiments, we may say that an approximately normal pattern of binocular input to cortical cells is already established in kittens at the time the eyes first open. Interference with the normal pattern of binocular excitation over the first few months, by monocular occlusion, abnormality of the relationship between the visual axes or alternate eye occlusion, leads to a permanent loss of the normal binocularity of cortical cells. Thus while binocular interaction is not, apparently, necessary for the establishment of the appropriate functional connections, it is necessary for their maintenance. We still do not know what factors lead to the initial organization of these connections.

Summary

THE CONTROL OF THE FORMATION OF INTERTECTAL CONNECTIONS IN THE IPSILATERAL VISUAL PROJECTION OF THE FROG

The visual projection to the ipsilateral tectum in the frog involves an intertectal pathway, as described in the previous chapter. Since my present argument relates to the formation of these intertectal connections it will be

electrolytic lesions, L' and L″ indicated approximately to scale by circles. To the left of the figure the track is reconstructed, each cell being indicated by a short horizontal line placed in its appropriate ocular-dominance group. Two lines close together, or dots between pairs of lines, indicate two-unit recordings. Total numbers are shown for each group in the histogram on p. 232. Lines to the right within the circles indicate by their tilt the receptive-field orientations of the cells within the brackets. Note the strong tendency for cells of a particular ocular-dominance group to occur in sequence. From Hubel and Wiesel, 1965.

worthwhile to summarize here our understanding of the nature and structure of the ipsilateral projection.

The nature of the anuran ipsilateral visual projection

Despite the fact that anatomical studies show that the retinotectal fibres in anurans decussate completely at the chiasma, so that each eye connects directly, by means of its optic nerve fibres, only with the contralateral

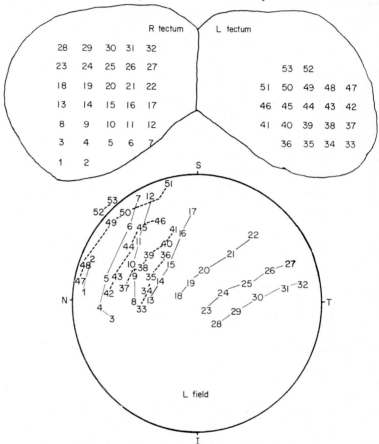

FIG. 5.6.   The contralateral and ipsilateral visual projections from the left eye in a normal frog. The numbers on the perimeter chart which are joined by continuous lines indicate the field positions projecting to the contralateral (right) tectum; numbers joined by dashed lines indicate the ipsilateral projection. From Keating and Gaze, in preparation.

tectum (Wlassak, 1893; Cajal, 1898; Knapp *et al.*, 1965), yet electrophysiological recording from the rostral part of the optic tectum (*Rana*, *Xenopus*) enables responses to be picked up following visual stimulation within the nasal part of the visual field of the ipsilateral eye (Gaze, 1958b; Gaze and Jacobson, 1962). The nasal part of the monocular visual field which gives rise to these ipsilateral tectal responses is coextensive with the

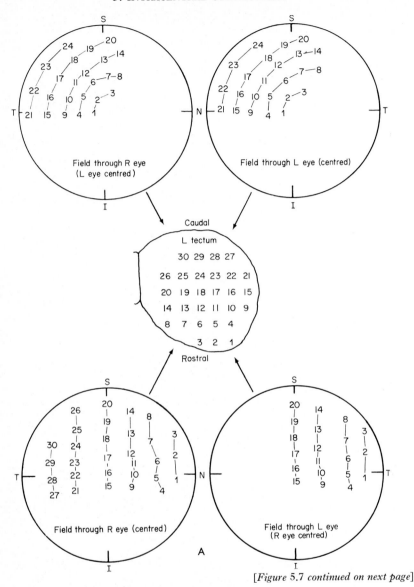

FIG. 5.7. Normal visual projections in *Xenopus*. (A) The projection of the visual field through both eyes to the left tectum. The numbers on the tectal diagram represent electrode positions. For each tectal position the corresponding field position is indicated by the appropriate number on the perimetric charts. N, nasal pole; S, Superior (dorsal) pole; I, inferior (ventral) pole. The field projections through both eyes are plotted with the left eye centred on the perimeter in the two upper charts in the figure and with the right eye centred on the perimeter in the two lower charts. When both contralateral and ipsilateral projections to one tectum are mapped with the same eye centred it can be seen that any one position on the rostral tectum is excited via *both* eyes from only one field position. The two perimeter charts are superimposable. Such a double map is made by placing the electrode at one position on the tectum, covering one eye with an opaque shield and determining the field position via the other eye; then the shield is transferred to the other eye and the process repeated;

[*Figure* 5.7 *continued on next page*]

binocular visual field. The ipsilateral visual projection is retinotopically organized and Fig. 5.6 shows the nature of the ipsilateral field map in the

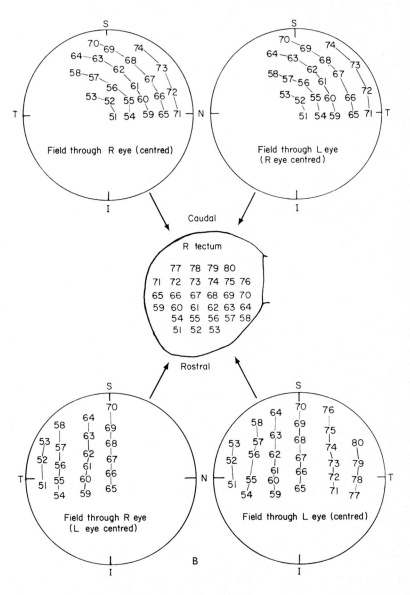

FIG. 5.7. (B) The projection of the visual field through both eyes to the right tectum. In this case the two upper field plots represent the projections via both eyes with the right eye centred on the perimeter and the two lower field plots the projections via both eyes with the left eye centred on the perimeter. These maps are somewhat diagrammatic representations of data combined from several animals. From Gaze, Keating, Székely and Beazley, 1970.

frog. In *Xenopus* the ipsilateral projection is similar; but owing to the greater overlap of the visual fields it is somewhat more extensive (Fig. 5.7).

In the direct contralateral retinotectal projection, nasal field (temporal retina) projects to rostral tectum and temporal field (nasal retina) to caudal tectum; and since the nasal extremity of the field for the right eye lies to the left of the animal while the nasal extremity of the field for the left eye lies to the right of the animal, any object extended in the horizontal direction in the binocular visual field must be represented, in its contralateral projections, extended in one direction rostrocaudally on the left tectum and in the opposite direction on the right tectum (Fig. 5.8).

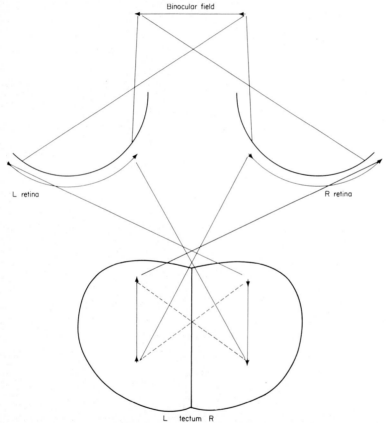

FIG. 5.8.   Diagram representing the projection, rostrocaudally on the two tecta, of the nasotemporal binocular field axis for each eye. For both right and left eye the nasal aspect of the field projects rostrally on the tectum, with more temporal field represented more caudally. The contralateral tectal representation of the field arrow thus points in a different direction on each tectum. Since one point in binocular visual space projects via both eyes to one tectal point on one side and to a different tectal point on the other, the intertectal connections effectively existing are indicated, in outline, by the dashed lines. The representation of the intertectal connections indicates merely the overall result of the connections, not the pathway. From Gaze and Keating, 1970b.

Gaze and Jacobson (1962) observed that one point in the binocular field projects via *both* eyes to one point on the left tectum and to another point on the right tectum. In view of what I have just said, this indicates that, through one eye, the ipsilateral projection of the nasotemporal field axis will have the reverse orientation to the contralateral projection of this axis. And since the second stage of the ipsilateral projection involves an intertectal linkage, this linkage must connect rostral contralateral tectum with more caudal ipsilateral tectum, and more caudal contralateral tectum with rostral ipsilateral tectum (Fig. 5.8).

The evidence relating to the ipsilateral visual pathway

The experimental observations leading to the conclusion that the ipsilateral pathway involves an intertectal linkage are the following:

(1) Ipsilateral responses are always of longer latency than contralateral responses elicited from the same field position. This suggests a longer pathway for the former (Gaze and Jacobson, 1963a; Gaze and Jacobson, 1963c).

(2) From one point in the visual field, both contralateral and ipsilateral paths converge on *one* point on one tectum and another point on the other tectum. These points on the two tecta are only symmetrically arranged for stimuli in the midsagittal plane of the animal.

(3) Localized destruction of the appropriate place on the contralateral tectum, from which a response is being recorded to stimulation at one place in the binocular field, selectively abolishes the ipsilateral response, at the functionally-corresponding point on the other tectum, to stimulation from the same point in visual space, without interfering with the contralateral input to this other tectum from the same field position (Fig. 5.9). This strongly suggests that the ipsilateral pathway involves passage through the corresponding point in the contralateral tectum.

(4) Contrary to the original report of Gaze and Jacobson (1962), there is *no* part of the visual field which is only represented on the ipsilateral tectum; electrode penetrations made sufficiently far rostrally on the contralateral tectum give responses from the far nasal visual field of the contralateral eye. Thus all retinal positions projecting to the ipsilateral tectum also project to the contralateral tectum (Keating and Gaze, 1970).

(5) Section of one optic tract between chiasma and tectum results in abolition of the contralateral projection to that tectum and disappearance of the ipsilateral projection to *both* tecta (Keating and Gaze, 1970).

(6) Massive intertectal lesions separating the tecta down to the ventricle, and from cerebellum caudally to posterior commissure rostrally, do not interfere with the ipsilateral projection. Nor do lesions of the ventral tegmentum.

(7) The evidence under heading (5) above suggests that the fibres involved in the intertectal linkage enter or leave the tectum via the optic

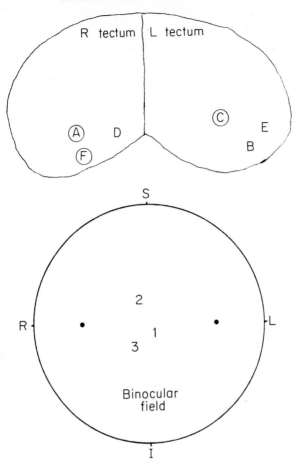

FIG. 5.9.   The effects of multiple, localized, tectal lesions on the ipsilateral projection in the frog. The electrode was first placed at position A on the right tectum and the corresponding field position was found to be position 1—for either eye. Field position 1 was then found to project to point B on the left tectum, again through either eye. A localized lesion (150 microns across) was then produced at tectal position A (indicated by the ring); all responses from this position naturally disappeared. When the electrode was replaced on tectal position B, it was found that stimulation at position 1 in the field evoked brisk responses via the right eye; the responses from tectal position B, previously evoked from field position 1 via the left eye were, however, no longer present. Thus a lesion at tectal position A abolished the ipsilateral response from the corresponding field position (1) at the other tectum. The left tectum itself was undamaged, as shown by the survival of the contralateral responses from the same field position at tectal position B. The abolition of the ipsilateral responses following a localized lesion of the contralateral tectum, is itself localized. Thus movement of the electrode about 100 microns away from B allowed ipsilateral responses to be evoked via the left eye.

   This procedure was repeated for two further field positions. Field position 2 projected via both eyes to C on the left tectum and D on the right tectum; localized destruction of position C (shown by the ring) abolished the ipsilateral projection from field position 2 via the right eye to the right tectum (D) but the contralateral projection via the left eye

[*Caption continued at foot of next page*]

tract. Localized lesions in the region of the postoptic commissures abolish *both* ipsilateral projections while leaving both contralateral projections intact (Keating and Gaze, 1970). These critical observations on the pathway of the ipsilateral projection are summarized in Fig. 5.10 and they

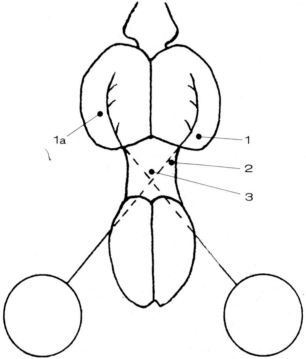

Fig. 5.10.   Summary of the evidence that the ipsilateral projection involves an intertectal linkage. (1) Localized tectal lesion abolishes the ipsilateral response at the other tectum (1a) from the same field position; (2) Tract lesion abolishes the contralateral projection on the same side, as well as *both* ipsilateral projections; (3) Localized destruction of the post-optic commissures abolishes *both* ipsilateral projections but leaves both contralateral projections intact.

indicate that the ipsilateral path involves passage first to the contralateral tectum as part of the normal contralateral retinotectal projection; then, presumably after a synapse, back down the optic tract, across the postoptic commissures and up the ipsilateral diencephalon to the ipsilateral tectum.

(8) The number of synapses on this intertectal path is unknown; but recently fibres have been demonstrated (Lázár, 1969; Rubinson, 1970)

---

to position D was unaffected. Field position 3 projected via both eyes to F and to E; localized destruction of F (shown by the ring) again abolished the ipsilateral projection from field position 3 via the left eye at tectal position E but the contralateral projection to this tectal point via the right eye remained.

In this experiment the perimeter was centred on the animal's nose. The approximate projection points of the right and left optic axes are indicated by the black dots on the perimeter charts. From Keating and Gaze (1970).

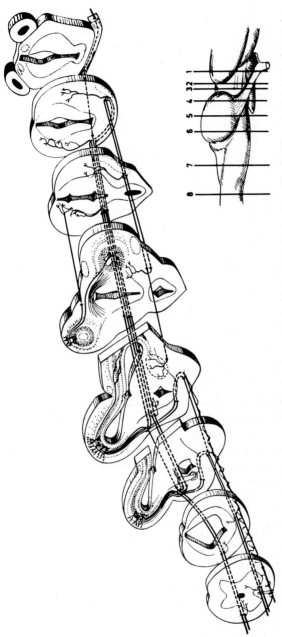

FIG. 5.11. Schematic representation of the efferent pathways of the optic tectum in the frog. Vertical lines in the inset figure show the planes of sectioning. In the sections the extent of the grey matter is outlined by thin lines, the tectal stratification is shown in detail. In sections 4 to 6 a few slightly magnified pyramidal neurones indicate the origin of the efferent pathways. The area occupied by the optic tract is indicated by dotted lines in sections 2 to 6. A round area encircled with broken lines in section 5 shows the place of the nucleus profundus lateralis, the nucleus isthmi is indicated by dots in section 6. Above the ventricle in section 4 the posterior commissure is represented by solid lines. Fibres are seen leaving the tectum, running rostrally and crossing in the postoptic commissures before going caudally again. From Lázár, 1969.

which leave the tectum, cross in the postoptic region and then course back towards the other tectum. These fibres do not go to the tectum but appear to end in the nucleus profundus lateralis (Fig. 5.11). Some of these fibres may be involved in the intertectal linkage of the ipsilateral projection; in which case there should be a further connection from the nucleus profundus lateralis to the tectum.

From these various observations we think that the ipsilateral visual path in the frog involves passage of the impulses through the contralateral tectum. The evidence suggests that the ipsilateral path in *Xenopus* is similar to that in the frog. The intertectal pathway concerned in the ipsilateral projection thus provides us with an excellent situation for the investigation of certain mechanisms involved in the genesis of central neural connections. The *contralateral* retinotectal projection is highly organized in a retinotopic fashion; and so also is the *ipsilateral* visual projection. Thus the intertectal connections that lead from the one to the other should also show order. Indeed, this follows from the observations already mentioned on the effects of localized lesions of one tectum on the ipsilateral projection to the other tectum.

There is, therefore, a retinotopically organized intertectal projection in anurans. We may then ask how this organized central projection is set up during development. If the operative mechanism is a form of neuronal specificity akin to that proposed by Sperry for the contralateral retinotectal projection, then we might assume that a localized region of one tectum, of a certain tectal specificity, would connect with a region on the other tectum of corresponding tectal specificity; and these intertectal connections should not, in this simple case, be affected by the optic input to either tectum.

A major advantage of the intertectal projection for our present purposes is that we can very easily alter the visual input from one eye, by rotating that eye. In this case, as discussed in the previous chapter, the *retinal* connections still go to their proper places on the contralateral tectum, and since the eye is now rotated with respect to the visual field, the projection of the *field* on the contralateral tectum is rotated correspondingly. On the simple assumption just made, that the intertectal connections are laid down on a specificity basis, the ipsilateral projection via the rotated eye should also be rotated. *This does not happen*; the ipsilateral projection in such a case is normal. Similarly, in animals with a NN compound eye, the contralateral projection from the appropriate part of the compound eye is reversed nasotemporally on the tectum. And thus, on the intertectal specificity hypothesis, the ipsilateral projection from such an eye should be reversed. *It is not.*

These considerations suggest that there is something worth studying in the mode of formation of the intertectal linkages. I will now present the evidence from various types of experiment, which leads us to think that, in this situation, a functional control, dependent on the visual input, gives rise to the ordered intertectal fibre projection.

The nature of the ipsilateral projections in animals with one compound eye

The contralateral retinotectal projection from a compound eye has been discussed in the previous chapter; each (similar) half of the compound eye appears to connect with the entire tectum as if it were a whole eye and the orientation of this projection is appropriate to the nature of the original half-eye, either nasal or temporal (Figs. 4.40 and 4.41). The contralateral retinotectal projection from the other, normal, eye in an animal with one compound eye, is normal.

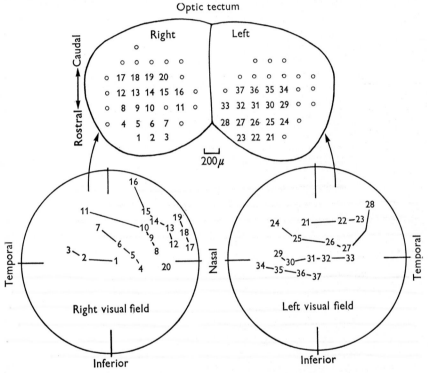

FIG. 5.12. Ipsilateral visual projections in a *Xenopus* with one NN compound eye. The right eye is NN and the left eye is normal. It may be seen that the ipsilateral projection from the compound eye is normal (compare 5.7) whereas that from the *normal* eye is inverted along the rostrocaudal tectal axis (as well as, in this case, being rotated some 45° clockwise). From Gaze, Jacobson and Székely, 1965.

The ipsilateral projection from a compound eye may show reduplication of field positions analogous to those seen in the contralateral projection; but more frequently there is only one set of field positions and these are essentially normal. The ipsilateral projection from the normal eye, in an animal which has one TT compound eye, is also normal. If the operated eye is NN, however, the ipsilateral projection from the *normal* eye shows consistently a peculiar abnormality (Gaze *et al.*, 1965; Gaze, Keating *et al.*, 1970); it is inverted in the way it projects along the rostrocaudal axis of the tectum (Fig. 5.12).

This abnormality of the ipsilateral projection from the *normal* eye in animals whose other eye was NN, was an unexpected finding. The abnormality was patterned, not random; the projection was systematically abnormal. The eye from which the abnormal ipsilateral projection arose was itself normal; the contralateral tectum through which this projection passed was also normal, as shown by the normal nature of the direct retinotectal projection to it. Seemingly the most likely site of abnormality was thus the ipsilateral tectum, which was the one receiving fibres directly from the compound eye. This suggests that, in some way, the presence of the NN compound eye had altered the receptivity of its corresponding tectum for fibres from the other tectum (Gaze *et al.*, 1965).

The nature of the ipsilateral projections in animals with one rotated eye

To make my further argument more readily comprehensible I must first discuss the nature of the ipsilateral projections found in animals in which one eye has been rotated during embryonic life, after the period of retinal axial polarization. As I have mentioned in the previous chapter, after such an operation the projection of the *field* via the rotated eye is correspondingly rotated on the contralateral tectum; and this is because each part of the retina connects with the tectum in a manner appropriate to its embryological origin and inappropriate to its new, rotated, position with respect to the field. The contralateral retinotectal projection from the other, normal eye is, of course, normal in such an animal. What about the ipsilateral projection from the rotated and the normal eye?

Before we examine the experimental results it will be as well for us to consider again what we might expect to find on the assumption that the ipsilateral visual projection, including its intertectal pathway, is established through the action of a neuronal specificity mechanism akin to that proposed by Sperry (see previous chapter) for the direct, contralateral, retinotectal projection. The intertectal connections that form the second stage of the ipsilateral visual projection are precise and retinotopically organized; we may represent the contralateral and ipsilateral projections of the nasotemporal field axis in the form of a linear diagram (Fig. 5.13a). If we assume that an intertectal specificity mechanism is operating in the formation of these intertectal connections, then rotation of an eye after the time of intertectal specification should, provided that the eye has already been specified, result in inversion of the ipsilateral projection. This is a necessary requirement of hypothesis; since with prespecified intertectal connections, inversion of the first stage of the ipsilateral projection must result in inversion of the second stage also (Fig. 5.13b).

The experimental findings in this situation are different. If the eye of a

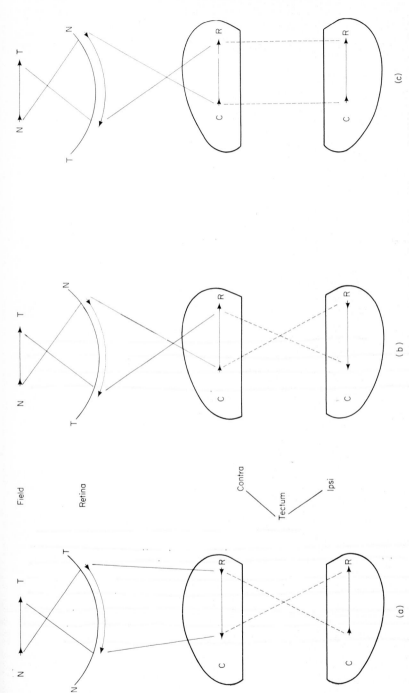

Fig. 5.13.   (a) Linear representation of the contralateral and ipsilateral projections of the field of the right eye; (b) Linear approximation to what might be expected in the case of an eye rotated by 180°, if the intertectal connections were determined by a specificity mechanism akin to that determining the contralateral retinotectal projection. In this case both contralateral and ipsilateral projections of the field are rotated; (c) Actual field projections found in animals with one eye rotated by 180°. The contralateral projection from the rotated eye is rotated while the ipsilateral projection is not. N, nasal; T, temporal; C, caudal; R, rostral. From Gaze and Keating, 1970b.

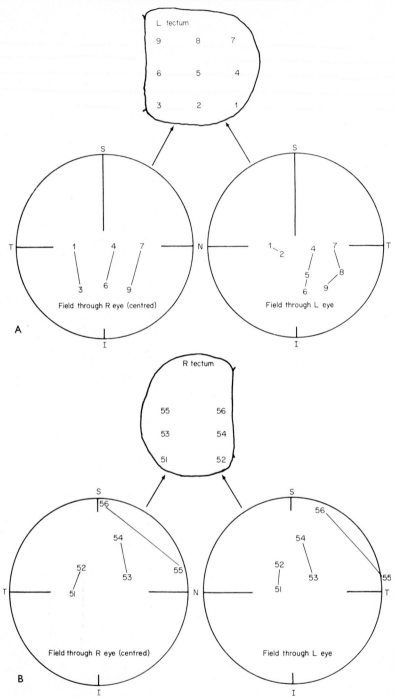

FIG. 5.14.   Visual projections in a *Xenopus* with one rotated eye. (A) Visual projections to the left tectum from both eyes, mapped with the right eye centred on the perimeter. The right eye was rotated approximately 180° clockwise, as seen from in front of the animal, and the left eye was normal; (B) Visual projections to the right tectum from both eyes, mapped with the right eye centred on the perimeter. Same animal as A. These projections may be compared with those from a normal *Xenopus* in Fig. 5.7. From Gaze *et al.*, 1970.

Xenopus is rotated during larval life, after retinal axial determination has occurred, its contralateral field projection is, of course, rotated; but its ipsilateral field projection is *normal* (Fig. 5.13c). And moreover, the contralateral projection from the normal eye in this situation is, naturally, normal, whereas the ipsilateral field projection from the *normal* eye is *rotated*, and to the same extent as the rotation of the operated eye (Fig. 5.14). These findings (Gaze *et al.*, 1970) thus show that a simple prefunctional specificity system cannot be the mechanism responsible for the elaboration of the retinotopically organized ipsilateral projection in this animal.

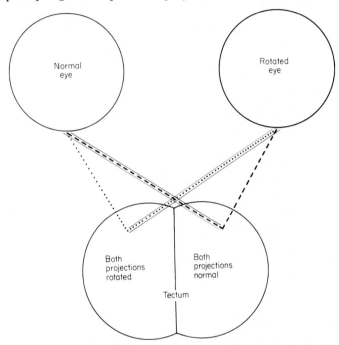

FIG. 5.15. Summary of the projections formed following rotation of a larval amphibian eye. Contralateral projections are shown within tramlines. Projections to the left tectum are shown by dots, those to the right tectum by dashes. The ipsilateral connections merely show the effective functional link, not the pathway. From Gaze and Keating, 1970b.

The situation in an animal with a rotated eye may be summarized in Fig. 5.15. Both projections to one tectum are rotated (and congruent); that is, the contralateral projection from the rotated eye and the ipsilateral projection from the normal eye both go to one and the same tectum and are both rotated to the same extent; and both projections to the other tectum, that is, the contralateral projection from the normal eye and the ipsilateral projection from the rotated eye, are normal. This means that the pattern of intertectal connections seen in an animal with a rotated eye is different from that seen in a normal animal (Fig. 5.13c). And moreover the extent of this systematic abnormality in the intertectal connections can be altered in a predictable direction and in a precise fashion merely by altering the extent of rotation of the operated eye.

The origin of the abnormality in the ipsilateral projection from the normal eye; and the normality of the ipsilateral projection from the operated eye

We may now return to a consideration of the abnormality of the ipsilateral projection from the normal eye in an animal with one compound NN eye. We may note that this abnormality is similar in some respects to that found in the ipsilateral projection from the normal eye in animals with one eye rotated by 180°. In both cases the ipsilateral projection from the normal eye is inverted (rotated 180°) in the way it projects along the rostrocaudal axis of the tectum. In both cases the eye giving rise to the abnormal ipsilateral projection is itself normal; the tectum contralateral to that eye is

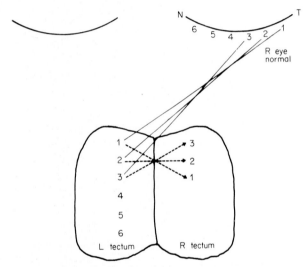

FIG. 5.16. The normal visual projection to the ipsilateral tectum in *Xenopus*. The ipsilateral projection involves, first, passage of impulses from retina to the contralateral tectum, then passage back to the ipsilateral tectum via an intertectal linkage. From Gaze *et al.*, 1970.

normal; and the likely site of abnormality is the ipsilateral tectum, which is the one receiving fibres directly from the *abnormal* eye. In both cases the abnormality in the ipsilateral projection from the normal eye reflects quantitatively and qualitatively the abnormality in the *contralateral* projection to the same tectum from the operated eye. For it will be recalled (Chapter 4) that the peculiarity of a NN compound eye is that the temporal half of the retina (being, in fact, a nasal half) projects *in reverse order* rostrocaudally on the contralateral tectum; and it is the temporal half of the retina which is mainly concerned with producing the ipsilateral projection since it is topographically temporal retina which looks out at the binocular field.

The ipsilateral projection in a normal *Xenopus* arises mostly from the nasal visual field (temporal retina) and projects first to the contralateral tectum and then back, via an intertectal linkage, to the ipsilateral tectum. In summary diagram this may be shown in Fig. 5.16 which shows again that the ipsilateral representation of the field (or retina) is reversed along the nasotemporal axis in comparison with the contralateral projection. Positions 1, 2, 3 run rostrocaudally on the contralateral tectum and caudorostrally on the ipsilateral tectum.

If we assume (what is reasonable) that the ipsilateral pathway from the compound eye involves passage through the contralateral tectum, as is the case with the path from a normal eye, we may represent the ipsilateral projection from a NN compound eye in diagrammatic form in Fig. 5.17.

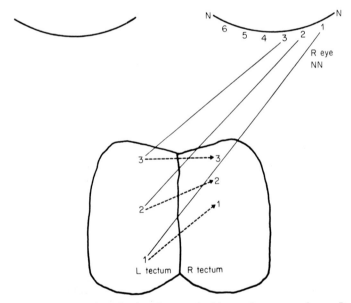

FIG. 5.17. The ipsilateral projection from a double-nasal compound eye. It may be seen, that although the end result, on the ipsilateral tectum, is normal (compare Fig. 5.16), the intermediate stage, on the contralateral tectum, is abnormal. From Gaze *et al.*, 1970.

The temporal part of the retina, which is embryologically of nasal origin, projects across its contralateral tectum in an order appropriate to its embryological origin and inappropriate to its temporal position. The temporal extremity of the retina should normally project to the *rostral* pole of the tectum (see Fig. 4.14). With a compound NN eye the projection of the temporal part of the retina (and thus of the nasal or binocular part of the visual field) is back to front on the tectum and moreover has covered

9

the whole rostrocaudal extent of the tectum rather than just half, as in a normal animal. Figure 5.16 shows that, despite this abnormal contralateral projection, the projection to the ipsilateral tectum is normal; this may be seen when we compare Fig. 5.17 with Fig. 5.16.

Two points emerge from these considerations: firstly the ipsilateral visual projection, which normally arises from temporal retina (nasal field) may in fact arise from nasal retina as in the case of a compound NN eye; embryologically specified temporal retina is not required. Secondly, the observation that the first stage (contralateral) of the ipsilateral projection from a NN eye is reversed rostrocaudally on the tectum while the final result (ipsilateral) is normal, enables us to argue, as was the case with the rotated eye, that the organization of the intertectal linkage cannot be due to the action of any simple intertectal specificity mechanism. This also

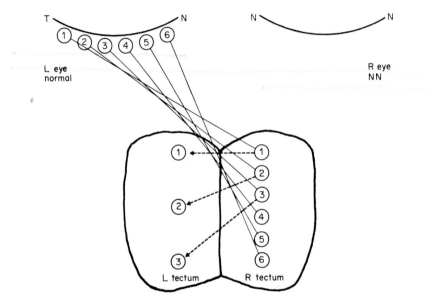

FIG. 5.18.   The ipsilateral projection from the normal eye in an animal with one double-nasal compound eye. In this case, while the contralateral projection from the normal eye is normal, the ipsilateral projection is not (compare Fig. 5.16). From Gaze *et al.*, 1970.

follows from the observation that, in an animal with one NN eye, the ipsilateral projection from the *normal* eye is abnormal (Fig. 5.18). Here, the first stage of the projection is normal but the subsequent intertectal part of the pathway is not.

The essential points which make possible an understanding of how the ipsilateral intertectal connections might be formed are, firstly, that in all the cases mentioned the ipsilateral projections, whether from operated or from normal eye, are *systematically* organized; not random. And secondly, in almost all cases (Gaze *et al.*, 1970) the abnormality in the projection ipsilaterally from the normal eye reflects the abnormality in the contra-lateral projection from the operated eye to the same tectum (Fig. 5.15), while the normality of the ipsilateral projection from the operated eye to its ipsilateral tectum reflects the normality in the contralateral projection from the normal eye to that tectum. Thus the ipsilateral projection from one eye appears to depend on the input to the same tectum from the contralateral eye; the ipsilateral projection seems to require an interaction, at tectal level, between the two eyes.

HYPOTHESIS 1: IMMEDIATE TECTAL RESPECIFICATION

We may now consider whether it is possible to account for these findings by invoking a form of transneuronal effect akin to "modulation" (Weiss, 1936; Sperry, 1951c; Jacobson and Baker, 1968; 1969). Perhaps the in-growing optic nerve fibres alter or modulate the tectal neurones on which they terminate contralaterally, thus altering the receptivity of these neurones to the intertectal fibres; in other words, the optic nerve fibres from the abnormal eye may respecify the contralateral tectum so that its ipsilateral input is altered appropriately.

According to this argument, in a normal animal, the intertectal fibres of the ipsilateral projection go mostly to the rostral tectum since this is where "temporally specified" tectal neurones are. However, again on this argument, in the tectum contralateral to an NN eye there will be *no* temporally specified neurones since both halves of the compound eye are nasal. So this modulation hypothesis does not help us to account for the findings. Similarly, in the case of an animal with a rotated eye, the respeci-fication hypothesis here considered would suggest that the intertectal fibres arrive at tectal neurones which have been appropriately specified as "temporal" by the incoming optic nerve fibres. However, we know that, following rotation of an eye after the time of axial polarization, the embryo-logically-specified temporal fibres still go to the rostral tectum (Fig. 5.19) as in a normal animal. Thus a respecification hypothesis of this nature should require that the intertectal connection in such a case should arrive on these neurones as they normally do. The pattern of intertectal connec-tion that is seen in such an animal is, however, quite different (Fig. 5.19 and 5.13).

HYPOTHESIS 2: DELAYED TECTAL RESPECIFICATION

The arguments of the previous section show that specification of tectal cells as "temporal" by the ingrowing optic nerve fibres is inadequate to account for the observations. We now consider the possibility of delayed respecification of the retinal ganglion cells. The original axial polarization of the eye occurs between stages 28–32 in *Xenopus* and tectal specification may occur independently and in parallel fashion (De Long and Coulombre,

1965). Let us suppose that, at some later stage, perhaps after metamorphosis, the structures surrounding the eye exert a further specifying effect on the ganglion cells, allowing the respecified "temporal" optic nerve fibres to instruct the tectal cells on which they terminate to give rise to and receive intertectal connections. In this case a rotation of the eye occurring before the final respecification could result in a normally oriented ipsilateral field projection via the rotated eye and a rotated ipsilateral field projection via the normal eye, as is found experimentally.

There appear to be two major objections to this hypothesis which make it unlikely. Firstly, such a respecification, in order to produce the results

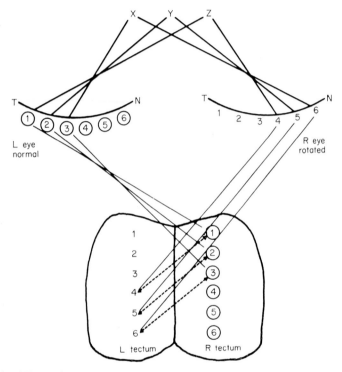

FIG. 5.19.   The ipsilateral projection from the normal eye in an animal with one eye rotated by 180°. See text. From Gaze *et al.*, 1970.

observed, would have to operate up to and including the time when the eye reaches its final position in the body; that is, after metamorphosis. This would be necessary to provide the binocular congruence found, where one point in visual space projects, via both eyes, to one (different) point on each tectum. At such a late stage of development the eye is freely movable in the orbit and it seems highly unlikely that the eye muscles or other orbital structures could exert an adequate respecifying influence on the ganglion cells. Secondly, while respecification could account for the overall field orientations, it could not account for the small individual variations in the ipsilateral projections, which are found to follow closely the variations in the contralateral projection to the same tectum (Gaze et al., 1970).

HYPOTHESIS 3: FUNCTIONAL INTERACTION

Since the experiments show that the ipsilateral projection is dependent on the contralateral projection in some fashion, and since we have shown that prefunctional mechanisms such as intertectal specificity and immediate respecification are inadequate to account for this dependence; and since even delayed respecification seems unlikely to fulfil our requirements, we now consider the case for functional interaction at the tectal level as the mechanism responsible for the organization of the ipsilateral projection.

The first point to note is the observation (Gaze and Jacobson, 1962; Keating and Gaze, 1970) that, within the binocular part of the visual field, a point in visual space projects to each tectum via both eyes; and furthermore one point in visual space projects through both eyes to the same point on the tectum (Fig. 5.20). The point X stimulates the retina of the right eye at position 1 and the left eye at position (3). Position 1 of the right eye projects contralaterally to position 1 on the left tectum, whereas position (3) of the left eye projects ipsilaterally to position (3) on the left tectum. Positions 1 and (3) on the left tectum are identical and point X thus projects to the same point on the left tectum through the two eyes. Similarly the contralateral projection from position (3) of the left eye to the right tectum and the ipsilateral projection from position 1 of the right eye to the right tectum are to the same tectal point. Similar arguments apply to the tectal projections of positions Y and Z of visual space.

Keating (1968) put forward the hypothesis that this feature of the ipsilateral projection, whereby the same point in visual space projects through both eyes to the same tectal point, instead of being the end result of various unknown processes of neural pathway organization may itself be the mechanism that produces the pattern of ipsilateral visual projection seen in the adult. Keating's hypothesis states that, at some stage of development, point X (Fig. 5.20) stimulates position 1 on the right retina and position (3) on the left retina; from these retinal positions impulses pass by the contralateral pathways to point 1 on the left tectum and point (3) on the right tectum. These two points, one on each tectum, thus receive similar spatiotemporal patterns of excitation. *The ipsilateral projection from point 1 of the right eye crosses to point 1 of the left tectum and then recrosses to that point on the right tectum (point (3)) which is simultaneously receiving a similar spatiotemporal pattern of excitation from the same point in visual space. Points on the two tecta receiving similar excitation patterns become specifically linked.*

This hypothesis can account for the formation of the ipsilateral projection in a normal animal. It could also account for the ipsilateral projections seen in animals with compound eyes. Thus if the contralateral projection from one eye is abnormal then the ipsilateral projection from the other eye should also be abnormal and the abnormality should be the same in both cases. This is what is found in animals with a double nasal eye (Fig. 5.21). Field position X will stimulate position (3) on the left (normal) retina, which projects contralaterally to point (3) on the right tectum. At the same time field position X will stimulate position 1 on the right retina, which projects contralaterally to point 1 on the left tectum. According to hypothesis, the ipsilateral projection from position (3) of the left

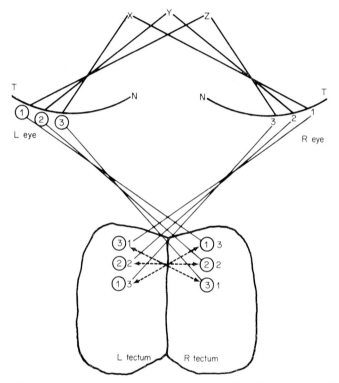

FIG. 5.20.   The binocular representation of the visual field in *Xenopus*. From Gaze *et al.*, 1970.

retina will be to point 1 of the left tectum. Similar considerations apply to stimulus positions Y and Z. Thus the hypothesis would predict that the ipsilateral projection from the normal left eye to the left tectum would reflect the abnormality in the contralateral projection from the right (NN) eye to the left tectum; and this abnormality is seen experimentally (Figs. 5.12 and 5.18). Similar arguments applied to the ipsilateral projection from the double-nasal eye (Fig. 5.22) lead to the prediction that the

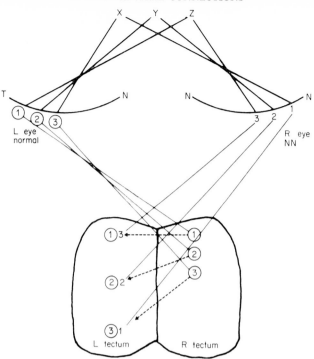

FIG. 5.21. The ipsilateral projection from the normal eye in an animal with one double-nasal compound eye: the field projection. From Gaze *et al.*, 1970.

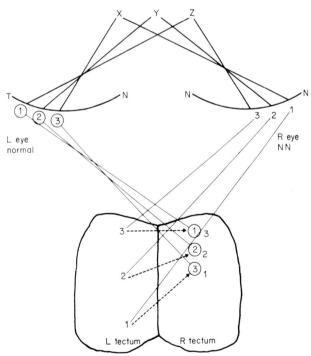

FIG. 5.22. The ipsilateral projection from a double-nasal compound eye: the field projection. From Gaze *et al.*, 1970.

ipsilateral projection from such an NN eye should reflect the normality of the contralateral projection from the normal eye to the same tectum; and, again, this is what occurs.

In animals with a double-temporal compound eye the contralateral projection from the operated eye (Fig. 4.41) shows the characteristic reduplication; the nasal (binocular) field projection through such an eye is, however, normally oriented on the tectum, since it involves temporal retina which is occupying its normal topographical position in the eye. Since the contralateral projection from the nasal field in TT eyes is normally oriented, the hypothesis would indicate a normal ipsilateral projection from the normal eye in these animals; and this is what is found experimentally.

In animals with one rotated eye the hypothesis would predict that, since the contralateral projection from the rotated eye is rotated, then the ipsilateral projection from the normal eye should be rotated; and to the same extent as the rotation of the other eye. Similarly, since the contralateral projection from the normal eye is normal, the ipsilateral projection from the rotated eye should also be normal. This is the case in such animals (Gaze et al., 1970).

In each of the cases considered so far the ipsilateral projection is seen to be dependent on the input to the same tectum from the contralateral eye. The ipsilateral projection appears to require an interaction, at tectal level, between the two eyes. And since it is one point in visual space that projects via both eyes to one point on the tectum, no matter what the relative positions of the retinae may be, it is the *field* that is of importance rather than the geography of the retinal point stimulated; the interaction that occurs appears to be a functional interaction.

If this is the case, then an animal which has had one eye removed early in embryonic life should not have a normal ipsilateral projection from its remaining eye since there is now no contralateral projection from the missing eye for the intertectal fibres to interact with. In fact such animals do have an ipsilateral projection from the remaining eye; but this projection is abnormal. The multi-unit receptive fields recordable at any given tectal position tend to be much wider than normal; multi-unit receptive fields of more than 50° diameter are commonly found, with no obviously better response in the centre than at the periphery (Gaze et al., 1970). This means that in many cases it is not possible to construct a meaningful projection map. It seems, therefore, that some growth process produces initially diffuse intertectal connections and that these diffuse connections require the functional modifying influence of the other optic input to narrow them down to specific connections.

Again, if the hypothesis of functional interaction is valid, the ipsilateral projection, in its adult state, should only be found in *Xenopus* when the eyes are in their final position in the head. Contralateral visual responses may be recorded from the tectum in *Xenopus* tadpoles, but ipsilateral responses only appear at metamorphosis (Gaze *et al.*, 1970). During larval life the eyes in *Xenopus* look out laterally and there is little or no binocular visual field. As metamorphosis approaches the eyes start to move relative to the head (Fig. 5.23) and by stage 66 or slightly later (the end of metamorphosis) the eyes have adopted their final adult position, looking upwards and outwards. Thus we may surmise that some metamorphic stimulus leads to the appearance of intertectal connections and that these are then focused by the functional mechanism postulated above.

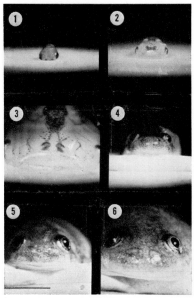

FIG. 5.23.   *Xenopus laevis* at various stages of development, photographed from directly in front of the animal. (1) Larva, stage 46; (2) Larva, stage 48; (3) Larva, stage 56; (4) Metamorphosing animal, stage 65; (5) Juvenile, 20 mm body length; (6) Juvenile, 34 mm body length. It may be seen that the larval eyes look out laterally and the process of movement of the eyes to their eventual adult position only occurs with metamorphosis. Bar, 5 mm.

The hypothesis of functional interaction is open to experimental invalidation; this alone, in view of the present generally unsatisfactory nature of such biological hypotheses, is almost enough to make it a good hypothesis. If, for instance, animals raised in the dark prove to have apparently normal contralateral visual projections, according to this hypothesis they should not have well localized ipsilateral projections; these should resemble the ipsilateral projections found in unilaterally enucleated animals. Moreover the presence of some artificially-induced optical abnormality in the input to one eye should lead to a corresponding positional abnormality in the ipsilateral projection from the other eye.

Such experimental tests of the hypothesis are in process at present and it is yet too soon to know whether the hypothesis as presently stated will stand up under investigation. Some form of binocular interaction is undoubtedly involved in the setting-up of the anuran ipsilateral visual projection; present evidence indicates that this mechanism depends on visual function in some way. The elucidation of the details of this process remains for future experimentation.

6. CONCLUSIONS

(1) "Histological studies show that no theory (of cortical organisation—R.M.G.), mathematical or other, relying on specific circuits can be maintained. The alternative approach must depend on statistical considerations in which the connections of individual neurons are of less concern and the connectivity pattern of the neuronal aggregate is studied" (Sholl, 1956).

(2) "The key to this organisation and the most fundamental principle of structure in the nervous system is given by the pattern of connections between cells. This pattern can be analysed in terms of the connections between groups of cells or between regions of the nervous system, a subject that has long occupied the attention of neuroanatomists and neurophysiologists. But there is a much more important level of analysis, at once more subtle and more fundamental: the detailed pattern of afferent terminals upon individual neurons and distribution of their efferents upon other cells. . . . Physiological studies of mammalian brain and invertebrate ganglia have demonstrated that individual neurons have unique and characteristic connections with other neurons. Anatomical analysis of a few regions in the brain and spinal cord have shown that afferent terminals from specific sources are arranged in precise displays over the surface of the neurons. . . . The nervous system is not a random net. Its units are not redundant. Its organisation is highly specific, not merely in terms of the connections between particular neurons, but also in terms of the number, style and location of terminals upon different parts of the same cell and the precise distribution of terminals arising from that cell" (Palay, 1967).

Thus two of the most eminent neuroanatomists of the present time offer views that are almost diametrically opposed, on the question of whether or not the brain is a precisely-connected structure. The truth is likely, as usual, to be more complex than suggested by such a statement of alternatives. Certain pathways in the nervous system are probably very precisely ordered and others may perhaps display a certain "randomness" of connection. In the absence of adequate histological information we are well advised to avoid what Austin (1962) calls the deeply ingrained worship of tidy dichotomies. Obviously, as I have previously argued, it is pointless to attempt to account for the formation of specific neural connections if these do not exist. In the present state of our knowledge of brain connections the most we can do is concentrate our attention on those few pathways about which we have fairly reliable information. This I have attempted to do for two intracentral systems, the binocular input to cat visual cortical cells and the anuran ipsilateral visual projection. However it is worthwhile emphasizing that the arguments presented in these cases depend on the assumption that the electrical activity recorded reveals the fibre pathways present. As I have said earlier this is not necessarily so. We are dealing, most of the time, with the electrical signs of neural *function*; we may, in certain circumstances, make the inference that these denote actual neuronal connections, but we do well to be wary. Such arguments may easily become circular.

I have repeatedly emphasized the futility of attempting to account for the organization of connections that may not be organized. A similar comment may be made about the detailed nature of the mechanisms involved; it is entirely premature to attempt to produce hypotheses concerning the cellular mechanisms giving rise to particular neural fibre projections. Thus our information on the development, maintenance, reactivity to insult, etc. of the anuran retinotectal projection is probably more extensive than for any other neural system yet studied. But even in this system we do not yet know enough of the limiting behaviour of the projection under various forms of experimental interference to make it worth while to produce a detailed explanatory hypothesis in terms of molecular ecology.

To the extent that neural connections are well-ordered, their development is a manifestation of pattern-formation. Where our study differs from the classical analysis of morphogenetic and individuation fields is that we are concerned not only with these phenomena but also with their manifestations at a distance. A developing organ such as the retina becomes axially polarized at a particular stage; by this we imply that its later behaviour, in terms of the connections it will form, becomes determined at this time. No means of analysis yet devised enables us to find differences between the various parts of a retinal axis at, or shortly after, determination. We infer that differences must exist because after axial determination the fibres which will later grow out to the tectum will only connect up in a certain way.

Our problem is thus always a double one; we have to disentangle the effects of *local* changes taking place in the tissue of origin, from other changes displaying themselves at a distance, at the sites where the fibres eventually terminate. This difficulty is well illustrated in the case of NN and TT compound eyes. In such cases (Chapter 4) the appearance of the retinotectal map led to the initial presumption that the fibres of each half-eye were spreading over the tectum; or conversely, that half the tectum was becoming overdeveloped to take the double input of similar fibres. The result of uncrossing the optic chiasma in such cases may lead to a different interpretation; each half of the compound eye is behaving as if it were a whole eye. This could be considered a good example of a differentiative "field" effect in the sense of Waddington (1966) and Wolpert (1969). If this is a valid interpretation of what is happening then the "specificities" of the retinal ganglion cells are being dramatically altered *after* the time of axial specification and the polarity of each half of the system is preserved in the face of operative interference. Individual ganglion cells appear to be changing their "positional information" (Wolpert, 1968; 1969) and they interpret this change in the way we detect as alteration in specificity.

Those of us whose main study is the vertebrate nervous system sometimes tend to think that the higher the animals in the phylogenetic scale the greater the complexity of the nervous system and the more freedom accorded to individual neurones in the organization of their connections. But here our understanding of the nature of nervous organization may suffer from our restricted point of view. A wider zoological viewpoint may suggest a different answer.

"Thus the evolution of progressively more complex functions has been made possible by the evolution of more complex connectivity patterns and greater differences between individual neurons. In the lower animals or in simpler situations we find nervous systems with many equivalent cells. In some of the higher forms in each major group, many of the neurons are anatomically different and appear to be 'recognisable' to each other at their terminations. Although little is known of the mechanisms controlling their growth, the neurons follow certain rules that decide their connectivity. From lower to higher animals there is a scale of increasing complexity in connectivity patterns, and this is made possible by progressively greater specificity and resolution in the morphogenetic mechanisms by which neurons avoid some contacts and form others. The nature of these mechanisms is almost entirely unknown, and an initial barrier to advance in their understanding is that diversity of the individual cells has proceeded to such an extent that one can almost say that every neuron is uniquely different from all others in an advanced adult animal such as a mammal or a crayfish" (Horridge, 1968).

It will be evident from the discussion presented in the previous chapters that much of the connection-pattern of the nervous system particularly in lower vertebrates (and invertebrates) is foreshadowed by the inheritance of the animal. This is not to imply, of course, that detailed instructions exist in the genome for each neural connection eventually to be formed; as Apter and Wolpert (1965) and Wolpert (1968) have pointed out, the development of a complex structure from an apparently structurally simple and undifferentiated egg, is perhaps more easily understood if the egg is considered to contain the programme for making the organism rather than the complete specification of the organism to which it will give rise; it may be much simpler to specify how to form a complex organism than to specify the organism itself.

Since so much of the organism's neural connectivity is ordered according to the running of its genetic programme, our task shows three separable aspects: (1) individuation (Waddington, 1956) of neuronal populations; (2) pathway control; (3) fibre to cell (or dendrite) matching. Early attempts to account for the development of neural connections (Sperry; see Chapter 4) emphasized cytochemical differentiation; individual neurones, pathways and matching were thought of as reflecting the distribution of various molecular species. This approach remains a viable one, but I would agree with Goodwin and Cohen (1969) that the belief that an understanding of global embryological problems will come with the application of the ideas and techniques of molecular biology to embryonic systems, is ill-founded. These ideas and procedures will be invaluable once we know what to look for; but they cannot tell us, for instance, what type of cellular phenomenon may be involved in the establishment of embryonic axes.

Goodwin and Cohen (1969) present a model for the spatial and temporal organization of developing systems wherein individual cells are supposed to be temporally organized in the sense that biochemical events essential for the control of development recur periodically; this temporal organization of an individual cell is converted by functional coupling between cells into a spatial ordering of the temporal organization of the different cells in a tissue, according to their positions; and the spatial organization of temporally-ordered cells provides the positional information necessary for developmental processes. Goodwin and Cohen point out that the parallels between the properties of their model of the epigenetic process and the behaviour of the central nervous system encourage the point of view that neural organization may be regarded as an elaboration and refinement of a communication process which is basic to the earliest spatial and temporal organization of the embryo.

Goodwin and Cohen (1969) consider that the major part of the problem of the retinotectal projection is the directional growth of fibres in response to information received locally, near the surface of the tectum (De Long and Coulombre, 1967); and they build their treatment of the fibre projection around this phenomenon. While the observations of De Long and Coulombre are, undoubtedly, of great interest and highly relevant to any postulated mechanism of connection-control, it is not obvious that the model of Goodwin and Cohen has any considerable advantages over other detailed realizations, for instance of a chemotactic gradient character.

The systems of neural connectivity that I have discussed have been deliberately restricted to neuromuscular, cutaneous and visual connections. I have ignored completely the observations that are beginning to be made on invertebrates and I have passed over most of the vertebrate nervous system as if it did not exist. Readers who have followed me thus far through the maze of observations and inferences on muscle, skin and eye, will perhaps feel relieved that my view has been somewhat narrow. It has been said that truth springs more readily from error than from confusion;

on this basis we have some way to go, for there is plenty of both in our present picture of neural development.

While we study connectivity in the nervous system, our overriding interest is, naturally, how the system works. Owing partly to the mere numbers of interacting units involved we are compelled to agree with Horridge (1968) that the complete physical state of the nervous system is not determinable; and we are reduced to making reductionist statements about how it *could* work; that is, we make models. From our models we then ask firstly, whether the nervous system could be working in this way; and secondly, whether it actually *does* work this way. Our reductionist arguments from the logical requirements of function may lead us very far astray here. Such an approach works very well when we are dealing with the mechanical or hydraulic aspects of life, as in cardiovascular and renal mechanisms, since in these cases we are dealing with phenomena that can be approximated, to any required degree of accuracy, by fairly simple artefactual set-ups. But in the case of the nervous system we are not dealing with a mechanical or hydraulic system but with a quite different *kind* of system, one involving control, the transformation of information. The tendency is to apply to the nervous system the same analytical and synthetic techniques that have been so successfully applied to the rest of the body. And here the historical shortness of our experience faults us; man has been familiar with mechanical phenomena for hundreds, if not thousands of years, but the technology of information machines has all grown up within the past 50 years or so and certainly since Babbage.

The difficulties and inadequacies of the logical-reductionist position are clearly illustrated in the work on regeneration within the visual system. What is the minimum requirement for spatial localization within this system? The control mechanism (brain, optic tecta) *must* be able to distinguish excitation of one part of the retina from excitation of another. Otherwise there is no possibility of making the appropriate move towards the prey; only a random selection of directions in which to jump. The animal jumps in a non-random fashion; it *does* distinguish between different parts of the retina. We know that, normally, the connection from eye to tectum is in the form of a retinotopically organized fibre projection. Is this a necessary requirement for visual localization? The answer, of course, is no: for *model* systems. It is quite simple to devise a system of linking the eye and the brain over a randomly-connected cable and still to preserve spatial localization. All we would need to do this is to have retinal position coded in some fashion at the eye and decoded at the tectum. Is this how the animal does it? We can say, with *almost* complete certainty that it is not. But the very fact that that this digression into communication bioengineering is still relevant, shows how little we know about the mechanisms of information transfer in the nervous system. And this system we have been considering is one of the simplest, involving a primary sensory input. How much less we know, and how much more open-ended the argument, about any more central connections.

It is true to say, as I argued in the introduction, that for any statements about nervous systems to have biological as well as logical validity, the premises must be correct; and this state of affairs is probably never achieved. Not only are we up against poorly-designed experiments and inaccurate observations but the system under study is changing with time. As most effectively expressed by Horridge (1968): "Any nervous system can perform actions that are not predictable from a set of descriptive explanations that up to that time is apparently complete." If the nervous system is considered as a form of computer, it is one that can change its mode of function (and, perhaps, its structure) as a result of experience. To what extent structural connections alter as a part of learning is an open question; functional connections certainly do. And this means, of course, that the process of investigation may alter that which is being investigated. Since it is impossible, in principle, to ask *all* relevant questions about nervous activity, perhaps our best strategy in this very difficult situation is to try to keep a few jumps ahead of the system by predicting, and attempting to build into our models, *classes* of functions; rather than to run behind the system all the time and attempt to explain individual observations as they occur.

To return finally to the subdivisions of the nervous system proposed in the introduction: the evidence discussed in the previous chapters would strongly suggest that the primary inputs and outputs of the nervous system are connected according to a predetermined plan; and so also may be a considerable part of the interneuronal system. Within the central nervous system proper, however, there is some fairly good evidence that attributes of function may play a major part in determining and maintaining certain connections. It remains one of the most exciting tasks ahead of us to determine to what extent this may be true of the higher centres of the nervous system.

REFERENCES

Adrian, E. D. (1926). The impulses produced by sensory nerve endings. Part 4. Impulses from pain receptors. *J. Physiol.* **62**, 33–51.

Adrian, E. D. and Zotterman, Y. (1926). The impulses produced by sensory nerve endings. Part 3. Impulses set up by touch and pressure. *J. Physiol.* **61**, 465–483.

Altman, J. (1967). Postnatal growth and differentiation of the mammalian brain, with implications for a morphological theory of memory. Pp. 723–743. *In* "The Neurosciences". (Eds. G. C. Quarton, T. Melnechuk and F. O. Schmitt). Rockefeller University Press, New York.

Andersen, P. O. (1966). Correlation of structural design with function in the archicortex. Pp. 59–84. *In* "Brain and Conscious Experience". (Ed. J. C. Eccles). Springer, Berlin.

Apter, M. J. and Wolpert, L. (1965). Cybernetics and development. I. Information theory. *J. Theoret. Biol.* **8**, 244–257.

Arbib, M. A. (1965). "Brains, Machines, and Mathematics". McGraw-Hill, New York.

Arora, H. L. (1963). Effect of forcing a regenerative optic nerve bundle towards a foreign region of the optic tectum. *Anat. Rec.* **145**, 202.

Arora, H. L. and Sperry, R. W. (1957). Myotopic respecification of regenerated nerve-fibres in Cichlid fishes. *J. Embryol. exp. Morph.* **5**, 256–263.

Arora, H. L. and Sperry, R. W. (1962). Optic nerve regeneration after surgical cross-union of medial and lateral optic tracts. *Am. Zool.* **2**, 389.

Arora, H. L. and Sperry, R. W. (1963). Color discrimination after optic nerve regeneration in the fish *Astronotus ocellatus*. *Devel. Biol.* **7**, 234–243.

Attardi, Domenica, G. and Sperry, R. W. (1960). Central routes taken by regenerating optic fibers. *Physiologist*, **3**, 12.

Attardi, Domenica, G. and Sperry, R. W. (1963). Preferential selection of central pathways by regenerating optic fibers. *Exp. Neurol.* **7**, 46–64.

Austin, J. L. (1962). "Sense and Sensibilia". Oxford University Press, London.

Barlow, H. B., Blakemore, C. and Pettigrew, J. D. (1967). The neural mechanism of binocular depth perception. *J. Physiol.* **193**, 327–342.

Barron, D. H. (1943). The early development of the motor cells and columns in the spinal cord of the sheep. *J. comp. Neurol.* **78**, 1–27.

Barron, D. H. (1946). Observations on the early differentiation of the motor neuroblasts in the spinal cord of the chick. *J. comp. Neurol.* **85**, 149–169.

Bernstein, J. J. and Guth, L. (1961). Nonselectivity in establishment of neuro-muscular connections following nerve regeneration in the rat. *Exp. Neurol.* **4**, 262–275.

Boell, E. J., Greenfield, P., and Shen, S. C. (1955). Development of cholinesterase in the optic lobes of the frog (Rana pipiens). *J. exp. Zool.* **129**, 415–451.

Bohm, D. (1969). Some remarks on the notion of order. Pp. 18–40. *In* "Towards a Theoretical Biology, 2. Sketches". (Ed. C. H. Waddington). Edinburgh University Press, Edinburgh.

Bone, Q. (1964). Patterns of muscular innervation in the lower chordates. *Int. Rev. Neurobiol.* **6**, 99–147.

Brown, A. G. and Franz, D. N. (1970). Patterns of response in spinocervical tract neurones to different stimuli of long duration. *Brain. Res.* **17**, 156–160.

Bruesch, S. R. and Arey, L. B. (1942). The number of myelinated and unmyelinated fibres in the optic nerve of vertebrates. *J. comp. Neurol.* **77**, 631–665.

Buller, A. J., Eccles, J. C. and Eccles, Rosamund, M. (1960a). Differentiation of fast and slow muscles in the cat hind limb. *J. Physiol.* **150**, 399–416.

Buller, A. J., Eccles, J. C. and Eccles, Rosamund, M. (1960b). Interactions between motoneurones and muscles in respect of the characteristic speeds of their responses. *J. Physiol.* **150**, 417–439.

Burgen, A. S. V. and Grafstein, Bernice. (1962). Retinotectal connections after retinal regeneration. *Nature, Lond.* **196**, 898–899.

Burns, B. Delisle. (1958). "The Mammalian Cerebral Cortex." Arnold, London.

Burns, B. Delisle. (1968). "The Uncertain Nervous System." Arnold, London.

Buser, P. and Dussardier, M. (1953). Organisation des projections de la rétine sur le lobe optique, etudiée chez quelques Téléostéens. *J. de Physiol.* **45**, 57–60.

Cajal, S. R. (1898). Estructura del kiasma óptico. *Rev. trim. microg.* **3**, 15–65.

Cajal, S. R. (1899). "Die Struktur des Chiasma opticum." Barth, Leipzig.

Cajal, S. R. (1952). "Histologie du Système Nerveux de l'homme et des vertébrés." Consejo Superior de Investigaciones Cientificas, Madrid.

Cajal, S. R. (1929). "Studies on Vertebrate Neurogenesis." Thomas, 1960 Springfield.

Carpenter, R. L. (1932). Spinal-ganglion responses to the transplantation of differentiated limbs in Amblystoma larvae. *J. exp. Zool.* **61**, 149–173.

Causey, G. and Hoffman, H. (1955). Axon sprouting in partially deneurotized nerves. *Brain*, **78**, 661–668.

Close, R. (1964). Dynamic properties of fast and slow skeletal muscles of the rat during development. *J. Physiol.* **173**, 74–95.

Close, R. (1965). Effects of cross-union of motor nerves to fast and slow skeletal muscles. *Nature, Lond.* **206**, 831–832.

Close, R. and Hoh, J. F. Y. (1968). Effects of nerve crossunion on fast-twitch and slow-graded muscle fibres in the toad. *J. Physiol.* **198**, 103–125.

Colonnier, M. L. (1966). The structural design of the neocortex. Pp. 1–23. *In* "Brain and Conscious Experience." (Ed. J. C. Eccles). Springer, Berlin.

Conel, J. Le Roy. (1939–63). "The Postnatal Development of the Human Cerebral Cortex." Vols. I to VI. Harvard University Press, Cambridge, USA

Coppoletta, J. M. and Wolbach, S. B. (1933). Body length and organ weights of infants and children. *Am. J. Pathol.* **9**, 55–70.

Cowan, J. D. (1962). The engineering approach to the problem of biological integration. Pp. 22–29. *In* "Symposium on Cybernetics of the Nervous System." (Eds. N. Wiener and J. P. Schadé). *Prog. Brain Res.* **2** (Elsevier, Amsterdam).

Cowan, J. D. and Winograd, S. (1963). "Reliable Computation in the Presence of Noise." M.I.T. Press, Cambridge, USA

Cragg, B. G. (1967). Changes in visual cortex on first exposure of rats to light. *Nature, Lond.* **215**, 251–253.

Crelin, E. S. (1952). Excision and rotation of the developing Ambylstoma optic tectum and subsequent visual recovery. *J. exp. Zool.* **120**, 547–577.

Cronly-Dillon, J. (1968). Pattern of retinotectal connections after retinal regeneration. *J. Neurophysiol.* **31**, 410–418.

DeCrinis, M. (1934). Aufbau und Abbau der Grosshirnleistungen und ihre anatomischen Gründe. Karger, Berlin.

De Long, G. R. and Coulombre, A. J. (1965). Development of the retinotectal projection in the Chick embryo. *Exp. Neurol.* **13**, 351–363.

De Long, G. R. and Coulombre, A. J. (1967). The specificity of retinotectal connections studied by retinal grafts onto the optic tectum in chick embryos. *Devel. Biol.* **16**, 513–531.

De Long, G. R. and Sidman, R. L. (1962). Effects of eye removal at birth on histogenesis of the mouse superior colliculus: an autoradiographic analysis with tritiated thymidine. *J. comp. Neurol.* **118**, 205–224.

Detwiler, S. R. (1920). Experiments on the transplantation of limbs in Amblystoma. The formation of nerve plexuses and the function of the limbs. *J. exp. Zool.* **31**, 117–169.

Detwiler, S. R. (1923). Experiments on the transplantation of the spinal cord in Amblystoma, and their bearing upon the stimuli involved in the differentiation of nerve cells. *J. exp. Zool.* **37**, 339–393.

Detwiler, S. R. (1924). The effects of bilateral extirpation of the anterior limb rudiments in Amblystoma embryos. *J. comp. Neurol.* **37**, 1–14.

Detwiler, S. R. (1925). Coordinated movements in supernumary transplanted limbs. *J. comp. Neurol.* **38**, 461–493.

Detwiler, S. R. (1928). Further experiments upon alteration of the direction of growth in amphibian spinal nerves. *J. exp. Zool.* **51**, 1–35.

Detwiler, S. R. (1936). "Neuroembryology." Reprinted 1964. Hafner, New York.

Detwiler, S. R. and Carpenter, R. L. (1929). An experimental study of the mechanism of coordinated movements in heterotopic limbs. *J. comp. Neurol.* **47**, 427–447.

Detwiler, S. R. and Van Dyke, R. H. (1934). Further observations upon abnormal growth responses of spinal nerves in Amblystoma embryos. *J. exp. Zool.* **69**, 137–164.

Diamond, Marian C., Krech, D. and Rosenzweig, M. R. (1964). The effects of an enriched environment on the histology of the rat cerebral cortex. *J. comp. Neurol.* **123**, 111–120.

Drachman, D. B. (1968). The role of acetylcholine as a trophic neuromuscular transmitter. Pp. 251–273. *In* "Growth of the Nervous System." Ciba Foundation Symposium. (Eds G. E. W. Wolstenholme and Maeve O'Connor). Churchill, London.

Dubowitz, V. (1967). Cross-innervated mammalian skeletal muscle: histochemical, physiological and biochemical observations. *J. Physiol.* **193**, 481–496.

Eakin, R. M. (1942). Determination and regulation of polarity in the retina of Hyla regilla. *Univ. Calif. Publ. Zool.* **51**, 245–287.

Eccles, J. C. (1963). *In* "The Effect of Use and Disuse on Neuromuscular Function," p. 164. (Eds. E. Gutman and P. Hnik). Elsevier, Amsterdam.

Eccles, J. C., Eccles, Rosamund M. and Lundberg, A. (1958). The action potentials of the alpha motoneurones supplying fast and slow muscles. *J. Physiol.* **142**, 275–291.

Eccles, J. C., Eccles, Rosamund M. and Magni, F. (1960). Monosynaptic excitatory action on motoneurones regenerated to antagonistic muscles. *J. Physiol.* **154**, 68–88.

Eccles, J. C., Eccles, Rosamund M. and Shealy, C. N. (1962). An investigation into the effect of degenerating primary afferent fibers on the monosynaptic innervation of motoneurones. *J. Neurophysiol.* **25**, 544–558.

Eccles, J. C., Eccles, Rosamund M., Shealy, C. N. and Willis, W. D. (1962). Experiments utilizing monosynaptic excitatory action on motoneurons for testing hypotheses relating to specificity of neuronal connections. *J. Neurophysiol.* **25**, 559–580.

Eccles, J. C., Ito, M. and Szentágothai, J. (1967). "The Cerebellum as a Neuronal Machine." Springer, Berlin.

Edds, Mac V. (1953). Collateral nerve regeneration. *Qu. Rev. Biol.* **28**, 260–276.

Feng, T. P., Wu, W. Y. and Yang, F. Y. (1965). Selective reinnervation of a "slow" or "fast" muscle by its original motor supply during regeneration of mixed nerve. *Scientia Sinica*, **14**, 1717–1720.

Fullerton, Pamela M. and Gilliat, R. W. (1965). Axon reflexes in human motor nerve fibres. *J. Neurol. Neurosurg. Psychiat.* **28**, 1–11.

Galambos, R., Norton, T. T. and Frommer, G. P. (1967). Optic tract lesions sparing pattern vision in cats. *Exp. Neurol.* **18**, 8–25.

Galbraith, J. K. (1958). "The Affluent Society." Penguin Books, 1962, London.

Gaze, R. M. (1958a). The representation of the retina on the optic lobe of the frog. *Qu. J. exp. Physiol.* **43**, 209–214.

Gaze, R. M. (1958b). Binocular vision in frogs. *J. Physiol.* **143**, 20 p.

Gaze, R. M. (1959). Regeneration of the optic nerve in *Xenopus laevis*. *Qu. J. exp. Physiol.* **44**, 290–308.

Gaze, R. M. (1960). Regeneration of the Optic Nerve in Amphibia. *Int. Rev. Neurobiol.* **2**, 1–40.

Gaze, R. M. (1967). Growth and Differentiation. *Ann. Rev. Physiol.* **29**, 59–86.

Gaze, R. M. and Jacobson, M. (1962). The projection of the binocular visual field on the optic tecta of the frog. *Qu. J. exp. Physiol.* **47**, 273–280.

Gaze, R. M. and Jacobson, M. (1963a). The path from the retina to the ipsilateral optic tectum of the frog. *J. Physiol.* **165**, 73–74 p.

Gaze, R. M. and Jacobson, M. (1963b). "Convexity-detectors" in the frog's visual system. *J. Physiol.* **169**, 1–3 p.

Gaze, R. M. and Jacobson, M. (1963c). A study of the retinotectal projection during regeneration of the optic nerve in the frog. *Proc. Roy. Soc. B.* **157**, 420–448.

Gaze, R. M., Jacobson, M. and Székely, G. (1963). The retinotectal projection in *Xenopus* with compound eyes. *J. Physiol.* **165**, 484–499.

Gaze, R. M., Jacobson, M. and Székely, G. (1965). On the formation of connexions by compound eyes in *Xenopus*. *J. Physiol.* **176**, 409–417.

Gaze, R. M. and Keating, M. J. (1969). The depth distribution of visual units in the tectum of the frog following regeneration of the optic nerve. *J. Physiol.* **200**, 128–129 p.

Gaze, R. M. and Keating, M. J. (1970a). Further studies on the restoration of the contralateral retinotectal projection following regeneration of the optic nerve in the frog. *Brain Res.* (in press).

Gaze, R. M. and Keating, M. J. (1970b). Functional control of nerve fibre connections. (In preparation).

Gaze, R. M. and Keating, M. J. (1970c). Regenerated visual units in the frog. *Brain Res.* (in press.)

Gaze, R. M., Keating, M. J. and Straznicky, K. (1970a). Retinotectal projections after uncrossing the optic chiasma in *Xenopus* with one compound eye. *J. Physiol.* (In press).

Gaze, R. M., Keating, M. J. and Straznicky, K. (1970b). The retinotectal projection from a double-ventral compound eye in *Xenopus*. (In preparation.)

Gaze, R. M., Keating, M. J., Székely, G. and Beazley, Lynda. (1970). Binocular interaction in the formation of specific intertectal neuronal connections. *Proc. Roy. Soc. B.* **175**, 107–147.

Gaze, R. M. and Peters, A. (1961). The development, structure and composition of the optic nerve of *Xenopus laevis* (Daudin). *Qu. J. exp. Physiol.* **46**, 299–309.

Gaze, R. M. and Sharma, S. C. (1968). Axial differences in the reinnervation of the optic tectum by regenerating optic nerve fibres. *J. Physiol.* **198**, 117 p.

Gaze, R. M. and Sharma, S. C. (1970). Axial differences in the reinnervation of the goldfish optic tectum by regenerating optic nerve fibres. *Exp. Brain. Res.* **10**, 171–181.

Gaze, R. M. and Watson, W. E. (1968). Cell division and migration in the brain after optic nerve lesions. Pp. 53–67. *In* "Growth of the Nervous System." Ciba Foundation Symposium. (Eds. G. E. W. Wolstenholme and Maeve O'Connor). Churchill, London.

Glücksmann, A. (1940). The development and differentiation of the tadpole eye. *Brit. J. Ophthalmol.* **24**, 153–178.

Glücksmann, A. (1965). Cell death in normal development. *Archs Biol.* **76**, 419–437.

Goodwin, B. C. and Cohen, M. H. (1969). A phase-shift model for the spatial and temporal organisation of developing systems. *J. Theoret. Biol.* **25**, 49–107.

Grafstein, Bernice. (1967). Transport of protein by goldfish optic nerve fibres. *Science,* **157**, 196–198.

Grafstein, Bernice and Burgen, A. S. V. (1964). Pattern of optic nerve connections following retinal regeneration. *Prog. Br. Res.* **6**, 126–138.

Grainger, Felicity, James, D. W. and Tresman, R. V. (1968). An electron-microscopic study of the early outgrowth from chick spinal cord in vitro. *Z. Zellforschung.* **90**, 53–67.

Gray, E. G. (1957). The spindle and extrafusal innervation of a frog muscle. *Proc. Roy. Soc. B.* **146**, 416–430.

Gyllensten, L. (1959). Postnatal development of the visual cortex in darkness (Mice). *Acta Morph. Néerl. Scand.* **2**, 331–345.

Gyllensten, L., Malmfors, T. and Norrlin, Marie-Louise. (1965). Effect of visual deprivation on the optic centers of growing and adult mice. *J. comp. Neurol.* **124**, 149–160.

Hamburger, V. (1934). The effects of wing bud extirpation on the development of the central nervous system in chick embryos. *J. exp. Zool.* **68**, 449–494.

Hamburger, V. (1961). Experimental analysis of the dual origin of the trigeminal ganglion in the chick embryo. *J. exp. Zool.* **148**, 91–123.

Harrison, R. G. (1921). On relations of symmetry in transplanted limbs. *J. exp. Zool.* **32**, 1–136.

Harrison, R. G. (1929). Correlation in the development and growth of the eye studied by means of heteroplastic transplantation. *Roux Archiv.* **120**, 1–55.

Harrison, R. G. (1936). Relations of symmetry in the developing ear of Amblystoma punctatum. *Proc. natn. Acad. Sci. USA.* **22**, 238–247.

Harrison, R. G. (1945). On relations of symmetry in the developing embryo. *Trans. Conn. Acad. Arts Sci.* **36**, 277–330.

Hecht, S. (1955). Theory of visual intensity discrimination. *J. Neurophysiol.* **18**, 767–789.

Herrick, C. J. (1930). Localization of function in the nervous system. *Proc. natn. Acad. Sci. USA.* **16**, 643–650.

Hess, A. (1960). The structure of extrafusal muscle fibres in the frog and their innervation studied by the cholinesterase technique. *Am. J. Anat.* **107**, 129–151.

Hibbard, E. (1959). Central integration of developing nerve tracts from supernumary grafted eyes and brain in the frog. *J. exp. Zool.* **141**, 323–352.

Hibbard, E. (1967). Visual recovery following regeneration of the optic nerve through the oculomotor nerve root in Xenopus. *Exp. Neurol.* **19**, 350–356.

Hnik, P., Jirmanová, Isa, Vyklicky, L. and Zelená, Jirina. (1967). Fast and slow muscles of the chick after nerve cross-union. *J. Physiol.* **193**, 309–325.

Holemans, K. C., Meij, H. S. and Meyer, B. J. (1966). The existence of a monosynaptic reflex arc in the spinal cord of the frog. *Exp. Neurol.* **14**, 175–186.

Holloway, R. L. (1966). Dendritic branching: some preliminary results of training and complexity in rat visual cortex. *Brain Res.* **2**, 393–396.

Horn, G. and Hill, R. M. (1969). Modifications of receptive fields of cells in the visual cortex occurring spontaneously and associated with bodily tilt. *Nature, Lond.* **221**, 186–188.

Horridge, G. A. (1968). "Interneurons." Freeman, London.

Hubel, D. H. and Wiesel, T. N. (1962). Receptive fields, binocular interaction and functional architecture in the cat's visual cortex. *J. Physiol.* **160**, 106–154.

Hubel, D. H. and Wiesel, T. N. (1963). Receptive fields of cells in striate cortex of very young, visually inexperienced kittens. *J. Neurophysiol.* **26**, 994–1002.

Hubel, D. H. and Wiesel, T. N. (1965). Binocular interaction in striate cortex of kittens reared with artificial squint. *J. Neurophysiol.* **28**, 1041–1059.

Hughes, A. (1957). The development of the primary sensory system in *Xenopus laevis* (Daudin). *J. Anat.* **91**, 323–339.

Hughes, A. (1961). Cell degeneration in the larval ventral horn of *Xenopus laevis* (Daudin). *J. Embryol. exp. Morph.* **9**, 269–284.

Hughes, A. (1964). Further experiments on the innervation and function of grafted supernumary limbs in the embryo of Eleutherodactylus martinicensis. *J. Embryol. exp. Morph.* **12**, 229–24..

Hughes, A. F. W. (1968). "Aspects of Neural Ontogeny." Logos, London.

Hughes, A. F. W. and Fozzard, J. A. F. (1961). The effect of irradiation on cell degeneration among developing neurones in *Xenopus laevis. Brit. J. Radiol.* **34**, 302–307.

Hughes, A. and Tschumi, P. A. (1958). The factors controlling the development of the dorsal root ganglia and ventral horn in *Xenopus laevis* (Daudin). *J. Anat.* **92**, 498–527.

Hunt, C. C. and Kuffler, S. W. (1954). Motor innervation of skeletal muscle: multiple innervation of individual muscle fibres and motor unit function. *J. Physiol.* **126**, 293–303.

Illis, L. (1964). Spinal cord synapses in the cat: the reactions of the boutons terminaux at the motoneurone surface to experimental denervation. Brain, **87**, 555–572.

Jacobson, M. (1962). The representation of the retina on the optic tectum of the frog. Correlation between retinotectal magnification factor and retinal ganglion cell count. *Qu. J. exp. Physiol.* **47**, 170–178.

Jacobson, M. (1966). Starting points for research in the ontogeny of behaviour. Pp. 339–383. *In* "Major Problems in Developmental Biology." (Ed. M. Locke). 25th Symposium of the Society for Developmental Biology. Academic Press, New York.

Jacobson, M. (1967). Retinal ganglion cells: specification of central connections in larval Xenopus laevis. *Science,* **155**, 1106–1108.

Jacobson, M. (1968a). Development of neuronal specificity in retinal ganglion cells of Xenopus. *Devel. Biol.* **17**, 202–218.

Jacobson, M. (1968b). Cessation of DNA synthesis in retinal ganglion cells correlated with the time of specification of their central connections. *Devel. Biol.* **17**, 219–232.

Jacobson, M. and Baker, R. E. (1968). Neuronal specification of cutaneous nerves through connections with skin grafts in the frog. *Science,* **160**, 543–545.

Jacobson, M. and Baker, R. E. (1969). Development of neuronal connections with skin grafts in frogs: behavioural and electrophysiological studies. *J. comp. Neurol.* **137**, 121–142.

Jacobson, M. and Gaze, R. M. (1964). Types of visual response from single units in the optic tectum and optic nerve of the goldfish. *Qu. J. exp. Physiol.* **49**, 199–209.

Jacobson, M. and Gaze, R. M. (1965). Selection of appropriate tectal connections by regenerating optic nerve fibres in adult goldfish. *Exp. Neurol.* **13**, 418–430.

Jehle, H. (1963). Intermolecular forces and biological specificity. *Proc. natn. Acad. Sci. USA.* **50**, 516–523.

Jenik, F. (1962). Electronic neuron models as an aid to neurophysiological research. *Ergebn. Biol.* **25**, 206–245.

Keating, M. J. (1968). Functional interaction in the development of specific nerve connexions. *J. Physiol.* **198**, 75–77 p.

Keating, M. J. and Gaze, R. M. (1970). *Qu. J. exp. Physiol.* (in press).

Kennedy, D., Selverston, A. I. and Remler, M. P. (1969). Analysis of restricted neural networks. *Science*, **164**, 1488–1496.

Kling, U. and Székely, G. (1968). Simulation of rhythmic nervous activities. I. Function of networks with cyclic inhibitions. *Kybernetik*, **5**, 89–103.

Knapp, Harriet, Scalia, F. and Riss, W. (1965). The optic tracts of *Rana pipiens*. *Acta neurol. scand.* **41**, 325–355.

Kollros, J. J. (1942a). Experimental studies on the development of the corneal reflex in amphibia. 1, the onset of the reflex and its relationship to metamorphosis. *J. exp. Zool.* **89**, 37–67.

Kollros J. J. (1942b). Localized maturation of the lid-closure reflex mechanism by thyroid implants into tadpole hindbrain. *Proc. Soc. exp. Biol. Med.* **49**, 204–206.

Kollros, J. J. (1943). Experimental studies on the development of the corneal reflex in amphibia. III. The influence of the periphery upon the reflex center. *J. exp. Zool.* **92**, 121–142.

Kollros, J. J. (1953). The development of the optic lobes in the frog. *J. exp. Zool.* **123**, 153–187.

Kornacker, K. (1963). Some properties of the afferent pathway in the frog corneal reflex. *Exp. Neurol.* **7**, 224–239.

Kuffler, S. W. and Gerard, R. W. (1947). The small-nerve motor system to skeletal muscle. *J. Neurophysiol.* **10**, 383–394.

Kuffler, S. W. and Vaughan Williams, E. M. (1953a). Small-nerve junctional potentials. The distribution of small motor nerves to frog skeletal muscle, and the membrane characteristics of the fibres they innervate. *J. Physiol.* **121**, 289–317.

Kuffler, S. W. and Vaughan Williams, E. M. (1953b). Properties of the "slow" skeletal muscle fibres of the frog. *J. Physiol.* **121**, 318–340.

Larsell, O. (1931). The effect of experimental excision of one eye on the development of the optic lobe and opticus layer in larvae of the tree-frog (Hyla regilla). II. The effect on cell size and differentiation of cell processes. *J. exp. Zool.* **58**, 1–20.

Lashley, K. S. (1929). "Brain Mechanisms and Intelligence." Reprinted 1964. Hafner, New York.

Lashley, K. S. (1950). In search of the engram. *Symp. Soc. exp. Biol.* **4**, 454–483.

Lawrence, P. A. (1966). Gradients in the insect segment: the orientation of hairs in the milkweed bug, *Oncopeltus fasciatus*. *J. exp. Biol.* **44**, 607–620.

Lawrence, P. A. (1970). *Adv. Insect. Physiol.* (in press).

Lázár, G. (1969). Efferent Pathways of the Optic Tectum in the Frog. *Acta Biol. Acad. Sci. hung.* **20**, 171–183.

Lázár, G. and Székely, G. (1967). Golgi Studies on the Optic Center of the Frog. *J. Hirnforschung.* **9**, 329–344.

Lázár, G. and Székely, G. (1969). Distribution of optic terminals in the different optic centres of the frog. *Brain Res.* **16**, 1–14.

Lele, P. O. and Weddell, G. (1956). The relationship between neurohistology and corneal sensibility. *Brain*, **79**, 119–154.

Lenneberg, E H.. (1967). "Biological Foundations of Language." Wiley, New York.

Lettvin, J. Y., Maturana, H. R., McCulloch, W. S. and Pitts, W. H. (1959). What the frog's eye tells the frog's brain. *Proc. I.R.E.* **47**, 1940–1951.

Liu, C.-N. and Chambers, W. W. (1958). Intraspinal sprouting of dorsal root axons. *Arch. Neurol. Psychiat.* **79**, 46–61.

Lopashov, G. V. and Stroeva, Olga G. (1963). "Development of the Eye." Moscow: Academy of Sciences of U.S.S.R. English Translation by B. Meytar, 1964, Israel Program for Scientific Translations, Jerusalem.

Mangold, O. (1931). Das Determinationsproblem. III. Das Wirbeltierauge in der Entwicklung und Regeneration. *Ergebn. Biol.* **7**, 193–403.

Mark, R. F. (1965). Fin movement after regeneration of neuromuscular connections: an investigation of myotypic specificity. *Exp. Neurol.* **12**, 292–302.

Matthey, R. (1925). Récupération de la vue après résection des nerfs optiques chez le triton. *C.r. Séanc. Soc. Biol.* **93**, 904–906.

Matthey, R. (1926). Récupération de la vue après greffe de l'oeil chez le triton adulte. *C.r. Séanc. Soc. Biol.* **94**, 4–5.

Matthey, R. (1927). La greffe de l'oeil. Étude expérimentale de la greffe de l'oeil chez le triton (Triton cristatus). *Roux Archiv.* **109**, 326–341.

Maturana, H. R. (1959). Number of fibres in the optic nerve and the number of ganglion cells in the retina of anurans. *Nature, Lond.* **183**, 1406–1407.

Maturana, H. R. (1960). The fine anatomy of the optic nerve of anurans—an electron microscope study. *J. Biophys. Biochem. Cytol.* **7**, 107–135.

Maturana, H. R., Lettvin, J. Y., McCulloch, W. S. and Pitts, W. H. (1959). Physiological evidence that cut optic nerve fibres in the frog regenerate to their proper places in the tectum. *Science*, **130**, 1709.

Maturana, H. R., Lettvin, J. Y., McCulloch, W. S. and Pitts, W. H. (1960). Anatomy and physiology of vision in the frog (Rana pipiens). *J. gen. Phys.* **43**, Suppl. 129–175.

May, R. M. and Detwiler, S. R. (1925). The relation of transplanted eyes to developing nerve centers. *J. exp. Zool.* **43**, 83–103.

McCulloch, W. S. (1950). Machines that think and want. *Comp. Psychol. Monog.* **20**, 39–50.

McCulloch, W. S. and Pitts, W. H. (1947). How we know universals. *Bull. Math. Biophys.* **9**, 127–147.

McMurray, Virginia M. (1954). The development of the optic lobes in Xenopus laevis. The effect of repeated crushing of the optic nerve. *J. exp. Zool.* **125**, 247–263.

Meij, H. S., Holemans, K. C. and Meyer, B. J. (1966). Monosynaptic transmissions from afferents of one segment to motoneurons of other segments in the spinal cord. *Exp. Neurol.* **14**, 496–505.

Melzack, R. and Wall, P. D. (1962). On the nature of cutaneous sensory mechanisms. *Brain*, **85**, 331–356.

Miledi, R. (1960). Properties of regenerating neuromuscular synapses in the frog. *J. Physiol.* **154**, 190–205.

Miledi, R. and Orkand, Paula. (1966). Effect of a 'fast' nerve on 'slow' muscle fibres in the frog. *Nature, Lond.* **209**, 717–718.

Miner, Nancy. (1956). Integumental specification of sensory fibers in the development of cutaneous local sign. *J. comp. Neurol.* **105**, 161–170.

Morrell, F. (1967). Electrical signs of sensory coding. Pp. 452–469. *In* "The Neurosciences." (Eds. G. C. Quarton, T. Melnechuk and F. O. Schmitt). Rockefeller University Press, New York.

Müller, J. (1840). "Elements of Physiology." Trs. W. Baly, 2 vols. London.

Narayanan, C. H. (1964). An experimental analysis of peripheral nerve pattern development in the chick. *J. exp. Zool.* **156**, 49–60.

Nicholas, J. S. and Barron, D. H. (1935). Limb movements studied by electrical stimulation of nerve roots and trunks in Amblystoma. *J. comp. Neurol.* **61**, 413–431.

Nieuwkoop, P. D. and Faber, J. (1956). Normal Table of *Xenopus laevis* (Daudin). North-Holland Publishing Co., Amsterdam.

Nikara, T., Bishop, P. O. and Pettigrew, J. D. (1968). Analysis of retinal correspondence by studying receptive fields of binocular single units in cat striate cortex. *Exp. Br. Res.* **6**, 353–372.

Palay, S. L. (1967). Principles of cellular organization in the nervous system. Pp. 24–31. *In* "The Neurosciences." (Eds. G. C. Quarton, T. Melnechuk and F. O. Schmitt). Rockefeller University Press, New York.

Pasquini, P. (1927). Ricerche di embriologia sperimentale sui trapianti omeoplastici della vesicola ottica primaria in *Pleurodeles waltlii*. *Boll. dell'-Ist. Zool. Roma.* **5**, 1–83.

Pettigrew, J. D., Nikara, T. and Bishop, P. O. (1968a). Responses to moving slits by single units in Cat striate cortex. *Exp. Br. Res.* **6**, 373–390.

Pettigrew, J. D., Nikara, T. and Bishop, P. O. (1968b). Binocular interaction on single units in Cat striate cortex: simultaneous stimulation by single moving slit with receptive fields in correspondence. *Exp. Br. Res.* **6**, 391–410.

Piatt, J. (1942). Transplantation of aneurogenic forelimbs in Amblystoma punctatum. *J. exp. Zool.* **91**, 79–101.

Piatt, J. (1952). Transplantation of aneurogenic forelimbs in place of the hindlimb in Amblystoma. *J. exp. Zool.* **120**, 247–286.

Piatt, J. (1956). Studies on the problem of nerve pattern. I. Transplantation of the forelimb primordium to ectopic sites in Amblystoma. *J. exp. Zool.* **131**, 173–202.

Piatt, J. (1957a). Studies on the problem of nerve pattern. II. Innervation of the intact forelimb by different parts of the central nervous system in Amblystoma. *J. exp. Zool.* **134**, 103–125.

Piatt, J. (1957b). Studies on the problem of nerve pattern. III. Innervation of the regenerated forelimb in Amblystoma. *J. exp. Zool.* **136**, 229–248.

Prestige, M. C. (1965). Cell turnover in the spinal ganglia of Xenopus laevis tadpoles. *J. Embryol. exp. Morph.* **13**, 63–72.

Prestige, M. C. (1966). The development of the nervous system to the hind leg of Xenopus tadpoles. Ph.D. thesis, University of Bristol.

Prestige, M. C. (1967a). The control of cell number in the lumbar spinal ganglia during the development of Xenopus laevis tadpoles. *J. Embryol. exp. Morph.* **17**, 453–471.

Prestige, M. C. (1967b). The control of cell number in the lumbar ventral horns during the development of *Xenopus laevis* tadpoles. *J. Embryol. exp. Morph.* **18**, 359–387.

Raisman, G. (1969). Neuronal plasticity in the septal nuclei of the adult rat. *Brain Research*, **14**, 25–48.

Roach, F. C. (1945). Differentiation of the central nervous system after axial reversal of the medullary plate of Amblystoma. *J. exp. Zool.* **99**, 53–75.

Rubinson, K. (1970). Projections of the tectum opticum in the frog. *Brain Behaviour Evolution.* (In press.)

Scalia, F., Knapp, Harriet, Halpern, Mimi and Riss, W. (1968). New observations on the retinal projection in the frog. *Brain, Behavior Evolution*, **1**, 324–353.

Schwind, J. (1933). Tissue specificity at the time of metamorphosis in frog larvae. *J. exp. Zool.* **66**, 1–14.

Shawe, G. D. H. (1955). On the number of branches formed by regenerating nerve-fibres. *Brit. J. Surg.* **42**, 474–488.

Sholl, D. A. (1956). "The Organisation of the Cerebral Cortex." Reprinted 1967. Hafner, New York.

Siebert, W. M. (1962). The description of random processes. Pp. 66–87. In "Processing Neuroelectric Data." Appendix A. (Ed. W. A. Rosenblith). M.I.T. Press, Cambridge, Mass., USA

Silver, P. H. S. (1961). Experimentally produced absence of the optic chiasma in the chick. J. Physiol. 155, 33–34 p.

Simpson, J. I. (1969). On how a frog is not a cat. Ph.D. thesis, M.I.T.

Sinclair, D. C. (1955). Cutaneous sensation and the doctrine of specific energy. Brain, 1955, 78, 584–614.

Sperry, R. W. (1941). The effect of crossing nerves to antagonistic muscles in the hindlimb of the rat. J. comp. Neurol. 75, 1–19.

Sperry, R. W. (1943a). Effect of 180° degree rotation of the retinal field on visuo-motor coordination. J. exp. Zool. 92, 263–279.

Sperry, R. W. (1943b). Visuomotor coordination in the newt (Triturus viridescens) after regeneration of the optic nerve. J. comp. Neurol. 79, 33–55.

Sperry, R. W. (1944). Optic nerve regeneration with return of vision in anurans. J. Neurophysiol. 7, 57–70.

Sperry, R. W. (1945a). The problem of central nervous reorganisation after nerve regeneration and muscle transposition. Qu. Rev. Biol. 20, 311–369.

Sperry, R. W. (1945b). Restoration of vision after crossing of optic nerves and after contralateral transplantation of eye. J. Neurophysiol. 8, 15–28.

Sperry, R. W. (1947). Nature of functional recovery following regeneration of the oculomotor nerve in amphibians. Anat. Rec. 97, 293–316.

Sperry, R. W. (1948). Patterning of central synapses in regeneration of the optic nerve in Teleosts. Physiol. Zoöl. 21, 351–361.

Sperry, R. W. (1950). Myotypic specificity in teleost motoneurons. J. comp. Neurol. 93, 277–288.

Sperry, R. W. (1951a). Mechanisms of neural maturation. Pp. 236–280. In "Handbook of Experimental Psychology." (Ed. S. S. Stevens). Wiley, New York.

Sperry, R. W. (1951b). Developmental patterning of neural circuits. Chicago Med. School Quarterly, 12, 66–73.

Sperry, R. W. (1951c). Regulative features in the orderly growth of neural circuits. Growth Symposia, 10, 63–87.

Sperry, R. W. (1958a). Developmental basis of behavior. Pp. 128–139. In "Behavior and Evolution." (Eds. Anne Roe and G. G. Simpson). Yale University Press, Newhaven, USA.

Sperry, R. W. (1958b). Physiological plasticity and brain circuit theory. Pp. 401–424. In "Biological and Biochemical Bases of Behavior." (Eds. H. F. Harlow and C. N. Woolsey). University of Wisconsin Press, Madison, USA.

Sperry, R. W. (1963). Chemoaffinity in the orderly growth of nerve fiber patterns and connections. Proc. natn. Acad. Sci. U.S.A. 50, 703–710.

Sperry, R. W. (1965). Embryogenesis of behavioral nerve nets. Pp. 161–186. In "Organogenesis." (Eds. R. L. De Haan and H. Ursprung). Holt, Rinehart and Winston, New York.

Sperry, R. W. and Arora, H. L. (1965). Selectivity in regeneration of the oculomotor nerve in the cichlid fish, Astronotus ocellatus. J. Embryol. exp. Morph. 14, 307–317.

Sperry, R. W. and Deupree, Norma. (1956). Functional recovery following alterations in nerve-muscle connections of fishes. J. comp. Neurol. 106, 143–161.

Sperry, R. W. and Miner, Nancy. (1949). Formation within sensory nucleus V of synaptic associations mediating cutaneous localisation. J. comp. Neurol. 90, 403–423.

Stone, L. S. (1930). Heteroplastic transplantation of eyes between the larvae of 2 species of Amblystoma. *J. exp. Zool.* **55**, 193–261.

Stone, L. S. (1944). Functional polarization in retinal development and its re-establishment in regenerating retinae of rotated grafted eyes. *Proc. Soc. exp. Biol. Med.* **57**, 13–14.

Stone, L. S. (1959). Experiments testing the capacity of iris to regenerate neural retina in eyes of adult newts. *J. exp. Zool.* **142**, 285–308.

Stone, L. S. (1960). Polarization of the retina and development of vision. *J. exp. Zool.* **145**, 85–96.

Stone, L. S. (1963). Vision in eyes of several species of adult newts transplanted to adult *Triturus v. viridescens. J. exp. Zool.* **153**, 57–68.

Stone, L. S., Ussher, N. T. and Beers, D. N. (1937). Reimplantation and trans-plantation of larval eyes in the salamander (*Amblystoma punctatum*). *J. exp. Zool.* **77**, 13–48.

Stone, L. S. and Zaur, I. S. (1940). Reimplantation and transplantation of the adult eye in the salamander (*Triturus viridescens*) with return of vision. *J. exp. Zool.* **85**, 243–269.

Straznicky, K. (1963). Function of heterotopic spinal cord segments investigated in the chick. *Acta Biol. Acad. Sci. hung.* **14**, 145–155.

Straznicky, K. (1967). The development of the innervation and the musculature of wings innervated by thoracic nerves. *Acta Biol. hung.* **18**, 437–448.

Straznicky, K. and Gaze, R. M. (1970). (In preparation).

Straznicky, K., Gaze, R. M. and Keating, M. J. (1970a). (In preparation).

Straznicky, K., Gaze, R. M. and Keating, M. J. (1970b). (In preparation).

Straznicky, K. and Székely, G. (1967). Functional adaptation of thoracic spinal cord segments in the newt. *Acta Biol. hung.* **18**, 449–456.

Ströer, W. F. H. (1940). Das optische System beim Wassermolch (Trit. taeniatus). *Acta Néerl. Morphologiae*, **3**, 178–195.

Swett, F. H. (1937). Determination of limb-axes. *Qu. Rev. Biol.* **12**, 322–339.

Székely, G. (1954a). Untersuchung der Entwicklung optischer Reflexmechanismen an Amphibienlarven. *Acta Physiol. Acad. Sci. hung.* **6**, Suppl. 18.

Székely, G. (1954b). Zur Ausbildung der lokalen funktionellen Spezifität der Retina. *Acta Biol. Acad. Sci. hung.* **5**, 157–167.

Székely, G. (1957). Regulationstendenzen in der Ausbildung der "Funktionellen Spezifität" der Retinoanlage bei *Triturus vulgaris. Arch. Entw. Org.* **150**, 48–60.

Székely, G. (1959a). Functional specificity of cranial sensory neuroblasts in urodela. *Acta Biol. Acad. Sci. hung.* **10**, 107–116.

Székely, G. (1959b). The apparent "corneal specificity" of sensory neurons. *J. Embryol. exp. Morph.* **7**, 375–379.

Székely, G. (1963). Functional specificity of spinal cord segments in the control of limb movements. *J. Embryol. exp. Morph.* **11**, 431–444.

Székely, G. (1965). Logical network for controlling limb movements in urodela. *Acta Physiol. Acad. Sci. hung.* **27**, 285–289.

Székely, G. (1966). Embryonic determination of neural connections. *Adv. Morphogen.* **5**, 181–219.

Székely, G. (1968). Development of limb movements: embryological, physiological and model studies. Pp. 77–93. *In* "Growth of the Nervous System." Ciba Foundation Symposium. (Eds. G. E. W. Wolstenholme and Maeve O'Connor). Churchill, London.

Székely, G. and Czéh, G. (1967). Localization of motoneurones in the limb moving spinal cord segments of Amblystoma. *Acta Physiol. Acad. Sci. hung.* **32**, 3–18.

Székely, G. and Szentágothai, J. (1962). Reflex and behavior patterns elicited from implanted supernumary limbs in the chick. *J. Embryol. exp. Morph.* **10**, 140–151.

Szentágothai, J. (1967). The anatomy of complex integrative units in the nervous system. Pp. 9–45. *In* "Recent Development of Neurobiology in Hungary," Vol. I. (Ed. K. Lissák). Akadémiai Kiadó, Budapest.

Szentágothai, J. and Kiss, T. (1949). Projection of dermatomes on the substantia gelatinosa. *Archs Neurol. Psychiat.* **62**, 734–744.

Szentágothai, J. and Székely, G. (1956). Zur Problem der Kreuzung der Nervenbahnen. *Acta Biol. Acad. Sci. hung.* **6**, 215–229.

Takeuchi, A. (1959). Neuromuscular transmission of fish skeletal muscles investigated with intracellular microelectrode. *J. Cell. comp. Physiol.* **54**, 211–220.

Taylor, A. C. (1943). Development of the innervation pattern in the limb bud of the frog. *Anat. Rec.* **87**, 379–413.

Thompson, J. D. (1936). Peripheral distribution of forelimb nerves in Amblystoma. *Science*, **84**, 310.

Turing, A. M. (1948). Intelligent machinery. N.P.L. Report 1–20.

Ungar, G. (1968). Molecular mechanisms in learning. *Perspect. Biol. Med.* **11**, 217–232.

Verzár, F. and Weiss, P. (1929). Untersuchungen über des Phänomen der identischen Bewegungsfunktion mehrfacher benachbarter Extremitäten. Zugleich: Direkte Vorführung von Eigenveflexen. *Pflügers Archiv. f.d. ges. Physiol.* **223**, 671–684.

Waddington, C. H. (1940). The genetical control of wing development in Drosophila. *J. Genet.* **41**, 75–140.

Waddington, C. H. (1956). "Principles of Embryology." Allen and Unwin, London.

Waddington, C. H. (1966). Fields and gradients. Pp. 105–124. *In* "Major Problems in Developmental Biology." (Ed. M. Locke). 25th Symposium of the Society for Developmental Biology. Academic Press, New York.

Weiler, I. J. (1966). Restoration of visual acuity after optic nerve section and regeneration, in *Astronotus ocellatus. Expl. Neurol.* **15**, 377–386.

Weiss, P. (1922). Die Funktion transplantierter Amphibienextremitäten. *Anz. Akad. Wiss. Wien*, **59**, 199–201.

Weiss, P. (1926). The relations between central and peripheral coordination. *J. comp. Neurol.* **40**, 241–251.

Weiss, P. (1930a). Funktionelle Transplantation Einzelner Muskeln bei Krotten. *Arbeiten Ungar. Biol. Forschungs. Inst.* **3**, 304–311.

Weiss, P. (1930b). Neue experimentelle Beweise für das Resonanzprinzip der Nerventätigkeit. *Biologisches Zentralblatt*, **50**, 357–372.

Weiss, P. (1931). Das Resonanzprinzip der Nerventätigkeit, dargestelt in Funktionspräfungen an transplantierten überzähligen Muskeln. *Pflügers Archiv f.d. Ges. Physiol.* **226**, 600–658.

Weiss, P. (1935). Homologous (resonance-like) function in supernumary fingers in a human case. *Proc. Soc. exp. Biol. Med.* **33**, 426–430.

Weiss, P. (1936). Selectivity controlling the central-peripheral relations in the nervous system. *Biol. Rev.* **11**, 494–531.

Weiss, P. (1937a). Further experimental investigations on the phenomenon of homologous response in transplanted amphibian limbs. I. Functional observations. *J. comp. Neurol.* **66**, 181–209.

Weiss, P. (1937b). Further experimental studies on the phenomenon of homologous response in transplanted amphibian limbs. II. Nerve regeneration and the innervation of transplanted limbs. *J. comp. Neurol.* **66**, 481–535.

Weiss, P. (1937c). Further experimental investigations on the phenomenon of homologous response in transplanted amphibian limbs. *J. comp. Neurol.* **66**, 537–548.

Weiss, P. (1937d). Further experimental investigations on the phenomenon of homologous response in transplanted amphibian limbs. IV. Reverse locomotion after the interchange of right and left limbs. *J. comp. Neurol.* **67**, 269–315.

Weiss, P. (1941). Self-differentiation of the basic patterns of coordination. *Comp. Psychol. Monog.* **17**, 1–96.

Weiss, P. (1942). Lid-closure reflex from eyes transplanted to atypical locations in Triturus torosus: Evidence of a peripheral origin of sensory specificity. *J. comp. Neurol.* **77**, 131–169.

Weiss, P. (1950a). Experimental analysis of co-ordination by the disarrangement of central-peripheral relations. *Symp. Soc. exp. Biol.* **4**, 92–111.

Weiss, P. (1950b). Central versus peripheral factors in the development of co-ordination. *Proc. A.R.N.M.D.* **30**, 3–23.

Weiss, P. (1955). Nervous System. Pp. 346–401. *In* "Analysis of Development." (Eds. B. H. Willier, P. A. Weiss and V. Hamburger). Saunders, Philadelphia.

Weiss, P. and Hoag, Ann. (1946). Competitive reinnervation of rat muscles by their own and foreign nerves. *J. Neurophysiol.* **9**, 413–418.

Weiss, P. and Litwiller, R. (1937). Quantitative studies on nerve regeneration in amphibia. II. Innervation of regenerated limbs. *Proc. Soc. exp. biol. Med.* **36**, 638–639.

Weiss, P. and Taylor, A. C. (1944). Further experimental evidence against "Neurotropism" in nerve regeneration. *J. exp. Zool.* **95**, 233–257.

Westerman, R. A. (1965). Specificity in regeneration of optic and olfactory pathways in teleost fish. Pp. 263–269. *In* "Studies in Physiology." (Eds. D. R. Curtis and A. K. McIntyre). Springer, Berlin.

Wickelgren, Barbara G. and Sterling, P. (1969). Effect on the superior colliculus of cortical removal in visually deprived cats. *Nature, Lond.* **224**, 1032–1033.

Wiersma, C. A. G. (1931). An experiment on the "resonance theory" of muscular activity. *Arch. Néerl. Physiol.* **16**, 337–345.

Wiesel, T. N. and Hubel, D. H. (1963a). Effects of visual deprivation on morphology and physiology of cells in the cat's lateral geniculate body. *J. Neurophysiol.* **26**, 978–993.

Wiesel, T. N. and Hubel, D. H. (1963b). Single-cell responses in striate cortex of kittens deprived of vision in one eye. *J. Neurophysiol.* **26**, 1003–1017.

Wiesel, T. N. and Hubel, D. H. (1965a). Comparison of the effects of unilateral and bilateral eye closure on cortical unit responses in kittens. *J. Neurophysiol.* **28**, 1029–1040.

Wiesel, T. N. and Hubel, D. H. (1965b). Extent of recovery from the effects of visual deprivation in kittens. *J. Neurophysiol.* **28**, 1060–1072.

Wlassak, R. (1893). Die optischen Leitungsbahnen des Frosches. *Arch. Anat. Physiol. Lpz., Physiol. Abt.* Suppl. 1.

Wolpert, L. (1968). The French Flag Problem. Pp. 125–133. *In* "Towards a Theoretical Biology. I. Prolegomena." (Ed. C. H. Waddington). Edinburgh University Press, Edinburgh.

Wolpert, L. (1969). Positional information and the spatial pattern of cellular differentiation. *J. Theoret. Biol.* **25**, 1–47.

Zelená, Jirina, Vylicky, L. and Jirmanová, Isa. (1967). Motor end-plates in fast add slow muscles of the chick after cross-union of their nerves. *Nature, Lond.* **214**, 1010–1011.

Author Index

279

Subject Index